Treatment and Pro...

Medicir

Treatment and Prognosis Series Editor: Richard Hawkins

Published simultaneously in 1986
  Medicine Richard Hawkins (ed.)
  Surgery Richard Hawkins (ed.)

In preparation
  Paediatrics GS Clayden (ed.)
  Obstetrics and Gynaecology JG Grudzinskas and T Beedham (eds.)

Treatment and Prognosis

MEDICINE

Edited by

Richard Hawkins MBBS, FRCS

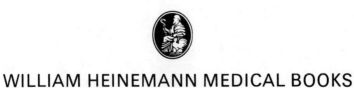

WILLIAM HEINEMANN MEDICAL BOOKS
London

William Heinemann Medical Books,
22 Bedford Square,
London WC1B 3HH

ISBN: 0-433-13395-3 (Medicine)
      0-433-13394-5 (Surgery)

First published 1986

Typeset and printed in Great Britain
by Butler & Tanner Limited, Frome and London

DEDICATION
Dedicated with the greatest affection to Dr Jane Foley

Contents

Forewords

A Breckenridge MD, MSc, FRCP
Professor of Clinical Pharmacology, University of Liverpool

For many years most medical textbooks have tended to concentrate on the pathogenesis and clinical features of disease rather than their treatment and prognosis. Yet it is in these latter areas where most progress has taken place recently. It is our intention and hope that both the young hospital doctor working for higher examinations and his more senior colleague requiring updating will be informed and helped by the *Treatment and Prognosis* series.

The main subject areas in each discipline are covered and while perforce large and important topics must be dealt with briefly, the editorial board is happy that the correct emphasis and balance has been given to the individual disease entities. Further, the distinguished panel of authors has been disciplined to adopt a reasonably uniform mode of presentation which will ease assimilation.

The *Treatment and Prognosis* series is written clearly to allow a succinct and up-to-date picture of those important aspects of modern disease management to emerge, which will be particularly appealing to the busy clinical doctor.

V W Michael Drury OBE, PRCGP
President of Royal College of General Practitioners and Professor of General Practice, University of Birmingham Medical School

Over the past thirty years the effectiveness of the doctor in treating disease has grown greatly. All doctors need now to have access to a much larger bulk of information and this includes not only treatment for the problems they see regularly, but also the problems dealt with in other branches of medicine so that they can advise or interpret advice for their patients appropriately. Nowhere is this more important than for the general practitioner and to be able to find at the same time an account of the prognosis associated with a variety of forms of treatment will greatly enhance his effectiveness.

These volumes set out to do just this and to ally it with advice about what might be seen as an appropriate follow-up regime by the hospital or the family doctor. I believe that my colleagues will find them as useful as I have.

Disease directory

7 Diseases of the skin   121

List of contributors

NC Allan MD, MB, ChB (Edin.), FRCP (Edin.), FRCPath
Director of Haematology Department, Western General Hospital, Edinburgh

JE Banatvala MA, MD, MRCP, FRCPath
Professor of Medicine, Department of Virology, St. Thomas' Hospital, London

I Barton MA, MRCP
Lecturer in Medicine, Department of Nephrology, St. Philip's Hospital, London

SR Bloom MA, DSc, MD, FRCP
Professor of Endocrinology, Royal Postgraduate Medical School, Hammersmith Hospital, London

IA Campbell MD, FRCP (Edin.)
Consultant in Thoracic Medicine, Llandough and Sully Hospitals, Cardiff

DL Cohen MBBS, MRCP
Unit for Metabolic Medicine, Guy's Hospital, London

JR Dawson MB, ChB, MRCP
Senior Registrar, Brompton Hospital, London

GE Forster MB, ChB, MRCOG
Consultant Venereologist, The London Hospital, Whitechapel

SK Goolamali MD, FRCP
Consultant Dermatologist, Northwick Park Hospital and Clinical Research Centre, Harrow

JRW Harris MB, BChir, MRCP
Consultant Physician, St. Mary's Hospital, London

GRV Hughes MD, FRCP
Consultant Rheumatologist, St. Thomas' Hospital, London

H Keen MD, FRCP
Director of Unit for Metabolic Medicine, Guy's Hospital, London

PJ Oldershaw MB, BChir, MRCP
Consultant Cardiologist, Brompton Hospital, London

S Parry MB, ChB, FRACP
Department of Surgery, School of Medicine, University of Otago, New Zealand

JP Patten BSc, MB, FRCP
Consultant Neurologist, The Royal Surrey County Hospital, Guildford

IW Pinkerton MB, ChB, FRCP (Edin.), FRCP (Glas.), FRFPS
Clinical Department of Infectious Diseases, Ruchill Hospital, Glasgow

RE Pounder MA, MD, FRCP
Reader in Medicine and Clinical Subdean, Royal Free Hospital School of Medicine, London

AE Read MD, FRCP
Professor of Medicine, Bristol Royal Infirmary

D Reid MD, FRCP(Glas.), FFCM, DPH
Director Communicable Diseases (Scotland) Unit, Ruchill Hospital, Glasgow

MA Reveley MD, MRCPsych
Senior Lecturer and Honorary Consultant Psychiatrist, The London Hospital (St. Clement's)

JM Welch BSc, MB, MRCP
Senior Registrar, St. Thomas' Hospital, London

G Williams MA, MD, MRCP
RD Lawrence Research Fellow and Honorary Senior Registrar, Hammersmith Hospital, London

Preface

General practitioners and hospital doctors necessarily have different perspectives, but there is an essential core of information common to both areas of practice, which serves as the basis for communication between them. This series of books concentrates on that core, bringing together a panel of distinguished authors with the aim of providing essential and up-to-date information in the areas of treatment and prognosis.

The format for each topic is identical and designed to enable the busy clinician to extract the maximum information in as short a time as possible. Each topic begins with a short account of the disease or condition with relevant details of pathology and epidemiology, followed by a section on prognosis. Some may consider that we are entering the proverbial lion's den by placing such emphasis on prognosis, yet the available information has improved and attitudes are changing. Most patients today ask questions about the likely outcome of their diseases and doctors need to be in as good a position as possible to evaluate the various management options open to them.

Prognosis is followed by sections on treatment, the heart of the book, and follow-up. This latter section aims to provide brief guidance for general practitioners and hospital doctors in out-patients as to further management of patients once initial treatment has begun. References are provided for further reading and more detailed enquiry.

A novel approach has been adopted to meet the needs of modern doctors. In particular it should appeal to general practitioners, and to junior hospital doctors with heavy clinical duties and examinations looming. Senior students should also benefit from these books. They are no substitute for the standard textbooks, since the authors have assumed a certain level of knowledge and sophistication in their readers. But they will give a perspective to each topic which is easily lost amidst the plethora of detail which some incorrectly imagine is needed to pass examinations and become good doctors.

Richard Hawkins

Acknowledgements

I would like to thank all members of the Editorial Board for their considerable assistance in the preparation of this volume and the Series in general. I would also like to thank Dr Richard Barling, Editorial Director of Heinemann Medical Books, for his imaginative enthusiasm for the Series; and Mr Stephen Bishop, Managing Editor, for his remarkably meticulous marshalling of the manuscripts.

1

Diseases of the Respiratory System

I. A. Campbell

Chronic Bronchitis and Emphysema

Chronic bronchitis is characterised by cough producing sputum on most days during at least three consecutive months for more than two successive years. Emphysema is defined in pathological terms as a condition characterised by increase beyond the normal in the size of the air spaces distal to the terminal bronchiole. Both conditions can result in persistent generalised airways obstruction. They frequently occur together, few patients having purely one or the other. Cigarette smoking is the single most important aetiological factor in chronic bronchitis and emphysema. The prevalence increases with age, cigarette consumption and atmospheric pollution. It is commoner among men than women and affects 10% middle-aged British males. Some 30 million working days per year are lost because of this disease. Acute exacerbations are usually caused by viral or bacterial infection and are commoner in winter months.

PROGNOSIS[1,2]

- Middle-aged patients whose FEV_1 is 1 l below the expected value are very likely to become disabled by airways obstruction unless they stop smoking.
- Stopping smoking returns the rate of deterioration of FEV_1 to that which would normally occur with advancing age, thus improving prognosis.
- Patients in whom the predominant pathology is mucus hypersecretion have a better outlook than those in whom airways obstruction predominates.
- Death rates approach 10% per year once the $FEV_1 < 1$ l.
- Once pulmonary hypertension and cor pulmonale develop the five-year survival is around 30%.

TREATMENT[2]

1. *Long-term treatment*

   a) Stopping smoking is important in prophylaxis and treatment. Currently doctors' advice achieves 5–10% success rate. It is important that the benefits to symptoms and lung function are emphasised. Nicotine chewing gum and other methods do not appear to increase success rate in patients.

   b) The reduction of atmospheric pollution has clearly been beneficial in the UK.

   c) Preventive antibiotics result in some reduction or curtailing of exacerbations but functional deterioration is not prevented.

   Sulphametopyrazine once weekly during the winter can halve exacerbations and time off work.

   d) Bronchodilator drugs (beta-sympathomimetic, anti-cholinergic, methyl xanthine) sometimes produce some improvement. Inhaler therapy is more effective than tablets provided inhaler technique is adequate. If no benefit reported or observed, bronchodilators should be stopped.

   e) Corticosteroids (tablets or inhaled) should not be used unless asthma also present

   f) Diuretics should be used for cor pulmonale. The place of digoxin is controversial but atrial fibrillation is a clear indication

   g) Domiciliary oxygen for 15 or more hours per 24 can prolong and improve quality of life in patients with chronic respiratory failure and $PaO_2 < 55$ mmHg[3]. Shorter periods result in no objective benefit but some patients derive subjective benefit.

   h) Autumn vaccination against influenza for patients with poor ventilatory reserve is recommended.

   i) Mucolytics are of little if any benefit.

2. *Treatment of acute exacerbations*

   a) Tetracycline or ampicillin, 250 mg 6 or 8 hourly for one week, is usually effective

   b) Adequate coughing and clearance of phlegm (home or hospital physiotherapy) is important.

   c) Hydration should be maintained.

   d) Bronchodilators, inhaled or systemic, are

usually prescribed. Dose for dose, nebulisers have no advantage over Nebuhalers.

e) Sedation should be avoided.

f) Cough suppressants should be avoided, or used only after careful consideration.

g) If the patient is cyanosed and/or has a $PaO_2 < 60-70$ mmHg, treatment should be with 24-28% oxygen depending on the degree of hypoxaemia and the $PaCO_2$. The hypoxic drive to breathing is important in patients with chronic CO_2 retention: too high an inspired oxygen concentration may remove this drive and lead to further CO_2 retention and narcosis. The clinical state and blood gases should be closely monitored when giving oxygen to patients known or likely to have chronic hypercapnia.

h) Bolus doses of nikethamide or doxapram may be necessary prior to physiotherapy for patients with drowsiness secondary to hypercapnia and hypoxia. The latter drug can also be used by constant infusion.

i) Assisted ventilation is indicated if, in spite of treatment, PaO_2 remains <40 mmHg and/or $PaCO_2$ climbs, with pH <7.25. It should not be undertaken in respiratory cripples.

FOLLOW-UP

Hospital out-patient review for those in respiratory failure until therapy is stabilised. GP review 3-6 monthly. Simple acute exacerbations in patients with mild/moderate disability do not require hospital follow-up. Anti-smoking advice should be repeated. Influenza vaccination in autumn for moderately/severely affected patients. Give supply of oxytetracycline or ampicillin to take at onset of exacerbation. Winter prophylaxis for those with frequent exacerbations.

[1] Fletcher C et al. (1976) The Natural History of Chronic Bronchitis and Emphysema. Oxford: Oxford University Press.
[2] Crofton J, Douglas A (1981) Respiratory Diseases 3rd edn. Oxford: Blackwell.
[3] Rees J (1984) Br. Med. J., 289, 1398.

Bronchial Asthma

Asthma is characterised by recurrent paroxysmal attacks of dyspnoea and wheezing due to generalised airways obstruction which changes in severity over short periods of time either spontaneously or as a result of treatment. Some patients have periods free of wheeze whilst others have chronic symptoms. Prevalence in Britain: 5–10% in children and 3–5% in adults. Allergy to house-dust mite or to grass pollen are the commonest causes. Atopy is commoner in asthma starting in childhood than in asthma starting in middle-age. Attacks are frequently precipitated by infection. Occupational exposure to toluene di-isocyanate, epoxy resins, platinum salts, colophony (solder flux), flour, red cedar dust and certain laboratory animals' urine can cause asthma.

PROGNOSIS[1,2]

- The mortality rate in Britain is 2–3 per 100 000 of total population.
- Childhood asthma has a good prognosis, the majority being free of symptoms in adulthood. It has a better outlook than adult onset asthma.
- Episodic asthma has a better prognosis than chronic asthma.
- Complicating bronchitis affects the prognosis adversely.
- Modern therapy has improved the quality of life but mortality has not been affected.

TREATMENT[1,2]

1. *Episodic asthma*

   a) Bronchodilators (beta-2 sympathomimetic or anti-cholinergic) via pressurised inhalers are safe and effective, and can be used regularly or as required. Teach and check inhaler technique.
   b) If symptoms demand frequent bronchodilater usage, i.e. >4–5 times/24 hours, regular prophylactic therapy should be started with inhaled cromoglycate or inhaled corticosteroids, continuing to use bronchodilator inhaler as required.
   c) Hyposensitisation to grass pollen for two successive years is effective in over 70% patients with pure grass pollen asthma.
   d) Hyposensitisation to house-dust mite helpful in selected children but benefit not conclusively shown in adults.
   e) Measures to reduce house-dust mite population at home, especially in the bedroom, are helpful to some extent. Occasionally exclusion of milk products from diet will help in childhood asthma.
   f) Allergenic pets should be avoided.
   g) Exercise-induced asthma is usually preventable by inhaled bronchodilator or cromoglycate 10–15 minutes before exercise.

2. *Chronic asthma*

   a) Regular inhaled bronchodilator 4–6 times/24 hours may control symptoms adequately but the majority will require regular inhaled cromoglycate (children) or inhaled corticosteroids (adults and children) as prophylaxis. The optimum dosage and interval between doses varies between patients. The bronchodilator inhaler should be continued either regularly or as required.
   b) Long-acting theophylline tablets are added if control is still not adequate; they often help to reduce nocturnal asthma. Side-effects are common and the therapeutic ratio is narrow.
   c) Short courses of prednisolone may be necessary from time to time for worsening symptoms not responding to increased bronchodilator therapy. Patients should be instructed to initiate or seek systemic corticosteroid therapy sooner rather than later in the face of deteriorating asthma.
   d) A minority require long-term therapy with prednisolone in addition to a), b) and c). The maintenance dose can usually be kept below 10 mg daily.
   e) Before committing a patient to long-term

corticosteroid therapy (inhaled or tablets) objective assessment of response should be made by monitoring ventilatory capacity before, during and at the end of three weeks' therapy, e.g. self-recording of peak expiratory flow rate (PEFR) on an out-patient basis.

f) Inhaler technique should be carefully taught and checked.

g) Inhaler therapy is preferable to tablets.

3. *Status asthmaticus*

a) Start with 35% oxygen, with or without humidification.

b) Corticosteroids: hydrocortisone 250 mg i.v. stat and 100 mg two hourly for 24–36 hours, plus prednisolone 40 mg stat and 10 mg six hourly until the patient is significantly improved. Thereafter the dosage is reduced over 2–4 weeks.

c) Bronchodilators: beta-2 sympathomimetic four hourly in large (2–5 mg) doses by Nebuhaler or nebuliser and/or aminophylline i.v. 250–500 mg six hourly. Aminophylline is better given by constant infusion, a loading dose or any bolus dose being administered slowly.

d) Rehydration should be vigorous, by mouth or by 5% dextrose i.v.; 2–3 l may be necessary in the first 12 hours.

e) Antibiotics: ampicillin or tetracycline if the history, temperature or sputum suggests infection.

f) Sedation is absolutely contraindicated.

g) The response is reviewed (clinically, pulse rate and paradox, PEFR and arterial blood gases) frequently in the first 12 hours.

h) Assisted respiration is indicated for exhaustion, persisting confusion, PaO_2 persistently <40 mmHg and $PaCO_2$ persistently >50 mmHg.

i) The intensity of therapy is reduced as the condition improves.

j) An attack of status asthmaticus is an indication for subsequent regular corticosteroid therapy (inhaled and/or tablets).

4. *Occupational asthma*

a) Avoid further exposure.

b) Treat symptoms—see 1) and 2).

FOLLOW-UP[3]

Moderate or severe asthma requires regular GP and hospital supervision, including PEFR measurement. Patients with exacerbations not responding to treatment should be admitted to hospital sooner rather than later.

---

[1] Crofton J, Douglas A (1981) *Respiratory Diseases* 3rd edn. Oxford: Blackwell.

[2] Clark TJH, Godfrey S (eds.) (1983) *Asthma* 2nd edn. London: Chapman and Hall.

[3] British Thoracic Association report (1982) *Br. Med. J.*, 285, 1251.

Pneumonia

Pneumonia is inflammation of the lung parenchyma characterised by exudation into the alveoli. It usually results from bacterial or viral infection and affects 1% of the population each year, most commonly in winter and spring. Among adults, 50% are aged < 50. Impaired clearance of secretions, inhalation of foreign material, pre-existing respiratory disease, immunosuppression, alcoholism and cigarette smoking are predisposing factors. Particular causal agents do not always produce the same anatomical pattern of consolidation. *Strep. pneumoniae* is the commonest cause of bacterial pneumonias (70–80%); *Staph. pyogenes* causes 5% (more during influenza epidemics) and Klebsiella 1%. *Mycoplasma pneumoniae* is responsible for 15% hospital admissions for pneumonia.

PROGNOSIS[1]

- Mortality rate is 5–10%. It is influenced by:

    a) Age—highest in very young and elderly.
    b) Organism—type 3 pneumococci, *Staph. pyogenes* and Klebsiella pneumoniae are the worst.
    c) Bacteraemia increases the mortality.
    d) Concomitant disease—chronic bronchitis/emphysema and persisting immunosuppression—adversely influences prognosis.

- Lung abscess (2%) or empyema (1%) may complicate inadequately treated pneumonia and worsen prognosis.
- Persistent or recurrent respiratory symptoms are more common after lobar than segmental pneumonia, especially in smokers and in lower socio-economic groups.

TREATMENT[1]

1. *Pneumococcal pneumonia*

    a) Benzyl penicillin 1 mega unit i.m. bd is given for 4–5 days, followed by phenoxymethyl penicillin 500 mg orally qds for 7–10 days. Ampicillin 250 mg qds for 10–14 days is an adequate alternative.
    b) 35% O_2 is administered if cyanosis is present, but if previous CO_2 retention is suspected 24–28% should be used and arterial blood gases monitored.
    c) The patient is rehydrated preferably orally but with i.v. 5% dextrose if too unwell to drink.
    d) Adequate analgesia is important for pleuritic pain. Opiates should be used with caution in CO_2 retainers.
    e) Supervised coughing and, later, chest physiotherapy to encourage expectoration is valuable.
    f) Patients allergic to penicillin should receive erythromycin or tetracycline.

2. *Staphylococcal pneumonia*

    a) Flucloxacillin 250–500 mg qds is given i.v. or orally for two weeks. Many physicians use this in combination with benzylpenicillin 1 mega unit qds, continuing with benzyl penicillin for a week even if organism is resistant *in vitro*.
    b) See 1b), c), d) and e).
    c) Postural drainage is important if a lung abscess develops.
    d) Lung abscess requires six weeks' chemotherapy.
    e) Patients allergic to penicillin should receive fusidic acid.

3. *Mycoplasma pneumonia, Rickettsial pneumonia (Q fever pneumonia), Chlamydial pneumonia (psittacosis)*

    a) Oxytetracycline or erythromycin 500 mg is given orally qds for 10–14 days.
    b) See 1b), c), d) and e).

4. *Haemophilus influenzae pneumonia* affects elderly and those with chronic bronchitis and emphysema, most com

monly as bronchopneumonia. Treatment is with ampicillin or tetracycline in addition to measures 1b), c), d), e) and f).

5. *Klebsiella pneumonia*

   a) Two drugs should be used to prevent emergence of resistance. Organism usually sensitive to gentamicin and chloramphenicol; continue this combination for two weeks at least. Halve dose of chloramphenicol if treatment continued longer or substitute other antibiotic.
   b) Measures 1b), c), d) and e).

6. *Legionella pneumophila pneumonia (Legionnaire's disease)*

   a) Erythromycin 500 mg–1 g i.v. or orally qds for three weeks.
   b) Measures 1b), c), d) and e), with particular reference to appropriate fluid and electrolyte balance.
   c) Rifampicin should be tried if there is no response to erythromycin.

7. *Viral pneumonias*

   a) Specific antiviral treatment is not available for those viruses causing pneumonia.
   b) Measures 1b), c), d) and e).
   c) Bacterial super-infection should be promptly treated. *Staph. pyogenes* pneumonia becomes more common during influenza epidemics.

8. *Fungal pneumonias*

   a) Actinomycosis is best treated with 10–12 mega units benzylpenicillin daily for 6–8 months. Lower doses of phenoxymethylpenicillin may suffice in later stages of treatment. Surgery may be necessary.
   b) Nocardiosis responds better to sulphonamides than to penicillin. Cotrimoxazole and cephalosporin are often used in combination for 6–8 months. Surgical treatment may become necessary.

   c) Intravenous amphotericin B offers the best hope of effective treatment of other fungal pneumonias, but is often unsuccessful because its use is limited by toxicity or because of other serious underlying illness. Histoplasma pneumonia usually responds well.

9. *Pneumonia caused by anaerobes.* These pneumonias usually occur in debilitated patients who may have aspirated and should be treated with metronidazole 400 mg tds.

10. *Pneumonia in immunocompromised patients*

    a) Try and restore immunocompetence if possible.
    b) For pneumocystis carinii high dose cotrimoxazole (8 tabs. twice daily), or pentamidine should be given.
    c) For cytomegalovirus no drug is available.
    d) For fungal infections see 8.
    e) For anaerobic infections see 9.
    f) Triple chemotherapy with rifampicin, isoniazid and ethambutol is used for tuberculosis.
    g) For the usual pneumonia pathogens see 1–7.

11. *Desperately ill patient*

    a) A combination of antibiotics sufficient to cover all the most likely organisms is given.
    b) Respiratory failure and peripheral circulatory failure should be corrected.

FOLLOW-UP[1]

The diagnosis or aetiological agent is reconsidered if the patient is not improving or is still febrile after five days. A chest x-ray should be performed at 6–8 weeks to confirm radiological clearing/resolution. Sputum cytology and/or bronchoscopy is indicated if x-ray resolution is delayed beyond 8–12 weeks.

---

[1] Crofton J, Douglas A (1981) *Respiratory Diseases* 3rd edn. Oxford: Blackwell.

Pulmonary Embolism

Pulmonary embolism (PE) occurs when an embolus, usually from a thrombus in veins of lower limb or pelvis, lodges in a main pulmonary artery or one of its branches. Pulmonary infarction usually ensues. Apart from pregnancy and the contraceptive pill sex distribution is equal. It is uncommon before age 40. It is among the commonest causes of death following surgery and is the main cause of death in 5% hospital patients. Routine autopsies reveal PE in 10–15% patients dying in hospital. Lowering the oestrogen content of the contraceptive pill has reduced the incidence in women.

PROGNOSIS[1]

- Massive PE (blockage of left or right pulmonary artery) carries a 50% mortality.
- >65% deaths occur within two hours, often before treatment can be started.
- Treatment reduces mortality and the chance of recurrence: the earlier it is started the better the prognosis.
- None of those leaving hospital after embolism are likely to die from recurrence although 5–10% recur.
- Most treated patients proceed to complete haemodynamic and angiographic resolution. Cor pulmonale is a very rare sequela.
- Resolution of the arterial obstruction can take place within two weeks and in over 60% occurs within four months.
- Emboli too small to cause symptoms do occur and, if repetitive, will eventually produce pulmonary hypertension and chronic cor pulmonale.

TREATMENT[1,2,3]

1. Prophylaxis influences mortality more than treatment. Deep vein thrombosis (DVT) in patients at risk can be reduced by:

   a) Continued ambulation/early mobilisation.
   b) Passive exercise of calf muscles using a motorised foot rocker or intermittent compression of the lower limbs by inflatable cuffs during operation reduces early postoperative DVT by 80%; electrical stimulation of calf muscles is favoured by some surgeons.
   c) Prompt treatment of cardiac failure.
   d) Avoidance of hypovolaemia or dehydration.
   e) Low dose subcutaneous heparin (5000–8000 i.u. 8–12 hourly) or anticoagulation with warfarin during risk period.
   f) Elastic stockings (doubtful value).

2. Prompt detection of DVT (clinical suspicion and examination, I^{125}–fibrinogen scan, ultrasound or venography) and prompt treatment will prevent PE.

3. *Massive pulmonary embolism*

   a) Pulmonary embolectomy under cardiopulmonary by-pass is indicated for desperately ill patients or patients who deteriorate during thrombolytic or heparin therapy.
   b) Morphine should be given for pain, apprehension or dyspnoea; and oxygen in high concentration (35–60%).
   c) Acidosis is corrected.
   d) Vasopressor drugs are sometimes necessary.
   e) After embolectomy heparin should be used for 1–2 weeks followed by warfarin for at least six weeks.

4. *Extensive embolism*

   a) In less desperate cases streptokinase 600 000 units i.v. is administered over 30 minutes followed by 100 000 units/hour for 72 hours; the value of laboratory monitoring/modulation of the dose is questionable; i.v. hydrocortisone and/or antihistamine should be given before starting streptokinase to prevent hypersensitivity reactions.
   b) Hypoxia or dyspnoea is relieved by oxygen (35–60%).

c) Pain, apprehension or dyspnoea is relieved by morphine.

d) Streptokinase therapy is succeeded by heparin, allowing thrombin time to fall to less than twice the control value before starting heparin (usually takes 3–4 hours).

e) Heparin is continued for 5–10 days, monitored by kaolin cephalin clotting time (KCCT).

f) Warfarin is begun after 3–8 days and continued for 3–6 weeks monitored by prothrombin time (BCR).

g) Streptokinase therapy should not be repeated until antibody levels fall, usually 3–6 months.

5. *Less extensive pulmonary embolism*

a) Heparin 5000 units i.v. loading dose is followed by 1000 units/hour by constant infusion for five days, using KCCT to govern infusion rate after 4–6 hours of treatment and daily thereafter (keep KCCT between 1½–2 times control).

b) Warfarin is begun on the evening of the third day, 10 mg loading dose and subsequent daily dosage monitored by BCR.

c) For the hypoxic patient oxygen should be given (24–35%).

d) Analgesia, even opiates, may be required.

e) Anticoagulation is continued for 3–6 weeks.

f) The underlying cause is treated if possible, e.g. the contraceptive pill is stopped or changed to the low oestrogen pill.

6. Recurrence of embolism is treated by warfarin for 3–12 months.

7. Chronic pulmonary embolism causing pulmonary hypertension needs permanent anticoagulation.

FOLLOW-UP

Follow-up is necessary at regular intervals while the patient is anticoagulated to check BCR and control dose. After stopping therapy the patient should be seen at 3, 6 and 9 months, then discharged from hospital or GP care if there is no evidence of recurrence clinically. The lung scan is repeated if there are doubts.

[1] Crofton J, Douglas A (1981) *Respiratory Diseases* 3rd edn. Oxford: Blackwell.
[2] Miller GH (1976) Pulmonary thromboembolism. In *Respiratory Disease Tutorials in Postgraduate Medicine* (Lane DJ ed.) vol. 5. London: William Heinemann Medical Books.
[3] Bell WR et al. (1982) Am. Heart J., 103, 239.

Lung Cancer

As cigarette smoking has increased so has lung cancer. In Western countries it is the commonest neoplasm in men, and among women only breast cancer kills more. In Britain over 30 000 men and 10 000 women die from lung cancer each year. It is commonest in the age range 50–70.

PROGNOSIS[1,2]

- Generally it is dismal: 5% overall five-year survival.
- The outcome is related to cell type and, for non small-cell tumours, operability.

  a) Squamous cell:
     i) Operable: 20–30% five-year survival.
     ii) Inoperable: median survival 9–12 months.
  b) Small cell: 1% five-year survival; median survival with chemotherapy: 12 months; limited disease better than extensive.
  c) Adenocarcinoma and alveolar cell:
     i) Operable: 20% five-year survival.
     ii) Inoperable: as for squamous cell.

- Operable patients: the smaller the tumour the better the prognosis. If hilar nodes are uninvolved the outlook is improved.
- If the tumour is resectable by lobectomy, the prognosis is better than if pneumonectomy is necessary.
- There is a 60% five-year survival for operable squamous carcinoma <3 cm diameter without lymph node invasion.
- The presence of weight loss, chest pain, or hypoalbuminaemia worsens the prognosis.

TREATMENT[2,3,4]

1. *Non small-cell tumours (squamous, adeno, alveolar cell)*

   a) Resection is the treatment of choice.
   b) Contraindications to surgery include:
      i) Advanced age: in patients over 70, surgery is usually inadvisable because the benefits are outweighed by operative morbidity and mortality.
      ii) Inadequate pulmonary function: An $FEV_1 > 1.21$ is necessary for lobectomy, and > 1.81 for pneumonec-
tomy. A raised $PaCO_2$ contraindicates surgery.
      iii) Local extension of tumour or metastases: tumour involving main bronchus to within 1 cm of carina on right or 2 cm on left; brachial plexus or chest wall invasion; Horner's syndrome; mediastinal or supraclavicular lymph node metastases; distant metastases; recurrent laryngeal or phrenic nerve involvement; malignant pleural effusion; superior vena cava (SVC) obstruction.
      iv) Other serious diseases may be relative contraindications.
   c) Preoperative work-up should include: physical examination, chest x-ray with or without hilar tomography or CT scan of thorax, measurement of FEV_1 and arterial blood gases, bronchoscopy, barium swallow, screening of diaphragm, liver function tests (if abnormal the liver should be scanned; if only alkaline phosphatase raised, check for liver or bone origin and then scan appropriately). Routine brain and bone scans or whole body computerised axial tomography are performed in some centres.
   d) At thoracotomy previously undiscovered metastases or local extension may render tumour unresectable.
   e) Intercostal nerve block at operation reduces post-thoracotomy pain and analgesic requirements.
   f) Physiotherapy and prompt treatment of chest infection are important postoperatively. Oxygen may be necessary initially.
   g) Apical and basal underwater sealed drains are removed in the first few days after thoracotomy, the patient is mobilised promptly and discharged home within 10–14 days.

h) If the tumour is inoperable management is directed towards palliation of symptoms. Radiotherapy (DXR) will normally relieve haemoptysis, pain from bone metastases and SVC obstruction; it is sometimes used to prevent blockage of the trachea or main bronchus. DXR to the primary can sometimes reduce non-metastatic effects. Few centres attempt 'curative' DXR. Prednisolone 10 mg bd removes malaise and restores appetite. Codeine is useful for cough. Pain must be adequately controlled. Opiates are likely to be required eventually in increasing doses at shortening intervals. Laxatives may be necessary. Phenothiazines and/or antidepressants are sometimes indicated. Care and understanding from staff are paramount for patient and relatives.

2. *Small-cell tumour*

a) Chemotherapy, with or without cranial irradiation, is currently regarded as the treatment of choice. Some surgeons resect small peripheral lesions prior to chemotherapy.

b) Trials of various regimens continue, aiming at increasing survival with minimum toxicity. Effective combinations include adriamycin, cyclophosphamide, etoposide and vincristine. Cisplatinum is effective but toxic. Treatment is given in pulses, with haematological monitoring to modulate doses and intervals. Anti-emetics are usually necessary. Treatment is usually discontinued if there is no response after four pulses.

c) For responders the optimum number of pulses and optimum intervals are still being researched.

d) Patients aged >70 are rarely offered treatment, especially if debilitated.

e) General measures of care: see 1.

3. *Malignant effusion*

a) Aspirate or drain dry. Insert 500 mg tetracycline, having given 10 mg lignocaine intrapleurally to reduce pain.

b) In the case of reaccumulation repeat aspiration or drainage, or perform talc pleurodesis (general anaesthetic is necessary).

c) Prednisolone 10 mg bd delays reaccumulation.

4. In a disease so difficult to treat, prevention by reducing prevalence of cigarette smoking is extremely important.

FOLLOW-UP

Regular review is necessary, usually by the GP and hospital.

[1] Clee MD *et al.* (1984) *Br. J. Dis. Chest*, **78**, 225.
[2] Crofton J, Douglas A (1981) *Respiratory Diseases* 3rd edn. Oxford: Blackwell.
[3] Hande KR *et al.* (1983) Non small-cell cancer of the lung. In *Recent Advances in Respiratory Medicine* (Flenley D, Petty L eds.) p. 205. Edinburgh: Churchill Livingstone.
[4] Spiro SG (1985) *Br. Med. J.*, **290**, 413.

Bronchiectasis

Bronchiectasis is a condition in which there is pathological dilation of bronchi. Secretions accumulate in the bronchiectatic bronchi, become chronically infected, cause cough and purulent sputum, and occasional haemoptysis. Whooping cough, measles and pneumonia in early childhood are the most common conditions leading to bronchiectasis. The prevalence in developed countries has declined considerably since broad spectrum antibiotics became available. Congenital causes include cystic fibrosis, immotile cilia (Kartagener's syndrome) and congenital hypogammaglobulinaemia.

PROGNOSIS[1]

- The majority of children can lead a normal life. 20–30% remain symptom free. The remainder will be improved or kept well by medical and/or surgical treatment.
- In adults, with modern medical or surgical treatment the prognosis is good: 80% 15-year survival and 70% of these have no social disability from bronchiectasis. Less than 10% become housebound.
- Patients with strictly localised bronchiectasis may become symptomless after surgery.
- With more diffuse disease symptoms can be reasonably well controlled medically.
- The mortality and morbidity is related to the amount of lung destruction, the severity of generalised chronic bronchitis and emphysema, and continued smoking.
- Empyema, lung abscess, cerebral abscess, and amyloidosis are rare complications.

TREATMENT[1]

1. Postural drainage. The patient is taught how to drain affected lobes and instructed to do this regularly for 20 minutes on waking and at bedtime.
2. Patients and relatives are taught simple physiotherapy techniques and told to use them at least twice daily.
3. Exacerbations of infection are treated promptly with antibiotics e.g. ampicillin for 10–14 days.
4. For those with frequent exacerbations prophylactic treatment throughout the winter or whole year is sometimes recommended e.g. doxycline once daily or sulphametopyrazine once weekly.
5. Influenza vaccination in autumn may help.
6. Smoking should be stopped.
7. Segmental resection or lobectomy is indicated in young or middle-aged patients with persistent troublesome symptoms from localised bronchiectasis.
8. In children surgery is best deferred until teenage because spontaneous improvement may occur.
9. Surgery will not relieve symptoms if residual areas of bronchiectasis remain.
10. Bronchial artery embolisation or surgery may be necessary for profuse haemoptysis.
11. Associated irreversible airways obstruction of moderate severity contraindicates surgery.
12. Associated sinusitis, asthma, respiratory failure and cor pulmonale require appropriate therapy.

FOLLOW-UP

Once the management is established (including postoperatively) the patient may be discharged from hospital review. At least bi-annual follow-up by the GP is advisable.

[1] Crofton J, Douglas A (1981) *Respiratory Diseases* 3rd edn. Oxford: Blackwell.

Pneumoconiosis

Pneumoconiosis is a disease caused by prolonged inhalation of an inorganic dust which accumulates in the lungs and causes tissue reactions. The three principal types in Britain are coal-workers' pneumoconiosis, asbestosis and silicosis[1,2].

Coal-workers' pneumoconiosis (Pn)

The overall prevalence is 4%. It varies geographically, depending on the method of coal production, total dust, dust composition (especially quartz content) and efficiency of dust suppression and ventilation.

PROGNOSIS

Pn may be subdivided into:

- Simple pneumoconiosis. This is characterised radiographically by minute opacities diffusely scattered throughout both lung fields and is subdivided into categories 0-3. The prognosis is related to continuation of dust exposure and category. It does not regress after exposure ceases. It is not usually progressive if further exposure is avoided and life expectancy is not directly affected unless complicated pneumoconiosis develops.
- Complicated pneumoconiosis (progressive massive fibrosis, PMF). Progressive complication of simple pneumoconiosis develops in 1% category 1 and 30% category 3. It is characterised by single or multiple homogeneous opacities > 1 cm in diameter, usually in the upper lobes and peripheral. Lesions enlarge causing destruction of lung parenchyma and emphysema. Chronic bronchitis adds to dysfunction. PMF reduces life expectancy, depending on the severity, rate of progression (variable) and concomitant cigarette smoking. Hypoxaemia, respiratory failure and cor pulmonale adversely affect outcome.

TREATMENT

1. No specific treatment is available.
2. Prevention is most important.

   a) Effective dust suppression.
   b) Early recognition of dust retention by routine radiography.
   c) Provision of alternative, low dust exposure employment.
3. Cigarette smoking must be discouraged.
4. Chest infections should be promptly treated with antibiotics.
5. Inhaled bronchodilator should be given for reversible airways obstruction.
6. Oxygen is indicated for hypoxaemia, with rest and diuretics (plus or minus digoxin) for cor pulmonale.

FOLLOW-UP

Radiological review is usually organised by the employer or Pneumoconiosis Panel. GP and hospital supervision is necessary for respiratory failure and cor pulmonale.

Asbestosis

Asbestosis is a pneumoconiosis from prolonged inhalation of asbestos dust. It is characterised by diffuse interstitial pulmonary fibrosis. Fibrosis is persistent and slowly progressive even though exposure may cease. There is a dose-response relationship. Prevalence depends on the at-risk occupation, fibre concentration and duration of exposure. About 120–150 new cases per year compensated in the UK. Relevant occupations are asbestos mining/manufacture, dock/shipyard work, electrical insulating, lagging, brake and clutch lining manufacture, builders and roofers. White, blue or brown asbestos can cause asbestosis. Blue asbestos can also cause mesothelioma (which has a very poor prognosis, the only treatment being palliative).
Contd.

PROGNOSIS

- The prognosis depends on the rate of progression which is variable and unpredictable, and the development of respiratory failure or cor pulmonale.
- Asbestosis predisposes to lung cancer, development of which considerably reduces life expectancy.
- The prognosis is adversely affected by cigarette smoking. There is synergistic interaction of carcinogenic risks.
- Asbestosis sufferers have 2.6 times the normal risk of death from all causes and 8.5 times the risk of death from lung cancer.

TREATMENT

1. No specific treatment is available. Corticosteroids do not slow progression.
2. Prevention is the most important aspect.

   a) Enforcement of statutory standards for working with asbestos in relation to production, storage, transport, use, monitoring fibre levels, protective clothing and respirators and disposal of waste.
   b) Production of safe alternatives to asbestos.

3. Further exposure to asbestos should be avoided.
4. Smoking should cease.
5. See 3, 4, 5 and 6 under *Coal-workers' pneumoconiosis Treatment*.

FOLLOW-UP

The Pneumoconiosis Panel reviews each patient to decide compensation. There should be regular GP or hospital follow-up with chest x-ray every 6-12 months to aid early detection of lung cancer.

Silicosis

Silicosis is a pneumoconiosis caused by inhaling dust containing silica particles 1–10 μm in diameter. Associated occupations include granite, slate and sandstone quarrying, mining, stone dressing, metal casting and sand blasting, pottery and ceramics, manufacturing/trimming of refractory bricks used in furnaces and boiler scaling. Approximately 100 new cases per year are compensated in UK.

PROGNOSIS

- Simple silicosis is progressive. May appear and progress after exposure ceases.
- More likely to progress to complicated silicosis (PMF) than is coal-workers' pneumoconiosis (see p. 13).
- Complicated silicosis more aggressive than coal-workers' PMF.
- Predisposes to pulmonary tuberculosis.

TREATMENT

1. No specific treatment is available.
2. Prevention is most important:

   a) Monitoring and reduction of dust levels.
   b) Adequate ventilation.
   c) Respirators should be worn.
   d) Regular chest x-rays.

3. Early detection and removal from exposure is important.
4. If tuberculosis develops treat promptly and adequately.
5. See 3, 4, 5 and 6 under *Coal-workers' pneumoconiosis Treatment*.

FOLLOW-UP

The Pneumoconiosis Panel regularly reviews each patient. GP review should occur every 6–12 months, with sputum check and chest x-ray. Specialist advice should be sought for treatment of tuberculosis or respiratory failure and/or cor pulmonale.

---

[1] Crofton J, Douglas A (1981) *Respiratory Diseases* 3rd edn. Oxford: Blackwell.
[2] Morgan K, Seaton A (1984) *Occupational Lung Disease* 2nd edn. Philadelphia: W. B. Saunders Company

Pneumothorax

Pneumothorax means air in the pleural cavity. Spontaneous pneumothorax occurs unexpectedly and is secondary to disease of the lungs/pleura (usually rupture of a sub-pleural bulla, rarely rupture of a lung abscess or TB cavity). Traumatic pneumothorax is due to rib fractures, crushed chest injuries or penetrating wounds (including medical procedures). Spontaneous pneumothorax is five times more common among men than women.

PROGNOSIS[1]

- Reabsorption of air and re-expansion of lung will occur over 3–12 weeks unless broncho-pleural fistula or tension pneumothorax develop.
- If respiratory function is poor pneumothorax may precipitate respiratory failure.
- If tension pneumothorax is not treated intrapleural pressure will increase, causing mediastinal shift, compression of great vessels and the other lung, and death from hypoxaemia and circulatory collapse.
- 20–30% spontaneous pneumothoraces recur, mostly within a year. Thereafter, if the patient is treated conservatively, the recurrence rate increases.
- For traumatic pneumothorax, the outlook depends on the cause and extent of injury.

TREATMENT[1,2,3]

1. If pneumothorax <20–30% and patient is not dyspnoeic, no treatment is necessary: the patient should be observed for 24 hours to make sure there is no progression.
2. If the patient is dyspnoeic or if the pneumothorax >30% it should be aspirated through a three-way tap or drained via an intercostal tube and underwater-sealed drain. The tube should be inserted through the 2nd intercostal space in the mid-clavicular line (men, older women) or the 5th intercostal space in the axilla (younger women) using local and/or systemic analgesia. It should be left in place for 24–48 hours after the lung is re-expanded. Failure to re-expand implies either pulmonary collapse due to blocked bronchi (secretions may be sucked away via a bronchoscope) and/or bronchopleural fistula for which surgical ligation is necessary. Adequate analgesia is important while the tube is *in situ*, for comfort and to facilitate respiratory movement/coughing.
3. *Tension pneumothorax* requires immediate treatment: intercostal insertion of a needle will suffice pending tube drainage.
4. Hypoxia is treated with oxygen.
5. Most physicians treat a 2nd pneumothorax on the same side by tube drainage, sometimes with intrapleural tetracycline to cause pleural adhesions.
6. A third episode is an indication for pleurodesis or pleurectomy, providing the patient's general condition permits it.
7. If pneumothorax occurs on different sides on separate occasions, surgical treatment is indicated.

FOLLOW-UP

A chest x-ray is advisable after three months to check on reabsorption and healing. The patient may then be discharged with advice to return if there is a recurrence.

[1] Crofton J, Douglas A (1981) *Respiratory Diseases* 3rd edn. Oxford: Blackwell.
[2] Archer GJ *et al.* (1985) *Br. J. Dis. Chest*, 79, 177.
[3] Spencer-Jones J (1985) *Thorax*, 40, 66.

Cystic Fibrosis

Cystic fibrosis (CF) is an autosomal recessive disorder. Birth prevalence ranges from 1 in 1600 to 1 in 7200. The carrier frequency in Caucasians is around 1 in 20. The chief clinical manifestations are bronchopulmonary infection, pancreatic insufficiency and raised sweat electrolytes. The basic biochemical defect is unknown[1,2].

PROGNOSIS[1,2]

- The prognosis has improved greatly over the last 50 years, especially since anti-staphylococcal antibiotics became available.
- 75% survive to adolescence and >50% to adulthood.
- In specialised centres average survival is now to the mid-twenties and of those who survive to sixteen >40% will survive to age 30.

TREATMENT[1,2]

1. Chest physiotherapy 2–3 times daily. First parents are taught and later the child/adolescent.
2. Antibiotics. In early childhood these are directed against *Staph. pyogenes*, e.g. flucloxacillin. But pseudomonas becomes a common pathogen later: therefore aminoglycoside (gentamicin or tobramycin) and an antipseudomonal penicillin (carbenicillin or azlocillin) are given in combination. Ceftazidime is sometimes used.
3. Larger doses than usual of antibiotics are necessary for CF patients and serum levels of aminoglycosides should be monitored to ensure adequate dosage.
4. Antistaphylococcal therapy usually given for 2–3 weeks but some physicians continue flucloxacillin permanently after the first staphylococcal infection.
5. Antipseudomonas therapy (intravenous) is usually given for 2–3 weeks. Older patients can learn to give their own injections via a sited canula, thereby shortening hospitalisation.
6. Bronchodilators are necessary for wheeze.

Those with asthma benefit from regular cromoglycate or inhaled corticosteroids.

7. Regular inhalation of nebulised antipseudomonal antibiotics is of value.
8. Pancreatic enzyme supplements should be taken with meals.
9. Regular vitamin supplements, in water soluble form if possible, are helpful.
10. The diet should be high in calories, protein and carbohydrates, with a moderate reduction of fat (use enteric coated microspheres).
11. A high fluid intake is important.
12. Acetylcysteine 20% (Airbron) or Gastrografin orally and/or rectally will usually relieve meconium ileus equivalent.
13. Haemoptysis usually stops spontaneously or with aminocaproic acid but bronchial artery embolisation may be necessary.
14. Respiratory failure and cor pulmonale will require rest, oxygen and diuretics. Eventually opiates may become appropriate.
15. This chronic progressive disease requires close liaison between doctors, nurses, physiotherapists, social workers and parents. Continuity of experienced and competent care is particularly important.

FOLLOW-UP

Ideally follow-up should be at specialist centres and should be regular. A policy of self-admission to hospital has much to commend it.

[1] Goodchild MC, Dodge JA (1985) *Cystic Fibrosis Manual of Diagnosis and Management*. London: Bailliere Tindall.
[2] Hodson ME, Norman AP, Batten JC (1983) *Cystic Fibrosis*. London: Bailliere Tindall.

Sarcoidosis

Sarcoidosis is a multi-system granulomatous disorder of unknown aetiology presenting most frequently with bilateral hilar lymphadenopathy, pulmonary infiltration erythema nodosum and uveitis. The prevalence is 10–60 per 100 000, with considerable geographic variation. Negroes are more commonly affected than whites. The incidence is highest in 20–40 age group, and women are slightly more affected than men[1,2]. Diagnosis is confirmed by the Kveim test.

PROGNOSIS[1,2]

- The 'sub-acute' form usually resolves spontaneously within two years while the 'chronic' form usually persists beyond two years.
- Hilar adenopathy clears spontaneously in a year in 60–80% and a further 10–15% clear in the next year.
- Pulmonary opacities clear spontaneously in 40–70%; the majority within two years, but in 20% resolution may take 3–7 years.
- About 10% are disabled from chronic pulmonary fibrosis.
- Central nervous system (CNS) sarcoidosis may progress despite treatment.
- The mortality is 5%.

TREATMENT[1,2]

1. Treatment is usually unnecessary because of the tendency for spontaneous resolution.
2. Indications for treatment include:

   a) Disabling breathlessness.
   b) Deteriorating pulmonary function tests (PFTs) after 3–6 months.
   c) Radiological progression after 3–6 months or failure to improve after 6–12 months (hilar enlargement alone, even if persistent, does not require treatment).
   d) Involvement of eyes, CNS, myocardium, parotid or lachrymal glands.
   e) Persistent hypercalcaemia or hypercalcuria.
   f) Disfiguring skin lesions.
   g) Persistent erythema nodosum with systemic upset.
   h) Symptomatic splenic involvement.

3. Corticosteroids suppress disease in most cases – prednisolone 20–40 mg daily.
4. The progress of the disease should be monitored clinically, radiographically and with PFTs.
5. After maximum improvement (usually 1–3 months) the prednisolone should be reduced in monthly 5 mg steps to 10 mg. If the disease is still suppressed (see 4) 7.5 mg or 5 mg daily dose can be tried. The higher dose is resumed if relapse occurs.
6. Suppression is maintained for 6–18 months, then gradual withdrawal in monthly 2.5 mg steps is attempted.
7. Suppressive doses are resumed if the patient relapses and continued for a year before re-attempting reduction.
8. A minority need lifelong treatment.
9. Oxyphenbutazone, chloroquine, chlorambucil, methotrexate and azathioprine have a suppressive effect, but toxicity is a problem. They are sometimes used in conjunction with prednisolone for refractory disease.

FOLLOW-UP

Specialist supervision with chest x-ray and PFTs is necessary. The patient may be discharged from hospital with GP follow-up after spontaneous resolution. Patients requiring corticosteroids need regular assessment (see 4–8) while on treatment and for a year after discontinuation.

---

[1] Crofton J, Douglas A (1981) *Respiratory Diseases* 3rd edn. Oxford: Blackwell.
[2] James DG, Williams WJ (1985) *Sarcoidosis and other Granulomatous Disorders*. Philadelphia: W. B. Saunders Company.

Pulmonary Tuberculosis

Pulmonary tuberculosis is declining in developed countries but remains common in developing countries where some 10 million cases occur per year. In Britain 6022 pulmonary cases were notified in 1983, with the highest rates in immigrants from the Indian subcontinent and middle-aged/elderly white males.

PROGNOSIS[1]

- The worldwide mortality is 25–30%.
- The mortality in Britain is 5%. Deaths are mainly among social drop-outs and the elderly, such patients usually presenting late and moribund; or, tuberculosis not being diagnosed ante-mortem.
- Proper chemotherapy cures virtually 100%.
- The relapse rate is 1–2%, usually in poor compliers.
- Residual pulmonary damage depends on pre-treatment extent and duration of disease.

TREATMENT[1,2,3]

1. Initially triple or quadruple chemotherapy, then continuation therapy with two drugs to which the organism is sensitive.

   a) Nine months isoniazid (H) and rifampicin (R) supplemented in the first two months by ethambutol or streptomycin.
   b) Alternatively, six months HR, supplemented in first two months by ethambutol and pyrazinamide, or streptomycin and pyrazinamide.
   c) If it is not possible to use HR (due to expense, intolerance or bacterial resistance) alternative treatment regimes should continue for 18 months.
   d) The tablets are taken all together once daily, before breakfast if possible.

2. Twice weekly streptomycin and high dose isoniazid (with pyridoxine) for 18 months is an effective form of supervised chemotherapy.

3. If renal function is reduced streptomycin and ethambutol are relatively contraindicated.

4. Biochemical disturbance of liver function, in the absence of clinical symptoms, may occur but is usually transient and resolves without interruption or change of therapy.

5. Prompt identification and treatment of cases is important in preventing community spread.

6. Smear-negative patients are a low infectious risk.

7. Infectivity wanes rapidly after starting chemotherapy: smear-positive patients are not infectious after three weeks and need not be segregated thereafter.

8. Contact tracing is best directed at close contacts of smear-positive patients: some 10% of these develop disease.

9. BCG confers 70–80% protection for 20 years.

FOLLOW-UP

Follow-up should be by a specialist during therapy. Thereafter it is unnecessary unless compliance with treatment was doubtful.

[1] Crofton J, Douglas A (1981) *Respiratory Disease* 3rd edn. Oxford: Blackwell.
[2] Horne NW (1983) Short course chemotherapy for tuberculosis. In *Recent Advances in Respiratory Medicine* (Flenley D, Petty L eds.) p. 223. Edinburgh: Churchill Livingstone.
[3] British Thoracic Society (1984) *Br. J. Dis. Chest*, 78 330.

Extrinsic Allergic Alveolitis

Extrinsic allergic alveolitis is a pulmonary hypersensitivity response (Type III) caused by inhalation of a variety of organic dusts. Farmers' Lung (reaction to *Micropolyspora faeni* in mouldy hay) and Bird Fanciers' Lung (reaction to antigens in pigeon or budgerigar serum/droppings) are the main types in Great Britain. Other types: Bagassosis (mouldy sugar cane bagasse containing *T. vulgaris*), Malt Workers' Lung (*Aspergillus clavatus* as antigen), Mushroom Workers' Lung (*M. faeni*, *T. vulgaris* as antigens). Malaise, fever, cough and dyspnoea occur 4–6 hours after exposure.

PROGNOSIS[1]

- The acute reaction is usually self-limiting, resolving within days or weeks with little residual fibrosis.
- With repeated exposure chronic pulmonary fibrosis develops. It may lead to respiratory failure and/or cor pulmonale.

TREATMENT

1. For an acute attack oxygen and prednisolone if the attack is severe. Some physicians always give a month's prednisolone from the time of diagnosis.
2. Further exposure should be avoided:

   a) Farmers' lung – change to silage; someone else should be employed; proper respirator should be worn if exposure is unavoidable.

   b) Bird fanciers' lung – dispose of pet pigeons or budgerigars.

3. Prevention: hay should be dried adequately, silage used and no birds kept.

FOLLOW-UP

Chest x-ray and pulmonary function tests are performed at one and three months. The patient can be discharged from hospital care if stable. GP follow-up to check for recurrence.

---

[1] Crofton J, Douglas A (1981) *Respiratory Diseases* 3rd edn. Oxford: Blackwell.

Fibrosing Alveolitis

The aetiology of fibrosing alveolitis is unknown. It is characterised by diffuse, chronic inflammatory process in the lung beyond the terminal bronchiole. It presents with breathlessness, cough, clubbing, cyanosis and crepitations. The prevalence is around 3 per 100 000 in UK and USA, onset being usually in middle age, with roughly equal sex representation.

PROGNOSIS[1,2]

- Survival varies from 1 month to 20 years; on average it is 3–12 years.
- <10% remain stable or improve spontaneously.
- The 'desquamative' type is more likely to respond to corticosteroids than the 'mural/usual' type (60% v. 10%).
- Younger patients are more likely to respond.
- 77% responders survive two years, against the two-year survival rate of non-responders of 56%.

TREATMENT[1,2]

1. Prednisolone 40–60 mg daily for 6–8 weeks should be tried.
2. Symptomatic, radiological and pulmonary function responses should be monitored.
3. In responders the dose of prednisolone can be reduced by 2.5–5 mg per month to 20 mg daily with careful monitoring (see 2). Thereafter the dose can be reduced in 1 mg steps to the lowest dose that will suppress the disease.
4. Non-responders: discontinue prednisolone or try adding azathioprine or chlorambucil.
5. Infection is promptly treated.
6. Dyspnoea is treated with oxygen, and with opiates terminally.
7. Diuretics (with or without digoxin) for cor pulmonale.

FOLLOW-UP

Regular review, frequency depending on stability/progression.

[1] Crofton J, Douglas A (1981) *Respiratory Diseases* 3rd edn. Oxford: Blackwell.
[2] Hance A *et al.* (1983) Idiopathic pulmonary fibrosis. In *Recent Advances in Respiratory Medicine* (Flenley D, Petty L eds.). Edinburgh: Churchill Livingstone.

2

Diseases of the Cardiovascular System

P.J. Oldershaw and J.R. Dawson

Hypertension

No completely satisfactory definition of hypertension exists. The World Health Organisation arbitrarily defines it as a single sitting blood pressure of 165/95 or over; values below 140/90 are considered normal and values between these two levels as borderline hypertension. Most cases of hypertension have no clearly definable cause, seeming to involve a complex interaction between a number of environmental and genetic factors, but a small proportion of cases is associated with coarctation of the aorta or with underlying endocrine disease (Conn's syndrome, Cushing's syndrome, phaeochromocytoma), or renal disease (renal artery stenosis, chronic pyelonephritis, chronic nephritis). Hypertension in itself produces few symptoms but its presence is associated with an increased incidence of renal disease, stroke and cardiovascular disease.

PROGNOSIS

- Life Insurance company tables show that the level of a subject's blood pressure is inversely related to their prospective survival. A large prospective community study[1] showed that hypertensive subjects had a sevenfold increase in the incidence of stroke, a fourfold increase in cardiac failure and a threefold increase in coronary heart disease.
- As a risk factor for cardiovascular disease the systolic blood pressure is equally as important as the diastolic blood pressure, irrespective of the patient's age or sex.
- A number of large well-designed studies[2,3,4] have shown that treatment of hypertension is effective in reducing mortality from stroke and renal failure, but there is much less compelling evidence that treatment is effective in reducing mortality from coronary events. The value of treatment, however, becomes increasingly clear cut with increasing levels of pretreatment blood pressure.
- The benefit of therapy in patients over 65 with sustained diastolic pressure in the range 95-115 mmHg has not been clearly established.
- Treatment of hypertensive patients who have had strokes reduces the incidence of further strokes.

TREATMENT

1. The principal problem in the management of a 'hypertensive' subject is deciding at which level of blood pressure to begin treatment. The risks of hypertension are related to the level of blood pressure and therefore in patients with only mildly elevated blood pressure the treatment risk/benefit relationships have to be considered. However evidence has accumulated from several large studies[4,5] that treatment is of benefit even in subjects with mildly elevated blood pressure.
2. General measures, such as stopping smoking and weight reduction by dieting and an increase in exercise are valuable.
3. Restriction of salt intake may be an effective means of lowering the blood pressure[6].
4. Beta blocking agents are now for many physicians the drug of first choice in treating hypertension. Recommended doses include atenolol 50-100 mg daily, metoprolol 100-200 mg daily and propranolol 160-320 mg daily. Cardioselective agents (e.g. atenolol and metoprolol) are safer to use in patient with asthma or diabetes mellitus but do not seem to have any advantages over non selective beta blockers in terms of blood pressure lowering effect. Beta blockers are less effective in black patients.
5. In most studies thiazide diuretics normally produce a reduction in blood pressure of 10-15 mmHg. Once daily dosage is normally sufficient and it should be remembered that full effect may not be reached until eight weeks after the onset of treatment. Loop diuretics e.g. frusemide, and potassium sparing agents e.g. spironolactone and amiloride, are less effective hypotensive agents than the thiazide group of diuretics and have little part to play in the treatment of hypertension. Long-term therapy with thiazide diuretics is frequently associated with significant hypokalaemia and

potassium supplementation is indicated in elderly patients particularly those on concurrent therapy with digoxin. Thiazide diuretics may also cause hyperuricaemia, glucose intolerance and also impotence in 20% male patients[7].

6. Calcium antagonist drugs (e.g. nifedipine 40–60 mg daily, verapamil 120–360 mg daily) are effective hypotensive agents and their use in the management of hypertension is increasing. Nifedipine may cause headache, palpitation, nausea and flushing although these adverse effects are less frequent when the delayed release preparation is used. Verapamil has a potent negative inotropic effect and delays atrioventricular conduction and therefore should be used with caution in patients with concomitant myocardial or conducting tissue disease.

7. Angiotensin converting enzyme inhibitors (e.g. captopril 25–150 mg daily, enalapril 10–20 mg daily) are powerful hypotensive agents that are useful in the management of moderate or severe hypertension.

8. Methyldopa and adrenergic neurone blocking drugs such as guanethidene, bethanidine, debrisoquine and clonidine are all effective hypotensive agents but have a high incidence of side-effects, principally affecting the central and sympathetic nervous systems, and therefore they have been superseded in recent years by drugs with fewer side-effects.

FOLLOW-UP

Once initiated on antihypertensive treatment, a patient's blood pressure should be checked at frequent intervals with no longer than three months between assessments.

[1] Kannel WB et al. (1969) Dis. Chest., 56, 43.
[2] Veterans Administration Cooperative Study (1970) J. Am. Med. Assoc., 213, 1143.
[3] Hypertension Detection and Follow-up Cooperative Group (1979) J. Am. Med. Assoc., 242, 2562.
[4] Report of the Management Committee: Australian Therapeutic Trial in Mild Hypertension (1980) Lancet, i, 1261.
[5] Medical Research Council Working Party (1985) Br. Med. J., 291, 97.
[6] MacGregor GA et al. (1982) Lancet, i, 351.
[7] Medical Research Council Working Party (1981) Lancet, ii, 539.

Coronary Heart Disease

Coronary heart disease is the commonest cause of death in the UK after malignancy and is almost invariably caused by narrowing or occlusion of the coronary arteries due to atherosclerosis. Important risk factors include heredity, cigarette smoking, systemic hypertension, hyperlipidaemia, diabetes mellitus and obesity. The incidence of the disease increases with age and is also related to occupation, stress, diet and gender (males more than females). In most cases coronary heart disease presents either as angina pectoris or as acute myocardial infarction but a significant proportion of patients present with ventricular arrhythmias (including the sudden death syndrome) or with symptoms of heart failure due to ischaemic myocardial damage.

Angina pectoris

PROGNOSIS

- The annual mortality of patients with angina is approximately 4%.
- In 33% patients with recent onset angina the symptoms will spontaneously remit.
- The presence of concomitant systemic hypertension adversely affects the prognosis.

TREATMENT

1. General measures: stop smoking, treatment of hypertension, treatment of hyperlipidaemia, weight reduction in the obese patient.
2. Glyceryl trinitrate administered either sublingually (0.5 mg) or by spray is the drug of choice in the treatment of acute anginal attacks.
3. Long-acting nitrate preparations (e.g. isosorbide dinitrate 30–120 mg daily, isosorbide mononitrate 20–60 mg daily, Transiderm Nitro 5–10 mg daily) increase the anginal threshold and reduce the frequency of anginal attacks. In general they are well tolerated particularly when formulated as a slow-release preparation.
4. Beta adrenergic blocking drugs are the mainstay of therapy in chronic stable angina. They attenuate the cardiac response to adrenergic stimulation and thereby reduce the frequency of anginal attacks and raise the anginal threshold. Generally they are well tolerated but care should be exercised in patients with impaired left ventricular function in whom beta blockers can precipitate heart failure. Commonly used preparations are atenolol 50–200 mg daily, metoprolol 100–400 mg daily and propranolol 60–320 mg daily. First reports of the use of a combined alpha and beta blocker preparation (labetolol) are favourable[3].
5. Calcium antagonist drugs (e.g. nifedipine 30–60 mg daily, verapamil 120–360 mg daily, diltiazem 120–240 mg daily) are useful in the treatment of chronic angina. In general they are safe to use but verapamil should only be given cautiously in combination with beta blocking agents in view of its potent effects on atrioventricular node function.
6. The conventional policy in the medical treatment of patients with angina pectoris is to begin with glyceral trinitrate tablets and a beta blocker and then, if the response to these is inadequate, to add either a long-acting nitrate preparation or a calcium antagonist agent or both. If the patient continues to complain of angina coronary arteriography should be performed to document precisely the coronary anatomy and to determine the patient's suitability for either percutaneous coronary angioplasty (see 7) or coronary artery by-pass surgery (see 8).
7. Percutaneous coronary angioplasty (first reported in 1978) is a procedure being used with increasing frequency in patients with both single and multiple vessel coronary artery disease. Successful dilatation of the coronary stenosis is achieved in 60–80% cases with associated abolition or amelioration of the symptom of angina. Factors favourable to a successful outcome are short non-eccentric proximal stenoses in males with a short preceding history of angina. The mortality of the procedure is approximately 1% once th

surgeon has negotiated an initial learning curve. The complication of coronary occlusion with myocardial infarction occurs in approximately 5% cases.

8. Coronary artery by-pass surgery using either lengths of saphenous vein or the internal mammary artery is a palliative operation which is highly effective in relieving the symptom of angina in patients for whom triple medical therapy (beta blocker, calcium antagonist and long-acting nitrate) has been ineffective. The underlying atherosclerotic disease process is unaffected by, and in some patients appears to be accelerated by, the operation. The operative mortality is 1–2% but is increased in women and in patients with impaired left ventricular function. Approximately 90% patients are symptom free in the year following operation and by five years approximately 75% patients are still free of angina. Saphenous vein grafts have an initial immediate failure rate of approximately 10% followed by an annual attrition rate of approximately 5%. Long-term follow-up studies suggest that internal mammary artery grafts have a substantially higher patency rate than saphenous vein grafts[4]. Treatment with anticoagulant drugs (e.g. warfarin) or antiplatelet agents (e.g. aspirin or dipyridamole) has not been shown conclusively to alter graft patency rates.

9. The value of surgical versus medical therapy in the reduction of mortality from coronary heart disease remains unsure except in the circumstance of left main stem stenosis where surgical treatment is clearly advantageous. A European study[5] shows a reduction in mortality in surgically treated patients with triple vessel disease and in patients with two vessel disease in whom the left anterior descending artery is affected. However an American study[6] of patients with mild angina shows no advantage of surgical treatment in terms of mortality or infarction rates.

FOLLOW-UP

Assessment of the response to treatment should be made at regular intervals, the timings of which are determined by the patient's age, general condition and level of original symptoms. After coronary angioplasty patients should be reviewed regularly. The effectiveness of enhanced myocardial perfusion can be assessed by exercise testing or by thallium scanning. Restenosis of dilated coronary vessels occurs in 20–30% cases and therefore reassessment by coronary arteriography should be performed at some time between six and twelve months following angioplasty. Review following coronary artery by-pass surgery at six weeks, six months and then at annual intervals. Recurrence of angina should be investigated by stress testing and cardiac catheterisation, both to assess graft patency and to identify progression of disease in the native coronary vessels.

Myocardial infarction

PROGNOSIS

- The overall hospital mortality for patients with acute myocardial infarction is 5–15%.
- The overall annual mortality for patients surviving for one year following myocardial infarction is approximately 5%. Myocardial infarct size and the state of the coronary vessels perfusing residual functioning myocardium are the most important factors determining survival. Patients with high grade atrioventricular block or intraventricular conduction abnormalities have reduced survival rates.
- Infarct extension occurs in 10–30% patients in the first 10 days following acute myocardial infarction.
- Patients with non-Q wave infarction have reduced early mortality in comparison with patients with Q wave infarction, but have high reinfarction rates and comparable late mortality[1].
- Cardiogenic shock (low cardiac output with hypotension and oliguria) complicates approximately 10% acute myocardial infarctions and is associated with a 75–100% mortality rate.
- Myocardial rupture either of the septum or of the ventricular free wall complicates 3% myocardial infarctions and is most common in elderly women.
- Ventricular fibrillation (VF) occurs in 4–18%

Contd.

patients with acute infarction. There is an equal incidence of VF between inferior and anterior infarcts but it is rare in non-Q wave infarction. VF occurs in 40–83% cases without warning arrythmia but a significant proportion of cases are presaged by ventricular ectopic activity. Ventricular premature beats or ventricular tachycardia following hospital discharge is associated with increased incidence of sudden death.

- The presence of ECG manifestations of myocardial ischaemia on early post infarction stress testing is associated with an increased incidence of recurrent infarction and sudden death[2].

TREATMENT

1. The alleviation of pain by the use of adequate analgesia (e.g. diamorphine 5–10 mg) is crucial in the initial management.
2. If appropriate to their age, general medical condition and social circumstances patients should be admitted to a coronary care unit for monitoring of cardiac rhythm and haemodynamic performance.
3. Frequent or multifocal ventricular ectopic beats should be treated with lignocaine using an initial 100 mg i.v. loading dose followed by a continuous infusion of 1–4 mg/minute. Immediate d.c. cardioversion is indicated for ventricular fibrillation and most cases of ventricular tachycardia.
4. Left ventricular failure should be treated with frusemide (40–120 mg i.v.).
5. Cardiogenic shock has an appalling prognosis. Positive inotropic agents (e.g. dopamine, dobutamine) and vasodilator drugs (e.g. nitroprusside) may all produce short-term haemodynamic benefit but none has been shown to affect the ultimate outcome. Likewise the results of treatment with aortic balloon counterpulsation have been disappointing.
6. Mechanical causes of haemodynamic deterioration which are surgically remediable (e.g. mitral regurgitation due to papillary muscle rupture and left to right shunting due to rupture of the interventricular septum) are best treated by immediate operation.
7. Reperfusion of infarcting myocardium to limit infarct size and thus influence prognosis is a concept which has elicited much recent interest[7]. Intracoronary streptokinase recanalises 60–90% occluded vessels in acute myocardial infarction. Intravenous streptokinase is less effective producing recanalisation in 40–60% cases. Thrombolytic therapy is probably only effective when administered within four hours of the onset of chest pain. Treatment with streptokinase is associated with a substantial incidence of major haemorrhagic complications; recent reports suggest that therapy with human tissue-type plasminogen activating substances produced by the use of recombinant DNA technology is superior in this respect[8]. Recanalised coronary vessels have a high incidence of reocclusion; therefore successful thrombolytic therapy should be followed by some form of revascularisation procedure, either percutaneous coronary angioplasty or coronary artery by-pass surgery.
8. Evidence is accumulating from secondary prevention studies that in patients with uncomplicated myocardial infarction treatment with beta blocking agents is effective in reducing mortality and reinfarction rates[9]. Benefit has been shown with metoprolol, propranolol and atenolol but the most compelling evidence is provided by the results of the Norwegian study of timolol[10] in which active treatment was associated with a 45% reduction in mortality.
9. Secondary prevention with anti-platelet drugs (aspirin, dipyridamole, sulphinpyrazone) has not been conclusively shown to affect mortality or reinfarction rates.
10. Despite many years study the role of anticoagulation with warfarin following myocardial infarction has not been clearly established. Anticoagulation reduces the incidence of systemic embolus from mural thrombus from 10 to 4% and a recent study[11] suggests that mortality may also be reduced.

FOLLOW-UP

Younger patients should be investigated by coronary arteriography, particularly if the exercise electrocardiogram is positive. Older patients should be followed-up regularly but only investigated by coronary arteriography if they have recurrent angina which cannot be controlled medically.

[1] Hutter AM *et al.* (1981) *Am. J. Cardiol.*, **48**, 595.
[2] Theroux P *et al.* (1979) *N. Eng. J. Med.*, **301**, 341.
[3] Quyyum AA *et al.* (1985) *Br. Heart J.*, **53**, 47.
[4] Lytle BW *et al.* (1985) *J. Thorac. Cardiovasc. Surg.*, **89**, 248.
[5] European Coronary Surgery Study Group (1980) *Lancet*, **ii**, 491.
[6] CASS principal investigators and their associates (1983) *Circulation*, **63**, 939.
[7] Rentrop KP (1985) *Circulation*, **71**, 627.
[8] Collen MD *et al.* (1984) *Circulation*, **70**, 1012.
[9] Chamberlain DA (1983) *Br. Heart J.*, **49**, 105.
[10] Norwegian Multicenter Study Group (1981) *N. Eng. J. Med.*, **304**, 801.
[11] Report of the Sixty Plus Reinfarction Study Research Group (1980) *Lancet*, **ii**, 989.

Mitral Stenosis

Mitral stenosis usually results from rheumatic fever but rarely may be congenital or due to connective tissue disease. Most patients in temperate climates will remain asymptomatic for 10–20 years after the onset of acute rheumatic fever, symptoms beginning most commonly in the third to fourth decade. The commonest symptoms are of breathlessness, orthopnoea and haemoptysis.

PROGNOSIS

- There is a latent period of 10–20 years after an attack of acute rheumatic fever during which the patient is asymptomatic. It then takes 5–10 years to progress from mild to severe disability.
- In the pre-surgical era there was a 62% five-year and 38% 10-year survival for patients in the New York Heart Association[1] (NYHA) function class 3, but only a 15% five-year survival rate for patients in class 4[2].
- With the advent of valvular surgery survival has considerably improved but of course there is an operative risk which is 5–8% in most centres.

TREATMENT

1. Patients should receive penicillin prophylaxis for bacterial endocarditis (see p. 43).
2. In symptomatic patients with mitral stenosis oral diuretics are the first line of therapy (e.g. amiloride hydrochloride and hydrochlorothiazide (Moduretic) tablets 1–2 daily, or amiloride 5–10 mg daily). Frusemide up to 80 mg daily is added if necessary. If the patient is still symptomatic on maximum dosage there should be further evaluation including the possibility of surgery.
3. If the patient develops atrial fibrillation digoxin is given, the dosage (0.0625 mg–0.5 mg per day) depending on the weight of the patient. There is no point in giving digoxin if the patient remains in sinus rhythm.
4. If the patient develops atrial fibrillation anticoagulants (warfarin) should also be given. Some centres will anticoagulate patients with sinus rhythm if the left atrium is markedly dilated. Therapy is lifelong.
5. If symptoms progress despite appropriate medical therapy the patient should be referred for cardiac evaluation and cardiac surgery (either mitral valvotomy or valve replacement). Tissue valves in current use function normally for at least 10 years but then further surgery may be required. Mechanical valves have been in use for longer than tissue valves and many are still satisfactorily functioning 20 years after the original operation.

FOLLOW-UP

Follow-up is at yearly intervals whilst the patient is asymptomatic. Once symptoms develop, six monthly chest x-rays and echocardiograms are required.

---

[1] The Criteria Committee of the New York Heart Association. Diseases of the Heart and Blood Vessels (1964) *Nomenclature and Criteria for Diagnosis* 6th edn. Boston: Little Brown.
[2] Oleson KH (1962) *Br. Heart J.*, **24**, 349.

Mitral Regurgitation

Mitral regurgitation has many causes. It may result from: a) abnormality of the valve leaflets, e.g. rheumatic fever, bacterial endocarditis, lupus erythematosus; b) abnormality of the mitral annulus, e.g. secondary to left ventricular dilatation; c) abnormality of the chordae tendinae, e.g. myocardial ischaemia, hypertrophic cardiomyopathy; d) abnormality of the papillary muscles, e.g. ischaemia, myocardial disease. Patients with mild mitral regurgitation may remain asymptomatic for their entire lives. Symptoms, if they do develop, are of breathlessness and haemoptysis. Patients with severe mitral regurgitation may also complain of fatigue and exhaustion due to a low cardiac output.

PROGNOSIS

- The prognosis is variable and depends on:

  a) The volume of regurgitation.
  b) The state of the myocardium.
  c) The aetiology.

- In an unselected group of patients with mitral regurgitation treated medically, 80% survived five years and 60% 10 years[1].

- Patients with combined mitral regurgitation and mitral stenosis had a poorer prognosis with only 67% five-year survival and 30% 10-year survival[1].

- In severe cases, valve replacement has improved survival but the operative risk is 5–8%. Repair of the valve carries a slightly lower risk (mortality 3–5%).

TREATMENT

1. Patients should receive prophylaxis against bacterial endocarditis (p. 43).

2. The first line treatment is diuretic therapy as for mitral stenosis (p. 28).

3. If atrial fibrillation develops, digoxin is given and the patient is anticoagulated.

4. Afterload reduction is used in more advanced cases using oral hydralazine (25–50 mg tds) or prazosin (starting dose of 500 µg tds increasing to a maximum dose of 20 mg daily).

5. If symptoms fail to respond to medical treatment the patient is referred either for mitral valve repair or mitral valve replacement.

FOLLOW-UP

Follow-up is at yearly intervals for the asymptomatic patient and six monthly once symptoms develop. The disease process is monitored by serial chest x-rays and echocardiograms.

---

[1] Rapaport E (1975) *Am. J. Cardiol.*, **35**, 221.

Mitral Valve Leaflet Prolapse Syndrome

This syndrome may affect either cusp of the mitral valve and is characterised by an increase in cusp area with folding and upward doming into the left atrium during systole.

The mitral valve leaflet prolapse syndrome is one of the most prevalent cardiac valvular abnormalities affecting 5–10% of the population[1,2]. The commonest pathology is myxomatous change in the mitral valve and its apparatus. The overwhelming majority of patients are asymptomatic but patients may develop palpitations (due to supraventricular tachycardia) or chest discomfort. If the mitral regurgitation becomes severe the patient develops shortness of breath.

PROGNOSIS

- For most patients the prognosis is excellent.
- Only a minority of patients develop significant mitral regurgitation.

TREATMENT

1. Asymptomatic patients – no treatment other than prophylaxis against bacterial endocarditis (p. 43).
2. If supraventricular tachycardia develops – either a small dose of beta blocker (propranolol 40 mg bd/tds) or verapamil (40mg tds) is given.
3. Patients with chest pain are difficult to treat as the mechanism is ill understood. Simple analgesics, beta blockers and digoxin have all been tried in the past with variable effect. The chest pain does not reflect underlying coronary artery disease.
4. If mitral regurgitation becomes severe treatment is as for this condition (p. 29).

FOLLOW-UP

Two yearly assessment is required to identify development of significant mitral regurgitation.

[1] Deveraux RB et al. (1976) Circulation, 54, 3.
[2] Markiewicz W et al. (1976) Circulation, 53, 464.

Aortic Stenosis

Aortic stenosis may be rheumatic, congenital (bicuspid) or degenerative in origin. There is usually a long latent period during which there is gradually increasing obstruction while the patient remains asymptomatic. The cardinal symptoms, which most commonly appear in the sixth decade of life, are angina, syncope and congestive heart failure.

PROGNOSIS

- If aortic stenosis is haemodynamically significant medical treatment carries a 64% five-year survival[1].
- Once a patient develops angina or syncope the average survival is 2–3 years whereas with congestive heart failure it is 18 months[1].
- Aortic valve replacement carries a 5–8% operative mortality in most centres.

TREATMENT

1. The patient should receive prophylaxis against bacterial endocarditis (p. 43).
2. Asymptomatic patients require no specific therapy.
3. If the patient develops congestive heart failure diuretics are required and consideration should be given to early valve replacement.
4. Patients with angina need cardiac catheterisation to decide whether this is due to increased left ventricular mass or to coronary artery disease. Treatment will then depend on angiographic findings.
5. Syncope is an indication for invasive investigation and/or surgical intervention.
6. Surgery in patients with aortic stenosis usually implies aortic valve replacement with tissue or mechanical prosthesis, although in young patients valvotomy may be possible.

FOLLOW-UP

Asymptomatic patients are seen at 1–2 yearly intervals. Development of symptoms indicates need for urgent investigation by ECG, chest x-ray, echocardiogram and/or cardiac catheterisation.

---

[1] Frank S *et al.* (1973) *Br. Heart J.*, 35, 41.

Aortic Regurgitation

Aortic regurgitation may be caused by a primary disease of either the aortic valve leaflets or the wall of the aortic root. The commonest symptom is progressive breathlessness although patients may remain asymptomatic until late in the disease process.

PROGNOSIS

- Severe chronic aortic regurgitation has a good prognosis, approximately 75% patients surviving five years and 50% 10 years[1].
- Once the patient becomes symptomatic death usually occurs within 3–4 years of onset of angina or 1–2 years from onset of congestive heart failure[2]. With the advent of surgical intervention, however, survival prospects have improved considerably.

TREATMENT

1. First line therapy is diuretics (see *Mitral stenosis*, p. 28 for details).
2. More severe cases require afterload reduction with hydralazine (25–50 mg tds) or prazosin (starting dose 500 μg tds increasing to a maximum dose of 20 mg daily). The response to vasodilator therapy is often unimpressive.
3. If symptoms progress aortic valve replacement may be necessary.
4. If the aortic regurgitation is due to syphilitic aortitis the patient should receive a full course of penicillin therapy, i.e. benzathine penicillin G 2.4 mega units i.m. weekly for three weeks or aqueous procaine penicillin G 500 000 units i.m. daily for 15 days.

FOLLOW-UP

Follow-up should be at regular (six monthly to one yearly) intervals using chest x-ray and echocardiogram to identify left ventricular dilatation. Progressive left ventricular dilatation necessitates further invasive evaluation.

[1] Rapaport E (1975) *Am. J. Cardiol.*, **35**, 221.
[2] Masell BF *et al.* (1966) *Circulation*, **34** Suppl. 2, 164.

Tricuspid Stenosis

Tricuspid stenosis is almost always rheumatic in origin. Rheumatic tricuspid stenosis is usually accompanied by rheumatic mitral valve disease. Severe tricuspid stenosis produces fatigue due to low cardiac output and abdominal discomfort due to hepatomegaly.

PROGNOSIS

- The prognosis is dominated by coexisting lesions.

TREATMENT

1. The management of tricuspid stenosis is usually dominated by the management of accompanying lesions (usually mitral stenosis) (see p. 28).

2. Diuretics may be used in mild cases to reduce peripheral and hepatic congestion.
3. Severe cases will require surgical intervention – often commissurotomy, rarely valve replacement.

FOLLOW-UP

Follow-up is determined by coexisting lesions.

Tricuspid Regurgitation

The commonest cause of tricuspid regurgitation is not intrinsic disease of the valve itself but dilatation of the right ventricle and the tricuspid annulus secondary to right ventricular failure from any cause. Primary lesions of the valve causing tricuspid regurgitation include rheumatic fever and carcinoid syndrome.

PROGNOSIS

- The prognosis is determined by the underlying disease process in secondary tricuspid regurgitation and by associated lesions (e.g. mitral valve disease) in primary tricuspid regurgitation.

TREATMENT

1. Treatment for secondary tricuspid regurgitation is aimed at the underlying disease process.

2. Diuretics may be useful in the early stages but later surgical intervention (annuloplasty/ valve replacement) may be required.
3. In cases of carcinoid-induced tricuspid regurgitation, the disease itself should be treated by surgical excision of the tumour or, if this is possible, by cytoxic agents (e.g. cyclophosphamide) or by serotomin antagonists (e.g. methysergide).

FOLLOW-UP

Follow-up is determined by coexisting lesions.

Pulmonary Stenosis

The congenital form is the most common cause of pulmonary stenosis. Rheumatic disease is a rare cause.

PROGNOSIS

- Prior to the development of surgical treatment, survival beyond 50 years was unusual for cases of significant pulmonary stenosis.
- Surgical intervention now results in excellent survival prospects and patients with isolated pulmonary stenosis can expect a normal lifespan.

TREATMENT

Surgical intervention (or balloon dilatation of the valve at the time of cardiac catheterisation) is indicated if the right ventricular systolic pressure is greater than 75 mmHg. Surgery almost invariably takes the form of pulmonary valvo-tomy, although pulmonary valve replacement has been performed rarely. More recently[1] balloon dilatation of the valve (at the time of cardiac catheterisation) has been developed and this new technique is now considered the treatment of choice in patients with typical pulmonary stenosis and thin mobile valves.

FOLLOW-UP

Follow-up consists of two yearly visits. Assessment is by physical signs and echocardiography.

[1] Miller GAH (1985) *Br. Heart J.*, **54**, 285.

Pulmonary Regurgitation

Pulmonary regurgitation is usually secondary to pulmonary hypertension and associated pulmonary valve ring dilatation.

PROGNOSIS

- The prognosis is determined by the degree and cause of the pulmonary hypertension.

TREATMENT

1. Pulmonary regurgitation is seldom severe enough *per se* to require specific treatment.
2. Treatment is aimed at the disease process causing pulmonary hypertension.

Atrial Septal Defect

Defects in the atrial septum can be divided into ostium primum defects, defects in the floor of the fossa ovalis (secundum defects) and sinus venosus defects. Of these, the commonest is the ostium secundum defect which forms the commonest congenital cardiac defect found in adults. After the first year of life it is seen in approximately 10% children with congenital heart disease presenting for the first time. The information below is confined to ostium secundum lesions.

PROGNOSIS

- This malformation frequently permits survival into middle age and beyond[1]. Deterioration at this stage may be due to the development of pulmonary vascular disease[1].

TREATMENT

1. Unless the left to right shunt is minimal (pulmonary/systemic flow ratio less than 1.5:1) all defects should be closed surgically by direct suture or by means of a Dacron patch[1,2,3].
2. Even elderly patients with large shunts have been shown to benefit from operation[4,5], provided pulmonary vascular disease has not developed.
3. The operative risk is very low (<1%).

FOLLOW-UP

All significant defects are closed surgically and do not need long-term follow-up. Small defects are reviewed two yearly by chest x-ray and echocardiography.

[1] Breyar RH et al. (1979) J. Cardiovasc. Surg., 20, 583.
[2] Anderson M et al. (1976) Am. Heart J., 92, 302.
[3] Steele PM et al. (1983) J. Am. Coll. Cardiol., 1, 663.
[4] Nasrallah AT et al. (1976) Circulation, 53, 329.
[5] St John Sutton MG et al. (1981) Circulation, 64, 402.

Ventricular Septal Defect

The ventricular septum is a complex structure having three muscular components (the inlet, trabecular and outlet parts) and being completed by a fibrous component – the membranous septum. Defects can exist either because the membranous septum does not close the interventricular communication or because the muscular components themselves are improperly formed and fused. In childhood ventricular septal defect (VSD) is the commonest congenital cardiac anomaly accounting for approximately 20% all lesions; in adult life it is rare. The principal reason for this is that over 70% defects close spontaneously.

PROGNOSIS[1,2]

- Outcome depends on the size of the defect and associated anomalies.
- 70% isolated VSDs close spontaneously.
- Large VSDs, if not operated on, may result in pulmonary vascular disease and premature death.

TREATMENT[1,2]

1. All small defects (no evidence of right ventricular hypertrophy) require no therapy other than prophylaxis against bacterial endocarditis (p. 43).
2. Large defects resulting in heart failure in infants require digoxin, diuretics and consideration for surgical closure.
3. Indications for surgery are persistent heart failure despite therapy and a pulmonary artery pressure (at cardiac catheterisation) of greater than two-thirds systemic pressure.

[1] Hoffman JIE (1965) Am. J. Cardiol., 16, 634.
[2] Moulaert AJ (1978) In Paediatric Cardiology (Anderson RH, Shinebourne EA eds.) p. 113. Edinburgh: Churchill Livingstone.

Persistent Ductus Arteriosus (PDA)

The ductus arteriosus is that part of the sixth aortic arch present in the normal fetus which connects the junction of the main and left pulmonary arteries to the descending aorta. Postnatal ductal closure normally occurs in the first week of life in infants born at full term. Persistence of the ductus arteriosus is one of the commonest congenital cardiovascular anomalies constituting approximately 15% of the total congenital heart disease population.

PROGNOSIS

- Prognosis is dependent on the size of the ductus and the level of the pulmonary vascular resistance, a large ductus and increased pulmonary vascular resistance having an adverse effect on survival.
- If the ductus is small the child will be asymptomatic and prognosis is excellent.
- If the ductus is large, infants born at term present with heart failure, usually in the second month of life. These children usually require surgical intervention.

TREATMENT

1. Surgical closure by ligation, transection or direct suture is indicated in all older children. The reasons for closure in asymptomatic patients are:

   a) To prevent development of pulmonary vascular disease.

   b) To diminish the risk of bacterial endocarditis.

2. Heart failure in infancy should be treated with digoxin, diuretics and potassium supplements followed by surgical closure of the PDA.

3. Recently prostaglandin synthetase inhibitors[1] such as indomethacin or aspirin have been used to encourage ductal closure with variable success.

FOLLOW-UP

The great majority of ducts will be surgically ligated at the time of identification and should not require long-term follow-up.

---

[1] Heymann MA *et al.* (1976) *New Eng. J. Med.*, **295**, 530.

Coarctation of the Aorta

Coarctation is a localised narrowing of the lumen of the aorta usually occurring in the area of insertion of the ligamentum arteriosum. Depending on its relation to the ductus arteriosus coarctation is divided into long 'preductal' cases (between the left subclavian and the ductus) and localised 'postductal' (at the insertion of the ductus) types. Coarctation of the aorta may present in many ways from the extremes of heart failure in the first week of life to an incidental finding in late adult life.

PROGNOSIS

- Prognosis will depend on the nature of the coarctation (i.e. whether there is localised constriction at the level of the ligamentum arteriosum or whether there is tubular hypoplasia of the isthmus) and on associated intracardiac anomalies.
- Only 25% untreated patients will survive beyond the fourth decade[1]. The others die earlier from bacterial endocarditis, ruptured aorta or hypertensive vascular disease.

TREATMENT

1. Coarctation causing heart failure or symptoms in infancy must be relieved surgically as a matter of urgency.
2. Asymptomatic coarctation with any significant hypertension should also be resected at any time after six months of age and this should carry a negligible mortality.
3. If significant coarctation is not treated early hypertension in upper and lower limbs may persist despite adequate relief of obstruction.
4. Coarctation of the aorta detected in older children and adults should be treated by surgical resection and end-to-end anastomosis. The hospital mortality for this condition is 0–5%[2].

FOLLOW-UP

The majority of cases will be treated by surgery at the time of identification. After operation the patient's blood pressure both at rest and during exercise should be monitored and treated if elevated.

[1] Reifenstein GH et al. (1947) Am. Heart J., 33, 146.
[2] Shinebourne EA et al. (1976) Br. Heart J., 38, 375.

Fallot's Tetralogy

The features of Fallot's tetralogy are ventricular septal defect, overriding aorta, pulmonary infundibular stenosis and right ventricular hypertrophy. The lesion is common, accounting for approximately 10% of all congenital cardiac anomalies.

PROGNOSIS[1,2]

- Occasionally patients have severe anoxic episodes in the early months of life and death may occur in such an episode.
- If the unoperated patient survives early infancy death usually occurs late in the first decade or early in the second decade of life.
- An occasional unoperated patient lives into adult life with only moderate cyanosis; very few have survived into the fifth and sixth decades of life.

TREATMENT[1,2]

1. All patients with Fallot's tetralogy should undergo formal assessment in a cardiac centre.
2. In early life, if cyanosis is severe, a surgical systemic-pulmonary artery anastomosis is performed; such a procedure can be performed at any stage after birth.
3. Hypercyanotic attacks due to infundibular shutdown are treated by oxygen administration and a beta blocking agent (e.g. propranolol 0.1 mg/kg).
4. If a child over the age of one year is persistently cyanotic, total surgical correction on cardiopulmonary by-pass is undertaken. Operative mortality is 1–8% in children and 10–15% in infants.

FOLLOW-UP

The majority of cases are treated by surgical correction. After operation patients should be assessed at 1–2 yearly intervals in a cardiac centre.

---

[1] Becker AE *et al.* (1975) *Am. J. Cardiol.*, 35, 402.
[2] Shinebourne EA *et al.* (1975) *Br. Heart J.*, 37, 946.

Eisenmenger's Syndrome

Decreased cross-sectional area of the pulmonary arteriolar bed with irreversible pulmonary hypertension characterises Eisenmenger's syndrome. Wood[1] used the term to refer to patients with congenital cardiac lesions and severe pulmonary hypertension in whom reversal of a left to right shunt had occurred.

PROGNOSIS

- Death usually occurs in the second or third decade of life, despite medical management as outlined below.

TREATMENT

1. Medical management consists of the treatment of heart failure (using diuretics and/or digoxin) and the complications of left to right shunts (i.e. paradoxical emboli).
2. Short-term benefit may result from venesection of patients with secondary polycythaemia[2].
3. No specific treatment has proved beneficial for pulmonary vascular disease.
4. No conventional surgical treatment is appropriate in this group. Heart–lung transplantation may become a treatment option.

FOLLOW-UP

Follow-up involves six monthly to one yearly assessment of the cardiac status by ECG, chest x-ray and echocardiogram. More regular measurements of haemoglobin may be essential to determine the timing of venesection.

---

[1] Wood P (1958) *Br. Med. J.*, **2**, 755.
[2] Oldershaw PJ *et al.* (1980) *Br. Heart J.*, **44**, 584.

Ventricular Tachycardia

Ventricular tachycardia (VT) is paroxysms of ventricular ectopic beats occurring at a rate of 140–220 beats per minute and lasting in duration from a few seconds to several hours. VT most commonly occurs in association with myocardial ischaemia or infarction but it may also occur in hypertrophic cardiomyopathy, the long QT syndrome, with drugs notably digoxin, and occasionally in apparently healthy individuals. Patients normally complain of palpitations but hypotension, shock and death may swiftly intervene if the heart rate is rapid and the myocardium diseased.

PROGNOSIS

- The prognosis depends on the underlying aetiology.
- Patients with VT following myocardial infarction (see below) and patients with hypertrophic cardiomyopathy and VT on halter monitoring (see below) are both groups which have a high incidence of sudden death.

TREATMENT

1. Immediate d.c. cardioversion is frequently indicated, particularly when there is hypotension and shock or when VT follows recent myocardial infarction when it is a frequent precursor of ventricular fibrillation.
2. Lignocaine 100 mg i.v. stat followed by an infusion at a rate of 1–4 mg per minute may be given if the patient is haemodynamically stable.
3. Intravenous infusions of disopyramide or flecainide are alternative treatments if VT is resistant to lignocaine.
4. Phenytoin (3.5–5 mg/kg i.v.) is the therapy of choice if VT is related to digoxin toxicity.
5. In recurrent VT long-term oral therapy with either class I drugs (mexilitene, flecainide, disopyramide) or class III drugs (amiodarone, sotalol) may control the arrythymia but the efficacy of any one drug is not predictable and a therapeutic trial guided by 24 hour electrocardiographic monitoring is required in every case[1].
6. No single agent or combination of agents has been conclusively shown to alter survival in patients with VT following acute myocardial infarction.
7. In patients with drug-resistant VT electrophysiological studies may allow the ventricular ectopic focus to be identified, thus enabling treatment by surgical resection or cryoablation.
8. Division of the left stellate ganglion may be effective in patients with the long QT syndrome.

FOLLOW-UP

Patients should be assessed at regular intervals, the timings of which are determined by the patient's level of symptoms and underlying cardiac disease. Treatment efficacy should be objectively monitored using 24 hour ambulatory electrocardiography.

---

[1] Ward DE et al. (1985) Br. Med. J., 290, 1926.

Atrial Fibrillation

In atrial fibrillation (AF) purposeful atrial contraction is lost and replaced by chaotic atrial activity. The atrioventricular node becomes bombarded by a multitude of stimuli of varying intensity; most are blocked but some are conducted in a random fashion resulting in heart beats that are irregular in time and force. AF may occur in apparently healthy adults, as part of degenerative disease of cardiac conducting tissue (sick sinus syndrome), in thyrotoxicosis or as a complication of any cardiac condition which causes atrial dilatation due to pressure or volume overload (e.g. rheumatic, ischaemic and hypertensive heart disease). Patients complain of palpitations or may develop symptoms of heart failure.

PROGNOSIS

- The prognosis is dependent upon the underlying aetiology.
- AF tends to occur early in the natural history of patients with rheumatic heart disease and late in the natural history of patients with coronary heart disease.
- Atrial stasis often results in thrombosis, thus predisposing patients with AF to systemic and pulmonary embolus.

TREATMENT

1. d.c. cardioversion to restore sinus rhythm is indicated in acute myocardial infarction and treated thyrotoxicosis. It is successful in about 80% cases, but of these 60% relapse over the next year. It is normally unsuccessful in lone AF or if AF has occurred as part of the natural history of a chronic cardiac disease.
2. Digoxin (0.0625–0.25 mg daily) slows ventricular rate and is the drug of first choice in chronic atrial fibrillation. If required rapid digitalisation can be achieved using intravenous or intramuscular digitalis preparations.
3. Beta blocking drugs may be given concurrently with digoxin to control ventricular rate (particularly in thyrotoxicosis), but care must be taken if there is any element of heart failure.
4. Amiodarone (200–400 mg daily) is useful in 70–95% patients refractory to treatment with digoxin and is particularly useful in patients with recurrent paroxysmal AF.
5. Verapamil may be used to control ventricular rate but is contraindicated in the sick sinus syndrome where bradyarrhythmias may also be a feature.
6. Anticoagulation with warfarin should be considered to prevent thrombosis and embolus and is mandatory in patients with mitral stenosis.

FOLLOW-UP

The interval between assessments is determined by the patient's underlying cardiac disease and symptomatic status. Treadmill exercise testing and/or 24 hour ambulatory electrocardiographic monitoring may be required to determine whether treatment is effective.

Endocarditis

Infective endocarditis may be due to bacteria, fungi, *Coxiella* or *Chlamydia* and may be acute or subacute. The commonest variety is bacterial in origin and subacute in its course. Infective subacute endocarditis seldom affects a previously normal heart and is usually superimposed upon pre-existing valvular or congenital heart disease.

PROGNOSIS

- Recovery is rare unless effective and prolonged antibiotic treatment is given.
- Even with effective treatment the mortality is 15-20%.

TREATMENT

1. Prevention is better than cure. Antibacterial prophylaxis should be given for any procedure likely to be accompanied by bacteraemia when the patient is at known risk from endocarditis. Standard therapy[1] is 3 g of amoxicillin one hour before the procedure or, if the patient is penicillin sensitive, erythromycin 1.5 g orally one hour before and 0.5 g orally six hours after the procedure. If the patient is undergoing genitourinary instrumentation, amoxicillin (1 g i.m.) plus gentamicin (120 mg i.m.) is a better combination.
2. For established infective endocarditis, treatment depends on the organism responsible. Bacteriocidal agents should be employed.
3. *Steptococcus viridans* is the commonest organism and is treated using penicillin G 8 million units per day intravenously. If the patient is allergic to penicillin, intravenous cephalothin 2 g every four hours is given.
4. For *Streptococcus fecalis* a combination of penicillin G (dosage as above) and streptomycin 0.5 g i.m. every 12 hours is given.
5. Infections due to penicillin sensitive staphylococci will respond to penicillin but the more common penicillin-resistant strains demand flucloxacillin 2 g i.v. every four hours.
6. Blood culture negative endocarditis should be treated as for *Streptococcus fecalis* infections; infection with *Coxiella* and *Chlamydia* having first been excluded.
7. A minimum of four weeks therapy is necessary in all cases and most units would still prescribe six weeks of antibiotics.
8. Antibiotic therapy is constantly changing as new drugs become available and as organisms become resistant to those in current use.
9. During the course of treatment surgery may become necessary for replacement of damaged valves or correction of congenital heart disease, although this should if possible be deferred until the infection is under control.

FOLLOW-UP

After bacterial sterilisation review with chest x-ray, ECG and echocardiogram at intervals appropriate to the haemodynamic severity of the valvular lesion.

---

[1] Oakley CM *et al.* (1981) *Br. Heart J.*, 45, 343.

Acute Pericarditis

Pericarditis is inflammation of the pericardial lining of the heart. It has many pathologies including infection (viral, pyogenic or tuberculous), connective tissue disorders, allergic and auto-immune reactions and neoplastic processes. It may result in the formation of a pericardial effusion (see p. 45).

PROGNOSIS

- The prognosis is usually excellent, only rare cases going on to constrictive pericarditis (see p. 45).

TREATMENT

1. The first step in the management of acute pericarditis consists of establishing whether the pericarditis is related to an underlying problem that requires specific therapy.
2. Non-specific therapy begins with the use of non-steroidal anti-inflammatory agents such as aspirin (300–600 mg orally every four hours) or indomethacin (25–75 mg orally qds).
3. When pain is severe and does not respond to this therapy within 48 to 72 hours steroids may be employed. Prednisone 20 mg tds is standard therapy with gradual reduction of dose after 5–7 days at this level.
4. In some cases the patient develops recurrent episodes of pericardial inflammation at intervals of weeks or months after the initial episodes. These cases are normally treated using steroids.
5. Rarely, total pericardiectomy may be performed in patients with recurrent disabling pericarditis who cannot be weaned from steroids.

FOLLOW-UP

Regular review including echocardiography is required while the disease process is active.

Chronic Pericarditis

Chronic pericarditis, as opposed to recurrent acute pericarditis, is normally constrictive in nature and is often due to past tuberculous infection. In developed nations however, many cases now are of unknown aetiology. There is thickening of the pericardial lining of the heart resulting in impaired ventricular filling.

PROGNOSIS

- If not treated patients become progressively more disabled by weakness, ascites and peripheral oedema.

TREATMENT

Initial treatment is by use of diuretics but the majority of patients with haemodynamic upset will require pericardiectomy. Operative mortality for this procedure is 5%[1,2,3].

FOLLOW-UP

After pericardiectomy annual review is necessary with assessment by physical signs and echocardiography.

[1] Somerville W (1968) *Circulation*, **38** Suppl. 5, 102.
[2] Stalpaert G *et al.* (1981) *Acta Chir. Belg.*, **80**, 277.
[3] Wychulis AR *et al.* (1971) *J. Thorac. Cardiovasc. Surg.*, **62**, 608.

Pericardial Effusion

A pericardial effusion is a collection of fluid in the pericardial sac lining the heart and usually develops as a response to injury of the pericardium occurring with all causes of acute pericarditis. It may be clinically silent but if the accumulation of fluid causes intracardiac pressure to increase the symptoms of cardiac tamponade develop.

PROGNOSIS

- Small effusions without tamponade have an excellent prognosis.
- If the patient develops pericardial tamponade and is not treated there is a progressive decline in systemic arterial pressure with elevation of systemic venous pressure and the patient may die.

TREATMENT

Pericardial aspiration is indicated if there is any evidence of cardiac compression and haemodynamic upset or if analysis of pericardial fluid is essential to establish a diagnosis such as bacterial pericarditis.

Cardiomyopathy

The cardiomyopathies are a group of primary diseases of heart muscle. Conventionally they are divided into three groups which, in order of frequency of occurrence are: dilated (congestive) cardiomyopathy, hypertrophic cardiomyopathy and restrictive cardiomyopathy.

Dilated cardiomyopathy

Patients have an enlarged flabby heart and present with symptoms and signs of low cardiac output and fluid retention. Some cases are associated with viral myocarditis and others with toxins, notably alcohol, but in most cases the aetiology is unknown.

PROGNOSIS

- The one-year survival rate is approximately 50%. The course of the disease is very variable; some patients pursue an inexorable downhill path whilst others may remain stable for many years.
- Death is due to intractable heart failure, or is sudden presumably from dysrhythmias or pulmonary embolus.

TREATMENT

1. A loop diuretic, e.g. frusemide, is the initial treatment of choice and is normally given in combination with a potassium sparing diuretic, e.g. amiloride or spironolactone.
2. Metolazone (2.5–10 mg) powerfully potentiates the effect of frusemide.
3. Vasodilator drugs e.g. hydralazine, prazosin, isosorbide dinitrate and captopril, all confer acute haemodynamic and symptomatic benefits but unfortunately tolerance to these agents frequently develops and only captopril has been clearly shown in a placebo controlled study to produce long-term benefit[1]. Vasodilators have not been shown to reduce mortality rates.
4. Treatment with beta blockers has been reported to improve symptoms and reduce mortality[2] but the results of this study have not been confirmed by other researchers.
5. If a left ventricular biopsy shows evidence of acute myocarditis, immunosuppression (prednisolone and azathioprine) may improve symptoms and prognosis[3].
6. Cardiac transplantation, current five-year survival rate 70%, is now the treatment of choice in end-stage disease.

Hypertrophic cardiomyopathy

Hypertrophic cardiomyopathy is characterised by an overgrowth of abnormal myocardial tissue. Ventricular filling is deranged and there may also be obstruction to ventricular emptying (hypertrophic obstructive cardiomyopathy). The disease is familial (autosomal dominant inheritance) but many cases occur sporadically. Patients present with chest pain, dyspnoea and particularly, sudden death.

PROGNOSIS

- The mortality rate is 4% per year from time of diagnosis.
- Presentation at a young age, the presence of a family history and ventricular arrhythmia on halter monitoring are all associated with reduced survival rate.

TREATMENT

1. Beta blockers (e.g. propranolol 60–320 mg daily) alleviate symptoms but do not affect survival.
2. Calcium antagonist agents (e.g. verapamil 120–360 mg daily) may alleviate symptoms but have been associated with life threatening side-effects.
3. In patients with ventricular arrhythmia on halter monitoring, treatment with amiodarone (150–400 mg daily) has been reported to improve survival[4].
4. Ventricular myomectomy, preferably producing left bundle branch block on the ECG may relieve symptoms for a number of years

5. Cardiac transplantation is an option in patients with intractable symptoms.

Restrictive cardiomyopathy

Restrictive cardiomyopathy occurs in a variety of rare diseases (e.g. amyloidosis, endomyocardial fibrosis) in which the myocardium is infiltrated by abnormal tissue severely affecting ventricular diastolic properties but leaving systolic function relatively intact. Patients most commonly present with the symptoms and clinical signs of systemic venous congestion.

PROGNOSIS

- The prognosis is dependent on underlying disease process but overall five-year survival rate is low.

TREATMENT

1. Diuretics may relieve fluid retention but should be used cautiously because they may adversely affect cardiac output which in these patients is often unusually dependent on the presence of a high filling pressure.
2. Endomyocardial resection may benefit patients with endomyocardial fibrosis. Cardiac transplantation is an option but restrictive cardiomyopathies are often associated with a generalised or malignant disease process which itself has a poor prognosis.

FOLLOW-UP

Regular review at a frequency determined by the severity of the patient's symptoms. Assessment by physical signs, chest x-ray, echocardiography, treadmill exercise testing (for objective measurement of work capacity) and ambulatory 24 hour electrocardiography (if the patient has ventricular dysrhythmia).

[1] Captopril Multicenter Research Group (1983) *J. Am. Coll. Cardiol.*, 2, 755.
[2] Swedburg K *et al.* (1979) *Lancet*, i, 1374.
[3] Mason JW *et al.* (1980) *Am. J. Cardiol.*, 45, 1037.
[4] McKenna WJ *et al.* (1985) *Br. Heart J.*, 53, 412.

Rheumatic Fever

Rheumatic fever is a recurrent febrile illness which occurs in a variable proportion of children or young adults following severe pharyngeal infection with a group A streptococcus. The disease has five major manifestations: carditis, chorea, arthritis, erythema marginatum and subcutaneous nodules. The important clinical consequences are: firstly that of acute myocarditis during an attack which may be lethal; and secondly the chronic fibrosis of the heart valves which ultimately results in the clinical spectrum of chronic rheumatic heart disease.

PROGNOSIS

- The incidence of carditic involvement in an acute attack falls with increasing age of the patient.
- Patients without carditis during an acute episode of rheumatic fever in whom recurrence is prevented have a low incidence (6% at 10 years) of developing chronic rheumatic heart disease.
- If an attack of rheumatic fever is associated with carditis then the severity of subsequent chronic valvular disease is directly related to the severity of carditic involvement during the acute attack.
- Once five years have passed following an attack of acute rheumatic fever with carditic involvement females are much more likely than males to develop slowly progressive valvular disease.

TREATMENT

1. Bed rest is mandatory if there is clinical or laboratory evidence for inflammation.
2. A one week course of parenteral benzathine penicillin should be given to eradicate residual group A streptococcus in the pharynx.
3. Aspirin (2–12 g daily dependent upon body weight) produces symptomatic control but has not been shown to influence the natural history of the disease or subsequent development of chronic valvular disease. However, it is common practice to give continuous therapy with aspirin whilst there is clinical or laboratory evidence of acute inflammation.
4. Corticosteroids (prednisolone 40–80 mg daily) are potent in suppressing acute inflammation and should be given if aspirin is ineffective or is not tolerated but as with aspirin they have not been shown to alter the natural history of the disease.
5. Prevention of recurrent attacks is essential. Benzathine penicillin 1.2 million units i.m. monthly is the optimal prophylaxis; and is ten times more effective than continuous oral therapy with penicillin V. Most centres would now continue with prophylaxis until the patient has reached the third decade of life.

FOLLOW-UP

Continue prophylaxis through adolescence into early adult life. Thereafter, if the subject is asymptomatic, no formal follow-up is required

Raynaud's Disease

A disease of unknown aetiology affecting women five times more commonly than men, characterised by paroxysmal ischaemia of the fingers and toes induced by cold and relieved by warmth[1]. In a typical attack the digits blanch, then become cyanotic when they feel cold and numb, and then, at the termination of the attack, become bright red due to reactive hyperaemia at which time the sufferer experiences severe pain and throbbing. Disease progression is associated with the development of trophic changes in the digits and in severe cases gangrene requiring limited amputation may occur.

PROGNOSIS

- Most cases have an excellent prognosis, the disease either remaining stable with only occasional attacks or spontaneously remitting.
- In a small proportion of cases the disease inexorably progresses with recurring local gangrene leading to increasing disablement.

TREATMENT

1. Avoidance of vasoconstrictor stimuli by protection of the fingers and toes from cold exposure and by stopping smoking is essential.
2. Drugs such as reserpine, alpha adrenergic blocking agents and vasodilator agents have all been reported to produce benefit but there is no incontrovertible evidence that has established the effectiveness of any one drug.
3. Patients with the progressive form of the disease may benefit from regional sympathectomy but improvement is not normally sustained for more than two years.

FOLLOW-UP

Regular review is indicated whilst the patient is symptomatic or requires treatment.

---

[1] Coffman JD *et al.* (1975) *Prog. Cardiovasc. Dis.*, **18**, 123.

3

Diseases of the Gastrointestinal System

S. Parry and R.E. Pounder

Gastro-oesophageal Reflux and Hiatus Hernia

Gastro-oesophageal reflux occurs when gastric or duodenal contents enter the oesophagus without associated belching or vomiting. Short-lived episodes of reflux are recorded in asymptomatic, normal people. Increased frequency or duration of these episodes can result in regurgitation of food, a burning retrosternal discomfort (heartburn), or dysphagia. Decreased lower oesophageal sphincter pressure, impaired oesphageal peristalsis and delayed gastric emptying can all contribute to gastro-oesophageal reflux. A hiatus hernia and gastro-oesophageal reflux are not synonymous, but if both are present it is usually the latter that causes symptoms. The presence of reflux can be assessed by barium swallow or oesophageal pH monitoring, and its effect assessed by endoscopy.

PROGNOSIS

- Most require no therapy or alternatively intermittent antacid treatment (mild disease).
- A smaller group with significant oesophagitis require intensive, intermittent or continuing medical therapy (moderate/severe disease).
- A few require surgical intervention, especially if oesophagitis causes a benign oesophageal stricture.

TREATMENT

1. *Mild disease*

   a) Weight loss if appropriate.
   b) Elevate the head of the bed by six to eight inches.
   c) Avoid large meals, especially late in the evening.
   d) Avoid smoking – the latter decreases lower oesophageal sphincter pressure[1].

2. *Moderate disease*

   a) As above.
   b) Liquid antacid, e.g. Maalox, Gelusil 10–20 ml one hour after meals and before going to bed.
   c) Metoclopramide taken before meals results in good symptomatic improvement[2].

3. *Severe disease*

   a) Oral cimetidine 400 mg qds[3] or ranitidine 150 mg bd.
   b) Intermittent endoscopic dilatation for stricture formation.
   c) Surgery for a severe stricture, significant bleeding or pulmonary aspiration[4].

FOLLOW-UP

Follow-up is only necessary for those with moderate and severe reflux, the latter requiring regular review.

[1] Dennish GW *et al.* (1971) *New Eng. J. Med.*, **284** 1136.
[2] McCallum RW *et al.* (1977) *New Eng. J. Med.*, **296** 354.
[3] Behar J *et al.* (1978) *Gastroenterology*, **74**, 441.
[4] Levin G *et al.* (1983) *Clin. Ther.*, **6**, 4.

Gastrointestinal Haemorrhage

Gastrointestinal haemorrhage presents with haematemesis, melaena, rectal bleeding or sudden collapse. Occult bleeding may present with anaemia, angina or dyspnoea. There are many causes ranging from oesophagitis, oesophageal varices, Mallory–Weiss tears, gastritis, peptic ulceration, carcinoma, arterial-enteric fistulae, diverticular disease, angiodysplasia and haemorrhoids. Initial management is directed at resuscitation of the patient, but the cause of bleeding must then be established. Haematemesis and melaena are investigated by upper gastrointestinal endoscopy. If the endoscopy is normal and the patient continues to bleed, radioisotope labelled red cell studies and arteriography may help identify the source of bleeding. Melaena alone or brisk rectal bleeding are investigated with upper gastrointestinal endoscopy (bleeding from the upper gastrointestinal tract is still very common), and sigmoidoscopy, followed by colonoscopy and arteriography.

PROGNOSIS

- Overall mortality 8–10%[1], but is increased in patients over 60 years of age.
- 80–90% patients with upper gastrointestinal haemorrhage stop bleeding spontaneously[1].
- Duodenal and gastric ulcers are the cause in 40–50% patients with upper gastrointestinal bleeding.
  Mortality after urgent surgery is approximately three times greater than with non-surgical or elective surgical therapy.
  Mortality with bleeding varices is approximately 40–50%.
- Fewer than 10% patients with bleeding from diverticular disease of the colon require surgery.

TREATMENT

1. General

a) Resuscitation with intravenous normal saline, or blood. Blood loss of 1000 ml or more is generally reflected by a pulse rate over 120 beats per minute, a systolic blood pressure under 100 mmHg, or a postural drop in blood pressure of 10–15 mmHg[1].

b) Blood transfusion is appropriate for shock or anaemia. The initial haemoglobin does not accurately reflect the degree of blood loss.

c) Coagulation defects should be corrected with fresh frozen plasma or platelets.

2. Oesophageal varices. Temporising measures

include intravenous vasopressin infusion and balloon tamponade. Definitive treatment is by endoscopic sclerotherapy or oesophageal transection[2].

3. Mallory-Weiss tears

a) Most tears stop bleeding without specific treatment.

b) Persistent bleeding is treated by selective intra-arterial catheterisation with vasopressin infusion or administration of an embolising agent followed by suture of the tear if embolisation is unsuccessful[2].

4. Haemorrhagic gastritis

a) Most common in patients already hospitalised with serious underlying illness. Drug-induced gastritis accounts for approximately 5% gastrointestinal bleeding (usually due to NSAIDs).

b) Potent antacids alone do not stop bleeding. Maintenance of gastric pH above 4.0–5.0 by the combination of an oral antacid (e.g. Maalox, Gelusil, up to 60 ml per hour), with ranitidine or cimetidine, is effective as prophylaxis in patients at risk.

5. Peptic ulcer

a) H_2-blockade or antacids do not stop bleeding or rebleeding.

b) Laser photocoagulation and electro-photocoagulation may stop bleeding[2], but controlled trials are awaited.

Contd.

c) Continued bleeding or rebleeding during medical therapy requires surgery: resection for a gastric ulcer; ligation of the bleeding point with a truncal vagotomy and pyloroplasty for a duodenal ulcer.

6. *Diverticular disease of colon*

a) Bleeding is often massive and can be from the right colon.
b) Surgery with segmental resection is indicated for persistent bleeding, rebleeding or prior episodes of proven diverticular bleeding. The site of the bleeding may have to be identified preoperatively by angiography.

7. *Angiodysplasia.* Colonoscopy and coagulation biopsy of the colonic vascular abnormality may be undertaken. Arterial embolisation, or segmental colectomy are the alternatives. Blind right-hemicolectomy is sometimes performed since the arteriovenous malformations occur predominantly in the caecum and ascending colon.

FOLLOW-UP

Follow-up is dictated by the cause of bleeding and whether definitive measures to prevent recurrence were undertaken.

---

[1] Pingleton S (1983) *Med. Clin. North Am.*, **67**, 121.
[2] Larson DE *et al.* (1983) *Mayo Clin. Proc.*, **58**, 371.

Gastric Ulcer

Benign gastric ulcers have a similar incidence in males and females, and are particularly common between the ages of 55 and 65 years. Most patients with gastric ulcer secrete normal amounts of gastric acid. The use of non-steroidal anti-inflammatory drugs by elderly patients seems to increase the risk of gastric ulceration. Patients with gastric ulcer commonly present with upper abdominal pain, variably related to meals, anaemia and weight loss. Diagnosis is by upper gastrointestinal double contrast radiology or endoscopy. Because 3–7% radiologically benign gastric ulcers will be malignant, all gastric ulcers should be biopsied.

PROGNOSIS

- Untreated, 45% are healed by six weeks.
- Treated 60–80% are healed by six weeks[1,2,3].
- Recurrence rate 55–89% over a 6–12 month period.
- Bleeding and perforation are the most frequent complications of gastric ulcer.

TREATMENT

1. Medical

   a) Avoid alcohol, aspirin and smoking.
   b) Cimetidine 1 g/day in four divided doses or ranitidine 150 mg bd orally for 6–8 weeks. Tripotassium dicitratobismuthate (De-Nol) 1 tab. or 5 ml qds before meals may also be used.
   c) Cimetidine 400 mg nocte or ranitidine 150 mg nocte will prevent recurrence of gastric ulcers but maintenance treatment is usually reserved for elderly patients or where there is a contraindication to surgery.

2. Surgical

   a) Ulcers refractory to medical treatment, i.e. unhealed at three months.
   b) Recurrent gastric ulceration in a fit, young patient.
   c) Perforation, continuing haemorrhage, or gastric outlet obstruction.

FOLLOW-UP

Repeat endoscopy or barium meal at eight weeks to assess healing. Follow-up until healing complete. Once the ulcer has healed and the possibility of a malignant ulcer has been excluded, the patient need only be seen if there is a recurrence. If the patient's initial presentation was with anaemia the haemoglobin should be checked regularly.

[1] Littman A (1983) *New Eng. J. Med.*, **308**, 1356.
[2] Isenberg J et al. (1983) *New Eng. J. Med.*, **308**, 1319.
[3] Feely J et al. (1983) *Br. Med. J.*, **286**, 695.

Duodenal Ulcer

Duodenal ulcer is a common disease, affecting approximately 10% of the population[1]. It is becoming less common in men, but more common in women. Only one third of patients with duodenal ulcers have hypersecretion of gastric acid. Epigastric pain and night pain are common features but relief by food or antacids is variable. Some patients may be asymptomatic and present with either haemorrhage or perforation. Diagnosis is by upper gastrointestinal endoscopy or radiology: diagnosis by symptoms alone is not precise[2].

PROGNOSIS

- With no therapy 43% ulcers will heal within four weeks.
- Cimetidine, ranitidine, sucralfate or colloidal bismuth result in 70–95% healing in 4–8 weeks.
- Approximately 66% patients will have an ulcer recurrence in the year following ulcer healing.
- Approximately 5% duodenal ulcer patients fail to respond to initial therapy.
- Complications with haemorrhage, perforation or obstruction are rare, but bleeding duodenal ulcer remains the most frequent cause of massive upper gastrointestinal haemorrhage.

TREATMENT

1. Smoking should be stopped. Smoking impairs ulcer healing and increases the rate of ulcer relapse.
2. Aspirin and non-steroidal anti-inflammatory drugs should be avoided.
3. Cimetidine 800 mg nocte or ranitidine 300 mg nocte for eight weeks[3]. Sucralfate 1 g qds before meals or colloidal bismuth 1 tab. qds before meals can also be used.
4. Repeat endoscopy or barium meal is not indicated at the end of the treatment period if the patient is asymptomatic.
5. Maintenance treatment with cimetidine 400 mg nocte, or ranitidine 150 mg nocte, decreases the ulcer recurrence rate to less than 20% in a 12 month period.
6. Surgery

   a) Indications for emergency surgery include continuing haemorrhage, perforation and persistent pyloric obstruction.
   b) Few patients require elective surgery for unremitting ulceration, as most patients can be managed using maintenance H_2 blockade.

FOLLOW-UP

Symptomatic recurrences require 4–8 week full-dose treatment with an H_2-blocker. Endoscopy is indicated where symptoms are atypical, when a long time interval has elapsed and when clinical response to treatment is unsatisfactory. Maintenance treatment with low-dose H_2 blockers may be needed for patients with aggressive duodenal ulceration, the elderly, or those with another serious medical problem.

[1] Hirschowitz B (1983) *Gastroenterology*, **85**, 967.
[2] Conn HO (1981) *New Eng. J. Med.*, **304**, 967.
[3] Pounder RE (1984) *Pharm. Ther.*, **24**, 221.

Gastroenteritis

Acute gastroenteritis is characterised by the sudden onset of vomiting and diarrhoea. The majority of episodes have a viral cause, the Rotaviruses and Norwalk-like viruses being the most frequently implicated. Rotaviruses affect mainly infants and children, and have a seasonal occurrence[1]. Norwalk-like viruses affect children and adults, causing explosive epidemic outbreaks due to contaminated food or water, but person-to-person transmission is also important[1]. *Campylobacter jejuni* is now recognised to be the leading cause of bacterial gastroenteritis (less common pathogens being enteropathogenic and toxigenic *E. coli, Salmonella, Shigella*). The major reservoirs for *C. jejuni* are animals and products obtained from animals; transmission to humans occurs by direct contact with, or indirectly by ingestion of, contaminated food or water. Grossly bloody stools are common in *C. jejuni* infections, can occur in *Shigella* and *Salmonella* infections, but are uncommon if there is a viral cause.

PROGNOSIS

- Rotaviral infections have a recovery period of 5–7 days. Untreated infants can die from dehydration.
- Norwalk-like virus infection usually results in a shorter and milder illness lasting 12–24 hours.
- *C. jejuni* infections may produce symptoms for only one day but can also produce a fulminant illness. Most patients recover within a week but up to 20% have a prolonged illness[2].

TREATMENT

1. Maintenance of hydration, particularly in young children, is critical. Oral hydration with sugar-electrolyte solutions will suffice for the majority of patients.
2. Antidiarrhoeal agents are not recommended for acute diarrhoea.
3. Erythromycin does not appear to alter the natural course of *C. jejuni* infection but, in the presence of high fever and bloody diarrhoea, treatment with this antibiotic is advised.

FOLLOW-UP

No long-term follow-up is necessary. Those who handle food should be wary that they are not a source of contamination.

---

[1] Barnett B (1983) *Med. Clin. North Am.*, **67**, 1031.
[2] Blaser MJ et al. (1983) *Epidem. Rev.*, **4**, 157.

Coeliac Disease

Coeliac disease, or gluten-sensitive enteropathy, is a disease of the small intestine in which sensitivity to gliaden, the alcohol-soluble glycoprotein in gluten, results in severe damage to the enterocytes of the duodenum and proximal jejunum[1]. There is an increased familial incidence. The disease typically presents in infancy with diarrhoea and weight loss. A second peak in incidence occurs in the third decade of life, and such patients may have been previously asymptomatic[2]. Protein, carbohydrate, fat, fat-soluble vitamins, folic acid, vitamin B_{12} and iron can all be malabsorbed, but the consequences of an isolated deficiency may be the only presenting feature (for example, iron deficiency anaemia). The diagnosis must be secure and is established by a jejunal biopsy documenting the characteristic pathological lesion of sub-total villous atrophy, followed by a further biopsy showing improvement of the mucosa towards normal after three months on a gluten-free diet.

PROGNOSIS

- Excellent if correctly diagnosed and treated with a gluten-free diet.
- The incidence of gastrointestinal lymphoma and carcinoma appears to be increased in patients with coeliac disease (a twofold increase in invasive malignancies of the gastrointestinal tract, particularly of the small bowel, being reported in one study[3]). It is uncertain whether gluten restriction diminishes this risk.
- Refractory sprue occurs in a small percentage of patients. It is characterised by an initial response to a gluten-free diet followed by return of the symptoms and pathology despite strict adherence to diet. This condition may respond to treatment with prednisolone.
- Ulceration and stricture of the small intestine is a rare complication, occurring in treated and untreated patients, with a high mortality rate[4].

TREATMENT

1. Strict lifelong adherence to a gluten-free diet. This means avoiding wheat, rye and barley in all meals and foodstuffs. It is not easily achieved.
2. Specific deficiencies should be corrected: for example, folate deficiency, vitamin K deficiency. Patients with hypocalcaemia or evidence of osteomalacia should receive oral calcium and vitamin D.

FOLLOW-UP

Correction of all deficiencies needs to be ensured initially but once the patient is asymptomatic and gaining weight follow-up can be decreased to 6–12 month intervals with review of haemoglobin, MCV, albumin and alkaline phosphatase.

[1] Peters TJ et al. (1984) Gut, 25, 913.
[2] Falchuk ZM (1983) Clin. Gastroenterology, 12, 475.
[3] Swinson GM et al. (1983) Lancet, i, 111.
[4] Jewell DP (1983) Br. Med. J., 287, 1740.

Traveller's Diarrhoea

Traveller's disease is a growing problem. The illness usually begins 4–6 days after arrival in a hot foreign country with the abrupt onset of abdominal cramps followed by watery diarrhoea. Associated symptoms can include nausea and vomiting, fever, headache and arthralgia. Enterotoxigenic *Escherichia coli* have been isolated in 40–70% patients, with the next most frequently isolated pathogens being *Shigella* (5–20%) and *Salmonella* (0–15%). Infections involving more than one pathogen are found in 10–20%; 25–30% remain undiagnosed[1]. The risk of acquiring traveller's diarrhoea is higher in tropical or developing countries and is higher in visitors from Western Europe or America.

PROGNOSIS

- The median duration of the untreated illness is 2–5 days.

TREATMENT

1. Maintenance of hydration with sugar-electrolyte solutions is essential.
2. In mild illness without fever, anti-diarrhoeal drugs (such as codeine phosphate or loperamide) can be used.
3. Oral trimethroprim 160 mg/sulphamethoxazole 800 mg (co-trimoxazole) bd or trimethoprim 200 mg bd for 3–5 days have been shown to reduce the duration of illness by as much as 60 hours[2].
4. The above antibiotic regimens or daily doxycycline (100 mg), are also effective as prophylaxis for the prevention of diarrhoea but, in view of the incidence of side-effects and the development of resistance in the gut flora, it is recommended that this therapy be reserved for treatment, unless the traveller really cannot risk falling ill[2].
5. If diarrhoea persists a *Campylobacter* or parasitic infection should be excluded.

FOLLOW-UP

Stool microscopy and culture are indicated in the returned traveller who continues to have diarrhoea. *Salmonella* and *Shigella* infections are followed until stool cultures are negative.

---

[1] Garbach S (1982) *N. Eng. J. Med.*, **307**, 881.
[2] DuPont HL (1982) *N. Eng. J. Med.*, **307**, 841.

Crohn's Disease

Crohn's disease (or regional enteritis) is a chronic inflammatory disorder of unknown aetiology which can affect any part of the gastrointestinal tract, although the distal ileum, colon and perineum are the sites most commonly affected. The disease occurs with increased frequency in peoples of European origin, is 3–8 times more common among Jews and is much more common among whites than non-whites. The disease can begin at any age, but usually occurs at 15–30. 75% symptomatic patients have diarrhoea and abdominal pain. The inflammatory process extends through all layers of the gut wall and may be accompanied by non-caseating granulomata (65%). Normal intestine may separate involved areas of the bowel which are thus called 'skip lesions'. Exclusion of an infective cause and adequate radiological examinations play a crucial role in the diagnosis of patients suspected to have Crohn's disease. Colonoscopy and biopsy are helpful when x-ray appearances are not typical. Findings at sigmoidoscopy are frequently unremarkable but granulomata may be present in normal appearing tissue, therefore a rectal biopsy should always be performed when Crohn's disease is suspected.

PROGNOSIS

- 10–20% patients remain completely asymptomatic for as long as 20 years after the first episode of active Crohn's disease.
- 10–20% patients ultimately die of Crohn's disease and its complications.
- Fistula formation, particularly in the perianal and perirectal regions, occurs in up to 50% patients with small bowel and colonic disease.
- Approximately 50% patients will require surgery for complications, and 75–90% patients operated on for small bowel disease or ileocolitis need reoperation within 15 years.
- Malignant neoplasms of the bowel occur three times more frequently in patients with Crohn's disease when compared with the general population.
- Systemic manifestations in Crohn's disease are of the same nature and occur with about the same frequency as in ulcerative colitis, but clinically significant liver disease (sclerosing cholangitis) is very unusual. Arthritis is the most common epiphenomenon.
- Nephrolithiasis occurs in 25–35% patients with Crohn's disease, and may partly be attributed to the increased oxalate absorption associated with steatorrhoea. Other urological problems due to Crohn's disease include trapping of the right ureter, enterovesical fistulae and amyloidosis.

TREATMENT

1. Prednisolone 40–60 mg daily diminishes the activity of the disease process[1].
2. Sulphasalazine 2–4 g/day also appears to be effective in patients with symptomatic Crohn's disease, particularly if the colon is involved. For patients with quiescent disease neither sulphasalazine nor prednisolone appear to be superior to placebo in preventing recurrence[1].
3. Metronidazole 400 mg tds is at least as effective as sulphasalazine in diminishing disease activity[2]. Larger doses 20 mg/kg may result in dramatic healing of perineal Crohn's disease[3], but may cause a peripheral neuropathy.
4. Immunosuppressive agents such as azathioprine or 6-mercaptopurine, should be considered only for those patients with persistent disease unresponsive to medical or surgical management, and for those who experience severe side-effects from prednisolone.
5. In patients with malabsorption (due to enteric-enteric fistulae, extensive small bowel disease or resection) replacement of vitamins D and K, calcium, folic acid and iron is indicated if deficiency is demonstrated. Parenteral vitamin B_{12} (1000 μg i.m. every two months) should be administered to all patients with extensive ileal disease or after ileal resection.
6. Total parenteral nutrition can be used to allow fistulae to heal, during episodes o

acute inflammation with obstruction and in the peri-operative period.

7. Operative resection is reserved for the complications of the disease such as small bowel obstruction, free perforation, abscess formation, fistula formation or unequivocal failure to respond to medical treatment.

FOLLOW-UP

Patients with moderate to severe disease need to be followed at 3–6 monthly intervals, particularly if their nutritional status is marginal or continuing treatment with prednisolone is required. Minimum routine investigations should include a blood picture and ESR, and biochemistry profile.

[1] Malchow H *et al.* (1984) *Gastroenterology*, **86**, 249.
[2] Ursing B *et al.* (1982) *Gastroenterology*, **83**, 550.
[3] Bernstein LH *et al.* (1980) *Gastroenterology*, **79**, 357.

Ulcerative Colitis

Ulcerative colitis is a chronic inflammatory disease of unknown aetiology which causes superficial ulceration of the rectal and colonic mucosa. The disease is characterised by exacerbations evidenced by rectal bleeding and diarrhoea, and remissions. Diagnosis is made on the basis of history and the finding at sigmoidoscopy of an inflamed rectal mucosa. Faecal culture should be performed to rule out an enteric infection as a cause of the patient's symptoms. Rectal biopsy, barium enema or colonoscopy may confirm the diagnosis. Most exacerbations can be managed by topical or systemic steroids, but significant local and systemic complications can occur.

PROGNOSIS

- 60-75% patients experience intermittent attacks, with intervening complete remissions.
- 4-10% have one attack with no subsequent symptoms for up to 15 years.
- 5-15% are troubled by continuous symptoms.
- Toxic megacolon arises in 1-2.5% patients.
- There is an increased incidence (about 23 times) of carcinoma of the colon for patients with disease activity lasting 10-20 years. The risk is diminished if only the distal colon or rectum are involved.
- One third of colitis-related deaths are due to cancer of the rectum and colon.
- 7% have some evidence of liver disease (the most serious being sclerosing cholangitis).
- 25% develop arthritic manifestations[1].
- 5-10% develop iritis.
- 3% develop erythema nodosum.
- 1-4% develop pyoderma gangrenosum.

TREATMENT

1. *Mild* (less than four bowel motions per day with no fever, anaemia, hypoalbuminaemia or weight loss; usually involving only the rectum and distal colon):

   a) Steroid enemas or foam twice daily, reduced to daily as control is achieved. Total treatment period usually less than six weeks.

   b) Sulphasalazine 1 g bd once remission has been induced[2] reduces the frequency of subsequent relapses.

2. *Moderate:*

   a) Prednisolone 40-60 mg/day orally; once a response has been achieved reduce by 5 mg every 3-7 days.

   b) Rectal steroids can be started as the dose of prednisolone is reduced or if diarrhoea is troublesome.

   c) Maintenance treatment with sulphasalazine when remission has been induced.

3. *Severe* (more than six bowel motions per day, weight loss, fever, tachycardia, anaemia and hypoalbuminaemia):

   a) Hospital admission.

   b) Intravenous fluid replacement and parenteral feeding if necessary.

   c) Intravenous steroids (prednisolone 64 mg/day).

   d) Metronidazole 400 mg tds orally.

   e) Abdominal x-rays to detect megacolon or perforation.

4. Surgery is indicated for:

   a) Megacolon not responding to intensive medical treatment.

   b) Colonic perforation.

   c) Unremitting disease despite optimal medical treatment.

   d) Carcinoma.

FOLLOW-UP

All patients with a diagnosis of ulcerative colitis should receive maintenance treatment with sulphasalazine 1 g bd. During symptomatic recurrences or 3-6 monthly patients should undergo sigmoidoscopy and measurement of haemo-globin, sedimentation rate and serum albumin. Patients with pancolitis and disease of greater than 10 years' duration require assessment every one or two years with sigmoidoscopy and colonoscopy with multiple biopsies[3].

[1] Greenstein AJ et al. (1976) Medicine, 55, 401.
[2] Lennard-Jones JE et al. (1965) Lancet, i, 185.
[3] Lennard-Jones JE et al. (1977) Gastroenterology, 73, 1280.

Colonic Diverticular Disease

Diverticular disease is common in developed countries, being found at autopsy in 33–50% of those over 60 years of age. The basic abnormality is an acquired defect of the large bowel where the mucosa and submucosa herniate through the muscular coat of the bowel to lie within the serosa. The sigmoid colon is involved in 95% patients. The absence of unrefined cereal grain in the diet of Western countries has been implicated as a cause of this disease[1]. The majority of affected patients will be asymptomatic. If symptomatic, left-sided lower abdominal pain associated with diarrhoea or constipation is the most common presenting feature. The diagnosis is usually revealed by a barium enema. Sigmoidoscopy and colonoscopy may be necessary to rule out the presence of other pathology – the differential diagnosis including carcinoma of the colon or inflammatory bowel disease. Diverticulitis refers to the clinical manifestations that result from the spread of inflammation to the adjacent bowel wall or surrounding tissue.

PROGNOSIS

- 80% are asymptomatic.
- 4–5% (20% of those clinically recognised) will develop a complication[2].
- Bleeding from diverticulae is a common cause of lower gastrointestinal haemorrhage in the elderly.
- 1–2% patients will require hospital admission.
- 0.5% will require surgical intervention.

TREATMENT

1. Diets high in vegetable fibre have been shown to lower the intraluminal pressure in the sigmoid and relieve pain[3]. The amount of bran should be increased slowly over a period of six weeks.
2. Hydrophyllic colloid laxatives are an alternative to bran. Initially they are usually more easily tolerated.
3. Antispasmodics are usually used only as an interim measure.
4. Simple analgesics may be required.
5. Antibiotics (metronidazole 400 mg tds with amoxycillin 250 mg tds) are indicated when there is evidence of diverticulitis, but severe illness requires hospital admission.
6. Urgent surgical intervention is indicated for intra-abdominal abscess, bowel obstruction or generalised peritonitis. The presence of recurrent, disabling attacks, fistula formation or persistent partial obstruction are indications for elective surgery.

FOLLOW-UP

Uncomplicated patients need be seen only during symptomatic recurrences.

[1] Painter NS et al. (1975) Clin. Gastroenterology, 4, 3.
[2] Almy TP et al. (1983) Diverticular disease of the colon. In Gastrointestinal Disease (Sleisenger MD, Fordtran JS eds.) p. 896. Philadelphia: W.B. Saunders Company.
[3] Brodribb A (1977) Lancet, i, 664.

4

Diseases of the Renal System

I. Barton

Acute Renal Failure (ARF)

ARF is an abrupt cessation of renal function. Although oliguria may occur, in recent series over 50% patients have been non-oliguric[1]. The most common cause is acute tubular necrosis (ATN), but the primary lesion may also be in the glomeruli, vessels or tubulo-interstitium. The principles of management are, however, independent of the underlying pathology. Ultrasound should be performed to exclude obstruction, which is best treated by drainage of the upper tracts. If intrinsic pathology other than ATN is suspected a renal biopsy should be taken as specific therapy is available for some conditions.

PROGNOSIS

- Overall mortality approaches 50%. Most deaths are secondary to infection or the underlying illness.
- Poor prognostic factors include oliguria and a traumatic or surgical aetiology.
- Among survivors, recovery of renal function is usual, but often incomplete. Acute cortical necrosis, renal vascular occlusion, and some types of rapidly progressive glomerulonephritis are especially likely to result in persistent renal failure.

TREATMENT

1. Prophylaxis

   a) The increased risk of ARF in arteriopaths, diabetics, patients with myeloma, and the elderly may be reduced by adequate hydration, osmotic diuresis, and alkalinisation of the urine at the time of major surgery or injection of radio-opaque contrast media.

   b) If potentially nephrotoxic drugs are given avoidance of dehydration and overdosage is essential.

2. Initiating phase

   a) Before ATN is established renal function may be restored by correction of hypotension and withdrawal of nephrotoxins.

   b) Dopamine, mannitol and large doses of loop diuretics may accelerate initiation of diuresis in some cases. Mannitol should be used with great care as it is an extracellular solute and so may precipitate pulmonary oedema. If no diuresis occurs following a test dose of 12.5–25 g its use should not be continued. Frusemide in high doses is ototoxic and bumetanide is preferred.

3. Established phase

   a) Fluid: The daily allowance should replace the 24 hour urine volume, insensible losses (5–10 ml/kg), and any additional losses from the gut, skin, respiratory tract, or into local areas of inflammation. Daily weights are the most useful index of overall fluid balance.

   b) Sodium: The daily replacement of 0.5–1 mmol/kg should be modified according to the central venous pressure and clinical assessment of the degree of salination. Hyponatraemia and hypernatraemia usually reflect abnormalities of water balance and are best corrected by appropriate alterations in fluid intake.

   c) Potassium: If normokalaemic up to 1 mmol/kg/day may be given. Hyperkalaemia, if untreated, is fatal. If gross ECG abnormalities are present calcium is cardioprotective and 10 ml of 10% calcium gluconate is indicated. For short-term control of hyperkalaemia intravenous dextrose and soluble insulin (4 g/unit) is preferred to sodium bicarbonate (50–100 mmol) because the latter may cause sodium overload and decreased ionised calcium levels. Oral or rectal calcium resonium reduces total body potassium by approximately 1 mmol/g of resin but is slow to act.

   d) Calcium: Hypocalcaemia is almost invariable but requires no treatment unless symptomatic. If tetany develops 10 ml of 10% calcium gluconate may be given intravenously and repeated as required. Absorption of oral calcium is poor unless a one alpha-hydroxylated vitamin D derivative is added.

e) Magnesium: Hypermagnesaemia is usual but seldom clinically significant. Magnesium containing antacids should be avoided.

f) Phosphate: Hyperphosphataemia may be ameliorated by restricting dietary phosphate and giving an oral phosphate binder such as aluminium hydroxide 950 mg with each meal.

g) Acid-base balance: Metabolic acidosis is usually present, but correction is unnecessary in the absence of respiratory distress, hypotension or cardiac arrhythmias, and is potentially hazardous (see above). If necessary 50–100 ml of 8.4% sodium bicarbonate should be given cautiously over 1–2 hours but must not be repeated without a full reassessment of the patient. Metabolic alkalosis usually reflects excessive gastric acid losses which may be reduced with H_2-blockade. The alkalosis can be treated safely with 0.1 mmol/l hydrochloric acid given slowly through a central line[2]; ammonium chloride and arginine hydrochloride both generate urea and are contraindicated.

h) Diet: The daily allowance of protein is 0.6 g/kg if undialysed, 1 g/kg if haemodialysed and 1.2 g/kg if peritoneally dialysed. The high intake of non-protein calories advocated in the past tends to cause hepatic dysfunction due to steatosis, and the current recommendation is for 200 calories per gram of nitrogen.

i) Dialysis: Absolute indications include deterioration in conscious level, pericarditis, bleeding, refractory hyperkalaemia and pulmonary oedema. Commencement before complications have developed has the advantages of making the patient feel better, allowing 'space' for feeding and improving prognosis.

j) Bleeding: Haemostasis in renal failure is impaired owing to platelet dysfunction; this may be corrected by desmopressin 0.2–0.4 units/kg given slowly intravenously if a patient is bleeding or about to undergo an invasive procedure[3]. The incidence of upper gastrointestinal bleeding is reduced by prophylactic antacids and H_2-blockade. Ranitidine is preferred to cimetidine since cerebral toxicity may result from accumulation of the latter in renal failure.

k) Infection: As uraemic patients are immunosuppressed, strict asepsis is especially necessary. Urinary catheters should be removed unless there is a specific indication. If serious infection is suspected appropriate antibiotics may need to be started before results of relevant cultures are available.

3. Recovery phase

a) Transient excessive losses of water, sodium, potassium, magnesium, bicarbonate and phosphate are common and require replacement.

b) Hypercalcaemia is also common but treatment is rarely needed.

FOLLOW-UP

Those who recover completely may be discharged. Those with a residual deficit have chronic renal failure and should be treated as such.

[1] Anderson RJ et al. (1977) New Eng. J. Med., **296**, 1134.

[2] Abouna GM et al. (1974) Surgery, **75**, 194.

[3] Mannucci PM et al. (1983) New Eng. J. Med., **308**, 8.

Acute Allergic Interstitial Nephritis (AIN)

AIN usually occurs as an allergic response to drugs but may also be precipitated by infection, or be cryptogenic. The beta lactam antibiotics (especially methicillin), sulphonamides, rifampicin, diuretics and the non-steroidal anti-inflammatory drugs are most commonly implicated. Classically there is non-oliguric acute renal failure, fever, rash, eosinophilia and eosinophiluria. Nephrotic syndrome may also be present.

PROGNOSIS

- Continuation of the responsible drug leads to progressive renal failure. With correct management recovery of renal function is usual although occasionally incomplete[1].
- The disease frequently recurs on re-exposure to the same or a similar drug.

TREATMENT

1. Withdrawal of the precipitating agent generally induces remission. If further drug therapy is required, agents which are neither cross-reactive nor nephrotoxic should be used.
2. Steroids lead to a faster and fuller recovery[2].

FOLLOW-UP

Those who recover completely may be discharged. Those with a residual deficit have chronic renal failure and should be treated as such.

---

[1] Kida H et al. (1984) Clin. Nephrology, **22**, 55.
[2] Galpin JE (1978) Am. J. Med., **65**, 756.

Thrombotic Thrombocytopenic Purpura (TTP)

TTP appears to be initiated by inappropriate platelet activation and usually presents with fever, renal failure, neurological dysfunction, microangiopathic haemolytic anaemia, and thrombocytopenia. There is rarely an obvious precipitant. Haemolytic uraemic syndrome (HUS) is a similar but milder disease in which microangiopathy is confined largely to the kidney. HUS affects mainly children and frequently is precipitated by an infection.

PROGNOSIS

- Without treatment mortality approaches 100%.
- There is little correlation between disease severity and response to therapy.
- With induction of remission, return of normal renal function and resolution of neurological abnormalities are usual but relapses are not uncommon.

TREATMENT

1. Daily administration of 6–8 units of fresh frozen plasma (FFP) usually induces response within 48–72 hours[1].
2. Plasma exchange allows infusion of larger volumes of FFP and may remove circulating platelet aggregating factors.
3. Prostacyclin infusions, steroids, immunosuppressants and heparin have been of limited effectiveness.
4. Platelet transfusions usually exacerbate the condition and are contraindicated.
5. After the induction of remission oral antiplatelet agents (e.g. aspirin 300 mg twice weekly plus dipyridamole 400–600 mg daily) appear to reduce the incidence of relapse.

FOLLOW-UP

The blood film, platelet count, and serum lactic dehydrogenase are useful indices of microangiopathy and should be monitored regularly as well as renal function. The possibility of relapse necessitates lifelong follow-up.

---

[1] Machin S (1984) *Br. J. Haemat.*, **56**, 191.

Hepato-renal Syndrome

Hepato-renal syndrome is the development of renal failure in a cirrhotic patient, and results from reduced cortical perfusion secondary to the accumulation of an unidentified vasoactive substance which is normally cleared in the liver. The kidneys are not structurally damaged and will function almost immediately if transplanted into a recipient with a normal liver. These patients are characteristically oliguric with a daily urinary sodium excretion of less than 10 mmol.

PROGNOSIS

- The outlook is poor with a mortality in excess of 85%.
- Death is rarely directly attributable to renal failure since the plasma creatinine is frequently below 0.5 mmol/l when the patient dies.

TREATMENT

1. Management is supportive and is directed at improving hepatic function.
2. Plasma expanders, paracentesis with reinfusion of ascitic fluid, and vasoactive drugs all produce only transient improvement.
3. Long-term remission may, however, follow insertion of a LeVeen shunt[1] or liver transplantation[2].

FOLLOW-UP

The rare patient who is fit enough to go home will require full reassessment at frequent intervals.

[1] Pladson TR et al. (1977) Arch. Int. Med., 137, 1248.
[2] Iwatsuki S et al. (1973) New Eng. J. Med., 289, 1155.

Chronic Renal Failure (CRF)

CRF is a loss of the excretory, homeostatic and endocrine functions of the kidney which is permanent and usually insidious in onset. The most common causes in the UK are chronic glomerulonephritis (GN), chronic atrophic pyelonephritis, analgesic nephropathy, hypertension, diabetes mellitus, and polycystic kidney disease. Once glomerular filtration rate (GFR) falls below 20 ml/min, there is inexorable progression to end stage renal failure (ESRF), due to either continuing parenchymal destruction by the original disease or the development of focal sclerosis and hyalinosis of remnant glomeruli. The annual UK incidence of treatable ESRF is 6 per 100 000. Under 50% are treated[1].

PROGNOSIS

- The rate of loss of renal function is variable but may be predicted in the individual patient by a plot of the reciprocal of the serum creatinine against time; this is usually linear unless there is a superimposed problem such as desalination, obstruction, uncontrolled hypertension, or infection.
- Once ESRF has developed, sufficient recovery of renal function to allow discontinuation of dialysis is uncommon but may follow improved blood pressure control in patients with hypertensive nephrosclerosis.
- Two-year survival of patients with ESRF is only 80% even with renal replacement therapy[2]. Poor prognostic factors include relative old age, diabetes mellitus, left ventricular failure and previous myocardial infarction.
- Generalised atherosclerosis develops prematurely and is clinically significant in 60%. Hyperparathyroidism and oxalosis, if present, may exacerbate vascular occlusion by causing calcification within vessel walls. Ischaemic heart disease is the most common cause of death.
- Renal failure is immunosuppressive and infections are the second most common cause of death. There is also a high incidence of tumours affecting the gut, lung and breast; following transplantation lymphomas and skin tumours are more common.
- Pericarditis occurs in 25%. Pericardial constriction and tamponade are becoming increasingly common because of anticoagulation for dialysis.
- Hypertension is present in 90% patients reaching ESRF.
- Peptic ulceration is common; in terminal cases there is frequently mucosal ulceration throughout the gut.
- Over 80% patients with ESRF are anaemic.
- By the time ESRF has developed renal osteodystrophy is present histologically in 90%, biochemically (raised alkaline phosphatase) in 10%, radiologically in 5%, and clinically in 2%. Most long-term survivors of dialysis have severe clinical disease with pathological fractures and fibrosis of joints.
- A mixed sensorimotor peripheral neuropathy is present in 65% patients entering dialysis programmes. Carpal tunnel syndrome occurs in 15% haemodialysis patients.
- Multiple renal cysts develop in 40% haemodialysis patients and are now well described in other patients with CRF; neoplasms develop within cysts in 30%, and 10% of these are malignant[3].
- Loss of libido occurs in both sexes; 50% males are impotent. Most patients are infertile and in females anovulatory cycles also cause amenorrhoea or menorrhagia.
- Psychosocial problems are common. In home haemodialysis patients they are an important predictor of survival[4].

TREATMENT

1. Reversible factors such as desalination, hypertension, infection, and obstruction should be corrected.
2. Fluid and electrolytes
   a) Intakes should be individually adjusted to replace losses. The typical daily allowances for a haemodialysis patient are 750 ml of water, 60 mmol of sodium, and 60 mmol of potassium.

Contd.

71

b) High doses of loop diuretics increase excretion of water, sodium and potassium allowing a more liberal intake. The GFR is, however, unaffected[5].

c) Sodium bicarbonate (0.6–1.8 g tds) reduces symptoms of acidosis but its use is limited by the risk of sodium overload.

3. Diet

a) Restriction of dietary phosphate (6.5 mg/kg/day) and protein (0.6 g/kg/day) slows the decline of renal function[6].

b) Protein allowances in ESRF are as described for ARF (see p. 66).

c) High dietary fibre reduces ammonia synthesis by the gut flora and lowers blood urea[7].

d) Vitamin supplements should not be given indiscriminately as, for example, vitamin C excess exacerbates oxalosis and hypervitaminosis A causes hypercalcaemia and anaemia.

4. Haematological

a) Haematinics should be given for specific deficiencies. Haemodialysis patients require regular iron but not folate[8].

b) Patients with high transfusion requirements may benefit from either splenectomy[9] or androgens[10].

c) The haemostatic defect related to platelet dysfunction may be improved by correction of anaemia[11], desmopressin 0.2–0.4 units/kg i.v.[12], or conjugated oestrogens (such as Premarin 25 mg/day[13]).

5. Musculoskeletal

a) Hyperphosphataemia stimulates parathormone secretion and so the plasma phosphate concentration should be reduced into the normal range by combining dietary restriction with oral phosphate binders (see *Acute renal failure*, p. 66).

b) One alpha-hydroxylated vitamin D derivatives should also be given provided the patient is not hypercalcaemic.

c) Parathyroidectomy is indicated for severe hyperparathyroidism if hypercalcaemia is present[14].

d) Although hyperuricaemia is usual, gout does not occur and use of xanthine oxidase inhibitors is unnecessary.

6. Cardiovascular

a) Hypertension resolves in most patients with correction of sodium overload. The remainder frequently have inappropriately raised blood renin levels and so beta blockers and angiotensin converting enzyme inhibitors are the most useful hypotensive agents.

b) Postural hypotension may improve with either sodium supplementation or indomethacin 25–50 mg tds[15].

c) Premature development of atheroma may be delayed by adequate control of hypertension and hyperlipidaemia[16].

d) Pericarditis usually resolves with adequate dialysis. Non-steroidal anti-inflammatory agents are useful for pain relief. Haemodynamically significant effusions require urgent drainage.

7. Neurological

a) Severe peripheral neuropathy is best treated by transplantation since dialysis, even if intensive, only effects partial resolution.

b) Restless legs respond to clonazepam 0.5 mg prn[17].

c) Dementia in dialysis patients is usually the result of aluminium accumulation in the brain: cerebral aluminium content may be reduced with desferrioxamine, but significant clinical improvement is unlikely except in mild cases. Preventative measures, such as avoidance of high doses of aluminium-containing phosphate binders and reduction of dialysate aluminium concentration by deionisation and reverse osmosis, should make aluminium intoxication increasingly rare.

d) Carpal tunnel syndrome requires urgent decompression.

e) Itching is improved by oral antihistamine or topical steroids.

8. Sexual function

   a) Impotence should be treated with zinc if deficiency is present. Androgens and dopaminergic agonists such as bromocryptine are also of use. Insertion of a penile prosthesis may be necessary[18].
   b) Infertility responds poorly to treatment other than transplantation.
   c) Menorrhagia can be suppressed by progestogens such as norethisterone 5–20 mg daily.

9. Renal replacement therapy: Potentially suitable patients should be referred to a specialist centre early so that vascular access can be created and allow to 'mature' before dialysis is required.

   a) Haemodialysis: two-year patient survival is 90%. There is a 10% dropout rate usually because of loss of vascular access or poor compliance.
   b) Continuous ambulatory peritoneal dialysis: two-year patient survival is 80%. 40% have to switch to another form of treatment owing to recurrent peritonitis, soft tissue infections, loss of ultrafiltration or sclerosing peritonitis. Patients should have fewer than two episodes of peritonitis per year.
   c) Transplantation: two-year patient survival is 95% from live related donors and 50–80% from cadaveric donors. Corresponding graft survival rates are 90% and 50%. Early complications are related to rejection, infection, and myocardial ischaemia. Late complications include malignancy and aseptic necrosis of the hip. Factors improving survival are: close HLA A and B matching, close HLA DR matching, low dose steroid regimens, use of cyclosporin for maintenance immunosuppression, anti-lymphocyte globulin for acute rejection, pre-transplant blood transfusions, and absence of severe extra-renal disease.

FOLLOW-UP

Follow-up will be lifelong but the frequency and parameters of assessment will vary from patient to patient. Consultations are often patient-initiated.

[1] Challah S et al. (1984) Br. Med. J., 289, 1119.
[2] Wing AJ et al. (1983) Proc. Euro. Dialysis Transplant Assoc., 20, 5.
[3] Gardner KD et al. (1984) Am. J. Kidney Dis., iii, 403.
[4] Wai L et al. (1981) Lancet, ii, 1155.
[5] Keeton GR et al. (1981) Nephron, 28, 169.
[6] Barsotti G et al. (1984) Clin. Nephrology, 21, 54.
[7] Rampton DS et al. (1984) Clin. Nephrology, 21, 159.
[8] Swainson CP et al. (1983) Lancet, i, 239.
[9] Bengmark S et al. (1976) Scand. J. Urology Nephrology, 10, 63.
[10] Neff MS et al. (1981) New Eng. J. Med., 304, 871.
[11] Livio M et al. (1982) Lancet, ii, 1016.
[12] Mannucci PM et al. (1983) New Eng. J. Med., 308, 8.
[13] Liu Y et al. (1984) Lancet, ii, 887.
[14] Dawborn JK et al. (1983) Nephron, 33, 100.
[15] Leslie BR et al. (1982) Clin. Nephrology, 18, 50.
[16] Golper TA (1984) Nephron, 38, 217.
[17] Read DJ et al. (1981) Br. Med. J., 283, 865.
[18] Mooradian AD et al. (1984) Arch. Int. Med., 144, 351.

Glomerulonephritis (GN)

The term glomerulonephritis describes a group of diseases characterised by inflammation of the glomeruli and manifested by one or more of proteinuria, haematuria, uraemia, oliguria, oedema, hypertension and loin pain. Evidence from renal biopsies suggests that the various morphological types behave differently and has led to a histologically-based classification. Some of the more common types are described below. Although GN usually occurs in isolation, there is occasionally an associated systemic disease, e.g. Hodgkin's disease (minimal change GN), other tumours (membranous GN), infections (any histology), or SLE (any histology). In such individuals prognosis and treatment are determined by the underlying condition.

Minimal change GN (MCGN)

In MCGN the electron microscope is needed to identity glomerular abnormalities which are not seen under the light microscope. It affects children mainly and usually presents with nephrotic syndrome.

PROGNOSIS

- Overall mortality is 3%.
- Mild uraemia occurs in 30% due to contraction of the intravascular volume but is seldom sufficiently severe to warrant dialysis. Persistent renal failure is exceptional.
- Hypertension, present in 20% in the acute phase, is not sustained.
- Steroid dependence and resistance predispose to complications.
- The prognostic significance of diffuse mesangial proliferation and mesangial IgM deposition remains unclear.

TREATMENT

1. Steroids (oral prednisolone $60\,mg/m^2/day$ for four weeks followed by a low maintenance dose) induce remission in 92% at eight weeks[1]. Of these 25% remain in remission, 25% have infrequent steroid responsive relapses and the remainder are steroid-dependent, relapsing whenever steroids are stopped. Steroid-dependence persists into adult life in only 5% cases[2].
2. Methylprednisolone pulse therapy has been used successfully to reduce steroid related side-effects[3].
3. Cyclophosphamide $(1.5–2.0\,mg/kg/day)$ is steroid-sparing, improves response rate and prolongs the relapse-free interval. Its use is, however, limited by toxicity.

Focal segmental glomerulosclerosis (FSGS)

FSGS is regarded by many as a variant of MCGN with a poorer prognosis. Histologically most glomeruli appear normal but some have segmental sclerotic lesions. Nephrotic syndrome is the most common presentation, but 60% have haematuria, 50% hypertension and over 30% uraemia.

PROGNOSIS

- Spontaneous remission occurs in 20%.
- Over 60% develop end stage renal failure within 10 years. Poor prognostic factors are presentation with uraemia, nephrotic syndrome or gross haematuria, steroid resistance, and increasing age.

TREATMENT

1. A trial of steroids is warranted but 67% are steroid-resistant. A proportion of these will respond partially to cyclophosphamide[4].
2. Management is otherwise supportive.

Membranous nephropathy (MN)

In MN there is diffuse basement membrane thickening. Most present with nephrotic syndrome but many also have haematuria, hypertension, and uraemia.

PROGNOSIS

- Spontaneous remission occurs in 67% children but only 25% adults.
- Nephrotic syndrome develops in 50–80%, hypertension in 50% and renal failure in 25%.

TREATMENT

Controlled trials have suggested a marginal benefit from steroids and immunosuppressants[5].

Membranoproliferative glomerulonephritis (MPGN)

There is basement membrane thickening and cellular proliferation affecting principally the mesangium. Three subtypes are recognised on the basis of electron microscopic appearances but clinically they behave similarly. Common presenting features are proteinuria, haematuria, uraemia, and hypertension.

PROGNOSIS

- Clinical remissions are frequent but persist in under 10%.
- Nephrotic syndrome develops in 80%, hypertension in 50% and renal failure in over 40%.

TREATMENT

A cocktail of steroids, immunosuppressants, anticoagulants and anti-platelet agents appears to improve prognosis[6].

IgA nephropathy

This, the most common form of GN, is characterised histologically by focal segmental proliferation and mesangial deposits of IgA. It classically presents with recurrent episodes of macroscopic haematuria and loin pain precipitated by infection or exercise.

PROGNOSIS

- Haematuria tends to improve with time; however proteinuria often develops. This rarely exceeds 1 g/day and under 5% become nephrotic.
- Acute renal failure occurs in up to 3% cases.
- Hypertension develops in 50% patients.
- Progressive renal failure develops in 30%, being most likely in those with uraemia at presentation, severe haematuria, or heavy proteinuria.

TREATMENT

1. Resistance to steroids and immunosuppressants is usual.
2. Phenytoin reduces haematuria but has not been shown to retard the progression of renal failure[7].

FOLLOW-UP

Blood pressure, body weight, urine microscopy, renal function, and 24 hour urine protein should be reviewed regularly. Follow-up should be life-long because of the possibility of late sequelae.

---

[1] ISKDC (1981) *J. Paediatrics*, **98**, 561.
[2] Trompeter RS *et al.* (1985) *Lancet*, **i**, 368.
[3] Ponticelli C *et al.* (1980) *Br. Med. J.*, **280**, 685.
[4] Geary DE *et al.* (1984) *Clin. Nephrology*, **22**, 109.
[5] Noel LH *et al.* (1979) *Am. J. Med.*, **66**, 82.
[6] Kincaid-Smith P (1984) *Am J. Kidney Dis.*, **iii**, 299.
[7] Egido J *et al.* (1984) *Nephron*, **38**, 30.

Nephrotic Syndrome

In nephrotic syndrome a glomerular protein leak of over 5 g/day causes the plasma albumin concentration to fall to below 20 g/l and so leads to peripheral oedema. It may result from almost any glomerular pathology including most types of primary glomerulonephritis, lupus nephropathy, amyloidosis and diabetic glomerulosclerosis.

PROGNOSIS

- The outcome is largely determined by the causative disease.
- Most deaths result from infection, thromboembolic events, severe negative nitrogen balance, progression of the underlying illness or complications of therapy.
- Nephrotics have an increased clotting tendency and arterial and venous thrombi occur in 35% patients[1]. Renal vein thrombosis is common and often results in pulmonary embolism.
- Renal failure is usually due to intravascular volume depletion, but other potential causes are acute allergic interstitial nephritis complicating diuretic therapy, interstitial oedema causing tubular obstruction, and progression of the original glomerular lesion.

TREATMENT

1. The underlying glomerulopathy should be treated if possible.
2. Daily sodium intake should be reduced to below 1 mmol/kg; fluid restriction may also be needed to prevent hyponatraemia.
3. Increasing daily protein intake to 3 g/kg will maximise hepatic albumin synthesis.
4. Diuretics should not be given unless oedema is causing marked distress to the patient. If no response occurs with a small dose of a thiazide, loop diuretics should be used in increasing amounts. Malabsorption of drugs due to oedema of the gut wall may be circumvented by intravenous administration. The ideal regimen will achieve negative sodium balance without causing intravascular volume depletion and consequent exacerbation of uraemia or postural hypotension.
5. Diuretic resistance due to a contracted plasma volume may be overcome by infusion of 20–40 g of salt-poor albumin immediately before diuretics are given.
6. Negative nitrogen balance may become life threatening, particularly if other problems such as infection supervene. Ablation of the remaining renal tissue will diminish protein loss and is best achieved by percutaneous embolisation since the patient is usually too ill to undergo bilateral nephrectomy. Alternatively renal perfusion may be reversibly reduced by giving a prostaglandin synthetase inhibitor such as indomethacin[2].
7. Thrombosis is an indication for anticoagulation with warfarin; as hypoalbuminaemia is present the required loading dose is small. Heparin is contraindicated because most patients are antithrombin III deficient.
8. Hyperlipidaemia is invariable but does not appear to cause excess atheroma and so requires no specific treatment.
9. Infections are common and should be treated promptly. Prophylactic pneumococcal vaccine does not effectively prevent pneumococcal peritonitis[3].

FOLLOW-UP

Renal function, plasma albumin, 24 hour urine protein and blood pressure should be assessed at least every three months.

[1] Llach F et al. (1981) Am. J. Med., 69, 819.
[2] Donker AJ et al. (1978) Nephron, 22, 374.
[3] Primack WA et al. (1979) Lancet, ii, 1192.

Acute Nephritic Syndrome (Acute Nephritis)

In acute nephritis there is a sudden onset of haematuria, oliguria, oedema and hypertension. It usually follows pharyngeal or cutaneous streptococcal infection and occurs in epidemics particularly in children. Glomeruli show diffuse endocapillary proliferation.

PROGNOSIS

- Most features remit spontaneously within two weeks but proteinuria and microscopic haematuria may persist for up to two years.
- Under 1% die in the acute phase, usually from encephalopathy or pulmonary oedema.
- Under 1% develop rapidly progressive glomerulonephritis.
- Late sequelae are rare, but hypertension, proteinuria and uraemia may occur after a long interval especially in adults and sporadic cases[1].

TREATMENT

1. Treatment is supportive. Bed rest confers no benefit.

2. Hypertension and oedema usually resolve with sodium and water restriction; vasodilators and loop diuretics can be used if a rapid response is required.

3. Steroids are not indicated.

FOLLOW-UP

See *Glomerulonephritis* (p. 74). As it is not possible to predict which patients will have late sequelae, all patients should be reassessed at 1–2-yearly intervals.

---

[1] Rodríguez-Iturbe B (1984) *Kidney Int.*, **25**, 129.

Rapidly Progressive Glomerulonephritis (RPGN)

This syndrome is characterised clinically by an acute nephritic or nephrotic onset with rapid development of renal failure, and histologically by diffuse extracapillary proliferation with crescents affecting the majority of glomeruli. Anti-glomerular basement membrane (anti-GBM) disease is present in 30%. Underlying systemic disease, such as vasculitis, systemic lupus erythematosus, cryoglobulinaemia or malignancy is present in 30%, and the remainder are cryptogenic.

PROGNOSIS

- Most progress to end stage renal failure within three months.
- Mortality from extra-renal causes exceeds 50% within one year.

TREATMENT

1. Many treatment regimens involving different combinations of steroids, immunosuppressants, anticoagulants, anti-platelet agents, and plasmaphoresis have been used. Success has been variable and the ideal regimen is far from clear.

2. The renal function of anuric patients, especially those with anti-GBM disease, is unlikely to improve[1,2] and in such cases treatment should be withheld unless it is indicated for severe extra-renal disease.

FOLLOW-UP

Should be as for *Glomerulonephritis* (p. 74).

[1] Neild GH *et al.* (1983) *Q. J. Med., New Series*, L11, 207, 395.
[2] Hind CRK *et al.* (1983) *Lancet*, i, 263.

Urinary Tract Infection (UTI)

The urinary tract is the most common site of bacterial infection in the body. Risk factors include being female (especially if sexually active or pregnant), increasing age, and structural or neurological lesions of the urinary tract. Most infecting organisms come from the gut flora and ascend via the urethra. Renal involvement is often present even when symptoms suggest uncomplicated cystitis. Treatment for pyelonephritis should be more prolonged than for cystitis but, unfortunately, no currently available laboratory test is reliably predictive of renal involvement; the best guide is the initial response to single dose chemotherapy.

PROGNOSIS

- The excess mortality associated with bacteruria[1] probably reflects the high incidence of UTI in debilitated patients.
- Cystitis often resolves spontaneously and will respond promptly to appropriate antibiotic therapy without permanent sequelae.
- Acute pyelonephritis is frequently complicated by bacteraemia and, without correct treatment, mortality is high. In adults it does not cause renal scarring, hypertension or chronic renal failure unless there is associated obstruction.
- Bacteruria in pregnancy results in overt pyelonephritis in 25%[2]. The incidence of stillbirths and low birth-weight infants is increased.

TREATMENT

. General measures include high fluid intake, complete bladder voiding, and regular bowel habit.

. *Acute symptomatic bacteruria:*

a) Conventionally an appropriate antibiotic is given for 10–14 days. The response rate is 85%; side-effects occur in 30%.

b) Single dose therapy with co-trimoxazole 1.92 g (four normal strength tablets) or amoxycillin 3 g has a similar response rate but with side-effects in under 2%. Early experiences with cephalosporins have not been encouraging[3,4,5].

. *Recurrent infections*

a) Relapse within one week of single dose therapy suggests pyelonephritis or an abnormal urinary tract. A 4–8 week course of antibiotics is indicated.

b) Recurrence after a longer interval implies reinfection. 'Suppressive' low dose regimens such as co-trimoxazole 480 mg nocte continued for six months are effective in 90%. Urinary antiseptics are less effective and demand an unnatural degree of compliance.

4. *Severe pyelonephritis:* Patients will be ill enough to warrant admission to hospital and parenteral broad spectrum antibiotics including an aminoglycoside. Less toxic antibiotics may be substituted when the results of cultures are available.

5. *Asymptomatic bacteruria:* In children and pregnant women it is generally agreed that elimination of infection is mandatory. In others the risk of morbidity from antibiotic side-effects may exceed that associated with untreated infection and, although one attempt with a single dose regimen is justifiable, early relapse is common and not infrequently symptomatic.

6. *Acute urethral syndrome (symptomatic abacteruria)*

a) Associated pyuria usually indicates infection with either *Chlamydia trachomatis* or an 'insignificant' number of bacteria, which will respond to appropriate chemotherapy.

b) In the absence of pyuria true infection is unlikely. Treatable local problems such as atrophic vaginitis are present in some but there is a high incidence of psychosocial problems and treatment is notoriously difficult[6].

Contd.

7. Radiological investigation is expensive and potentially hazardous and should be reserved for those with suspected structural lesions or reflux, such as women with recurrent infection who fail to respond to appropriate antibiotics and children who do not respond to single dose chemotherapy.

FOLLOW-UP

The urine should be cultured one week after completion of treatment to exclude relapse and again six weeks later to exclude reinfection.

[1] Dontas AS *et al.* (1981) *New Eng. J. Med.*, **304**, 939.
[2] Brumfitt W (1975) *Kidney Int. (Suppl.)*, **8**, S113.
[3] Brumfitt W *et al.* (1970) *Postgrad. Med. (Suppl.)*, **46**, 65.
[4] McCracken GH Jr *et al.* (1981) *Paediatrics*, **67**, 796.
[5] Greenberg RN *et al.* (1981) *Am. J. Med.*, **71**, 841.
[6] Stamm WE *et al.* (1981) *New. Eng. J. Med.*, **304**, 956.

Chronic Atrophic Pyelonephritis

Chronic atrophic pyelonephritis is usually diagnosed radiologically by the presence of coarse cortical scars overlying clubbed calyces. The most widely accepted cause is intrarenal reflux of infected urine during childhood. Whether scarring can result from a similar process in later life or from reflux of sterile urine at high pressure remains controversial. Severe scarring may be complicated by hypertension, an associated glomerular lesion (focal and segmental hyalinosis and sclerosis), and progression to end stage renal failure (ESRF). It is the underlying pathology in 25% patients on renal replacement programmes.

PROGNOSIS

- Bilateral scarring is associated with hypertension in 15% and chronic renal failure in 10%.
- Poor prognostic factors include generalised scarring, impaired renal growth, associated obstructive abnormalities (e.g. posterior urethral valves), and the development of hypertension and proteinuria.

TREATMENT

1. Optimum management is preventative. Treatment of refluxing bacteruric children with a continuous suppressive dose of an appropriate antibiotic (e.g. co-trimoxazole 480 mg nocte) will arrest progression of renal scarring and re-establish normal renal growth in 95% cases[1]. Antireflux surgery should be reserved for those in whom this regimen fails but is rarely of benefit once hypertension and proteinuria have developed[2].
2. Early treatment of hypertension, obstruction and infection may retard progression to ESRF in established cases.

FOLLOW-UP

As for *Chronic renal failure* (p. 71). Children should also have monthly urine cultures and six-monthly technetium ^{99}m-labelled dimercaptosuccinic acid (DMSA) scans; this is the preferred method for regular imaging since the radiation dose is less than that of an intravenous urogram.

---

[1] Smellie J et al. (1981) *Kidney Int.*, **20**, 717.
[2] Torres VE et al. (1980) *Ann. Int. Med.*, **92**, 776.

Analgesic Nephropathy

Renal failure secondary to papillary necrosis and chronic tubulointerstitial nephritis develops in about 10% individuals ingesting over 2 kg of non-narcotic analgesics during a period of 1–2 years. In the UK it accounts for about 10% patients developing end stage renal failure (ESRF).

PROGNOSIS

- Renal function progressively deteriorates if analgesic intake is continued.
- Necrotic papillae may slough causing obstruction and acute renal failure (ARF).
- As extrarenal problems such as peptic ulceration and ischaemic heart disease are relatively common, these patients have a higher mortality than those with renal failure from other causes.
- Increased incidence of urothelial tumours.

TREATMENT

1. Stopping non-narcotic analgesic intake will stabilise or even improve renal function[1].
2. Abuse of purgatives, diuretics, alcohol, and tobacco is also common in this group and their use should be discouraged.

FOLLOW-UP

See *Chronic renal failure* (p. 71).

[1]Nanra RS *et al.* (1978) *Kidney Int.*, **13**, 79.

5
Diseases of the Liver and Pancreas

A. E. Read

Cirrhosis of the Liver

Cirrhosis is a chronic, generalised and irreversible disease of the liver characterised by liver cell damage, fibrosis and the formation of regeneration nodules. These nodules result from cellular regeneration in areas of liver cell necrosis and in them there is a disturbance of the normal regular relationship between the portal tracts and the centrilobular veins. A late complication of cirrhosis is the development of one or more malignant tumours of hepatocytes—hepatoma.

PROGNOSIS

- The prognosis in cirrhosis depends partly on the cause and also whether the disease is compensated or uncompensated. The latter is associated with liver cell failure, i.e. a syndrome accompanied by jaundice (due to liver cell dysfunction), fluid retention (ascites and/or oedema), hepatic encephalopathy and a bleeding tendency. Once these features appear the prognosis is grave, suggesting death within two years. Furthermore hepatoma – seen in 15–20% of cirrhotics – is always a risk and the prognosis is then on average only six months.

- *Alcoholic liver disease:* The prognosis is related to whether the patient can remain totally abstemious or not. The five-year mortality of those who continue to drink is 60% reducing to 40% in those who abstain[1]. In the acute stage when there may be prominent evidence of liver cell failure – deep jaundice and ascites – there is a 30–50% mortality.

- *Viral hepatitis:* Cirrhosis associated with Virus B infection usually follows an insidious or mild attack of Virus B hepatitis. It is commonly associated with the presence of the e antigen. If liver cell function is preserved, the prognosis may be good[2]. Hepatic cancer is an important complication.

- *Chronic active (auto-immune) hepatitis:* There is a good prognosis (65% 10-year survival). Acute liver cell failure and immune disease in other organs responds to corticosteroid therapy which significantly improves the mortality[3]. Without corticosteroids the 10-year survival is <30%.

- Cirrhosis associated with *haemochromatosis* responds favourably to venesection therapy. Provided cardiac disease does not cause early death the prognosis is good but there is a considerable (20%) risk of hepatoma which is not altered by treatment.

- In *Kinnier Wilson disease* effective treatment following early diagnosis is compatible with a good prognosis. However, severe liver cell failure accompanying an acute onset with marked neurological involvement signifies an extremely poor outlook.

- In *cystic fibrosis* the prognosis is poor due to progressive pulmonary disease and right heart failure. Complications of liver disease apart from portal hypertension are, however, unusual.

- In *heart failure* with cirrhosis the prognosis is poor unless congestive cardiac failure can be relieved. Death does not result from the liver disease which is usually mild.

- *Homozygous alpha₁ antitrypsin deficiency* accompanied by cirrhosis has a poor prognosis once liver cell failure occurs, but many patients with stable liver function have a reasonable long-term outlook. A rapidly progressive form in adults is described and hepatoma is always a threat[4].

- In *primary biliary cirrhosis* in patients with deepening jaundice the prognosis is bad[5] Death usually occurs within five years of the time of diagnosis. Portal hypertension with bleeding from varices significantly worsens the prognosis. In patients in whom the diagnosis is made on the basis of a compatible liver biopsy and a positive M antibody test and who lack any evidence of clinical liver disease the prognosis is very good and progression of the disease is minimal.

- In *secondary biliary cirrhosis* the prognosis depends on whether biliary obstruction can be completely relieved. If the underlying disease is progressive, e.g. sclerosing cholangitis this is not usually possible[6]. A mean survival of about seven years exists in this group but there are marked variations.

TREATMENT

1. The treatment of *alcoholic liver disease* is abstention from alcohol together with dietary support and vitamin supplements. Corticosteroids are rarely helpful. Prolonged cholestasis may be an indication for corticosteroids but propylthiouracil has been disappointing[7].

2. In cirrhosis following *Virus B and Non A, Non B hepatitis* treatment is usually not effective. Corticosteroids are not helpful and may promote viral replication. Agents that have have been used with partial success include the antivirals such as adenine arabinoside and interferons, as well as immunostimulants like levamisole and transfer factor.

3. *Chronic auto-immune hepatitis* responds to treatment with corticosteroids. Azathioprine is also effective but not by itself; it acts as a corticosteroid sparing agent. These drugs are given until liver function becomes normal when they are stopped. Relapse is an indication for restarting therapy and often means that it must be lifelong. Treatment controls liver cell disease but does not prevent the progression to cirrhosis if this has not already occurred. Disease of other organs, e.g. ulcerative colitis, is also controlled by treatment.

4. *Haemochromatosis* is treated by venesection, at first one unit being withdrawn every week then fortnightly, progress being monitored by estimation of serum ferritin. When serum ferritin levels are normal and liver biopsy confirms that hepatic vein stores are near normal, venesection frequency can be reduced to once per month. Diabetes may require standard treatment and may improve as iron stores fall.

5. *Kinnier Wilson disease* is treated by lifelong copper chelation using D penicillamine[8] (usual dose 1.2–2 g/day). Drug hypersensitivity is unusual but can be countered by cover with prednisolone. Pyridoxine supplements are also given. In non-responsive cases or where hypersensitivity to penicillamine occurs alternate therapy is with triline or zinc. Liver transplantation is a further possibility in severe cases.

6. There is no specific treatment for the cirrhosis of *fibrocystic disease* though variceal haemorrhage is treated by sclerotherapy and lung disease with continuous antibiotics and mucolytics. Pancreatic replacement therapy taken together with H_2 antagonists minimises malabsorption.

7. There is no specific therapy for the cirrhosis accompanying *chronic heart failure*.

8. No specific therapy exists for the cirrhosis of *alpha$_1$ antitrypsin deficiency*, though it is possible that synthetic alpha$_1$ antitrypsin might become available as a nebuliser which could be used to diminish the effects of pulmonary involvement. Hepatic transplantation has also been successfully used.

9. In *primary biliary cirrhosis* there is also no specific treatment. Therapy with azathioprine and D penicillamine is ineffective particularly when one considers the toxic side-effects. However, the prevention of complications is important. Chronic pruritis is treated with cholestyramine or aluminium hydroxide which bind intestinal bile salts. Night blindness can be prevented by vitamin A, and osteomalacia by supplements of vitamin D and calcium. Vitamin K prevents bleeding from prothrombin deficiency. A low fat diet may be required for troublesome steatorrhoea and calcium infusion may relieve acute bone pain associated with osteoporosis. Painful peripheral neuropathy due to xanthomatous deposits in peripheral nerves may require plasmapheresis. Bleeding varices are treated by sclerotherapy. Non-responsive disease in young patients physically and psychologically suitable for hepatic transplantation can be treated in this way. Corticosteroids are contraindicated.

10. *Secondary biliary cirrhosis* needs careful investigation to identify the cause and site of biliary obstruction. Anastomosis of patent bile ducts within the liver with a loop of small bowel is usually the only possible approach, and in the case of sclerosing cholangitis stenting of the biliary tree and hepatic transplantation are other approaches.
Contd.

85

FOLLOW-UP

Routine liver function tests and repeated clinical examination at three-monthly intervals to detect worsening liver function, liver cell failure and hepatoma. In addition, serum ferritin for haemochromatosis and urinary copper excretion in Kinnier Wilson disease. Barium studies or endoscopy to detect varices.

[1] Powell WJ Jr et al. (1968) Am. J. Med., 44, 406.
[2] Dudley FJ et al. (1972) Lancet, ii, 1388.
[3] Cook GC et al. (1971) Q. J. Med., 40, 159.
[4] Eriksson S et al. (1974) Acta Medica Scand., 195, 451.
[5] Shapiro JM et al. (1979) Gut, 20, 137.
[6] Chapman RWG et al. (1980) Gut, 21, 870.
[7] Orrego H et al. (1979) Gastroenterology, 76, 105.
[8] Walshe JM (1960) Lancet, i, 188.

Acute Liver Failure

Liver failure is a syndrome characterised by the presence of: jaundice due to liver cell dysfunction; fluid retention (ascites and/or oedema); hepatic encephalopathy – confusion, coma and basal ganglion signs etc.; and a bleeding tendency – due to impaired hepatic synthesis of hepatic coagulant factors. It occurs in two situations: due to severe hepatic dysfunction in patients with a previously normal liver; or in subjects with chronic liver disease in whom an acute incident e.g. intestinal bleed, infection, or the administration of diuretic or sedative drug produces a sudden deterioration in already compromised liver function. Acute liver cell failure in those with previously normal livers is due to: Virus hepatitis (A, B and Non A Non B); hepatotoxic drugs and poisons, e.g. halothane, paracetamol; acute fatty liver in pregnancy; Reye's syndrome in children; or unknown causes.

PROGNOSIS

- In acute liver cell disease arising in a patient with a previously normal liver the prognosis is poor. Bad signs include deep coma, the presence of renal failure, hypotension and a bleeding tendency. Respiratory infection and septicaemia resulting from i.v. lines are further hazards. Most centres even with meticulous clinical care record a mortality of about 80%[1].
- In acute liver failure complicating chronic liver disease the prognosis is fair if a precipitant feature like bleeding or infection can be controlled. The prognosis is, however, that of the underlying liver disease, and, for example, liver failure in cirrhotics following a gastrointestinal bleed still carries a mortality of 25–50%.

TREATMENT

In either type of situation the principles of treatment are:

1. Careful identification and isolation of patients with Virus A and B infection.
2. Cessation of all protein feeding by mouth; calories are supplied in the form of i.v. glucose (20–40%) into a large vein.
3. The gut is sterilised with neomycin 1 g tds and the colon washed out to remove faecal residue.
4. All sedative, diuretic, constipating and nitrogen-containing drugs are stopped.
5. Lactulose by a gastric tube ensures soft, frequent stools and combats encephalopathy.
6. Vitamin K_1, fresh blood or fresh frozen platelets and platelet infusion help to correct a bleeding tendency.
7. Cerebral oedema may require treatment with corticosteroids.
8. Monitoring of the serum electrolytes, amylase (complicating pancreatitis), blood glucose and exclusion of sepsis are vital, and these aspects must be vigorously treated.
9. The following treatments are of no value:

   a) Corticosteroids – which potentiate intestinal bleeding, oedema and hypokalaemia (but see cerebral oedema above).
   b) Various types of exchange transfusion, and cross circulation (using a normal subject) etc.

10. Improved survival is claimed for haemoperfusion using a polyacrylonitrile membrane[2] to remove toxins up to MW 5000. The improved mortality is not great and improved intensive care methods may account for some of this.
11. In patients with acute or chronic liver failure, treatment is along the same lines but ascites and fluid retention may need treatment with diuretics and sodium restriction. L-dopa and bromocryptine are useful in the treatment of chronic encephalopathy. Liver transplantation may be possible for the occasional patient with liver failure who has underlying chronic liver cell disease.

Contd.

FOLLOW-UP

Fulminant failure cases who survive do not need long-term follow-up. Chronic cases need routine clinical follow-up and studies of electrolytes, liver function etc. Hepatitis B vaccine is essential for staff attending Virus B cases.

[1] Saunders SJ et al. (1975). In *Artificial Liver Support* (Williams R, Murray Lyon IM eds.) p. 217. London: Pitman Medical.
[2] Silk DBA et al. (1977) *Lancet*, ii, 1.

Portal Hypertension

A raised portal venous pressure (>14 cm) water is seen in a variety of clinical situations: complicating chronic liver disease, e.g. cirrhosis (intrahepatic); resulting from portal venous obstruction with a normal liver (extrahepatic); resulting from hepatic venous hypertension or obstruction (suprahepatic). The clinical effects arise from the presence of oesophageal varices and other porto-systemic vascular anastamoses, and include intestinal bleeding and ascites. Liver cell failure may complicate the picture, particularly where there is diffuse liver disease present (intrahepatic portal hypertension).

PROGNOSIS

- The outlook for the patient with bleeding oesophageal varices depends on whether there is underlying liver disease or not. In patients with bleeding varices complicating cirrhosis the mortality in those who develop liver cell failure is 25–50% depending on the severity of the underlying liver disease. In those with extrahepatic portal venous occlusion with normal liver function the prognosis is fairly good[1].

- In patients with portal hypertension complicating hepatic venous outflow in whom alimentary bleeding occurs (Budd Chiari syndrome) the prognosis is extremely bad, over 80% dying from accompanying liver cell failure[2].

TREATMENT

1. The basis of the treatment of variceal bleeding is:

   a) Replacement of blood – often required in large amounts and preferably some of it fresh.

   b) i.v. drip infusion of vasopressin to produce splanchnic arterial constriction with consequent reduction of portal venous outflow (i.v. glypressin may be a suitable alternative, as may i.v. somatostatin).

   c) If bleeding does not stop then a Sengstaken tube (quadruple lumen) is passed by mouth and the gastric and oesophageal balloons inflated – gentle traction is maintained on the apparatus and skilled and constant nursing care are essential.

   d) A full anti-liver failure regime is indicated (see p. 87).

   e) Once bleeding has stopped the patient is endoscoped and the source of bleeding identified. It is stressed that not all patients who have varices actually bleed from them, and it would be important to identify those with other lesions such as acute and chronic peptic ulcer, and acute haemorrhagic gastritis.

   f) Sclerotherapy of varices is carried out via an endoscope and 5 ml of phenylethanolamine is injected in two or three sites within varices. Provided bleeding stops, repeat injections are carried out every two or three weeks until varices have thrombosed.

   g) If bleeding continues despite the above manoeuvres, surgical treatment must be considered. The minimal surgery compatible with the patient's condition and degree of liver cell dysfunction is employed. The varices in the oesophagus may be directly attacked:

      i) By a staple gun introduced into the lower oesophagus to transect and occlude varices[3].

      ii) A plastic (Boerema) button is inserted into the lower oesophagus and a tight ligature allows separation of the mucosa and occluded varices[4].

      iii) A formal variceal ligation or oesophageal transection is performed.

      iv) Alternatively a graft may be placed between the superior mesenteric vein and inferior vena cava (meso-caval shunt)[5].

2. In patients with repeated bleeds an elective shunt (porto-caval or spleno-renal) may be done, but this demands accurate radiological visualisation of the portal venous system and

the long-term complications of hepatic encephalopathy and worsening liver cell failure must be considered. Shunting does not improve the life span which is determined by the degree of hepatic dysfunction.

3. In extrahepatic portal obstruction operation is avoided if at all possible because of the otherwise good long-term prognosis.

FOLLOW-UP

Following sclerotherapy check endoscopy is performed every six months to make sure varices have not reappeared. If they have, sclerotherapy is repeated. Blood tests are performed to check for anaemia and occult blood in faeces to detect bleeding.

[1] Webb LJ et al. (1979) Q. J. Med., 48, 627.
[2] Powell-Jackson PR et al. (1982) Q. J. Med., 51, 79.
[3] Johnston GW (1978) Br. Med. J., i, 1388.
[4] Boerema I et al. (1970) Surgery, 67, 409.
[5] Cameron JL et al. (1979) Surgery, 85, 257.

Drug-induced Jaundice

Jaundice associated with the use of drugs and toxins can be due either to liver cell disease (necrosis, fatty infiltration) or to intrahepatic cholestasis. Sometimes a combined picture is produced. The term predictable is used where the liver lesion is dose-related, and non-predictable where it is not. In the latter, either altered patient susceptibility or abnormal drug biotransformation seems to be responsible for liver damage.

PROGNOSIS

- Liver cell damage causing jaundice has a worse prognosis than cholestasis. Drugs producing hepatic necrosis such as paracetamol, halothane, sodium valproate, carbon tetrachloride, isoniazid etc. can produce a mortality ranging from 5–50%[1].
- Cholestatic liver disease has a much better outlook – though some drugs e.g. chlorpromazine may cause chronic liver disease.
- In those patients with a mixed picture prognosis is affected by the degree of liver cell dysfunction rather than the cholestasis.
- Drugs may also cause chronic parenchymal disease including cirrhosis. It is particularly important that such cases are recognised early so that the drug can be stopped. Considerable improvement may then occur. Drugs in this category include: methyldopa, nitrofurantoin, perhexiline, isoniazid, paracetamol and amiodarone.

TREATMENT

1. Apart from some hepatic drug reactions where specific therapies are indicated, the treatment is generally supportive using a regime as outlined under *Acute liver failure* (p. 87).
2. In patients with cholestatic problems the symptomatic treatment of itching with cholestyramine, and replacement of fat soluble vitamins by i.m. injection is important.
3. Cessation of drug therapy is obviously the lynchpin of treatment though recovery may not occur for some time after doing this and indeed liver cell failure may be progressive even after offending drugs (like halothane and anti-tuberculous drugs) have been withdrawn.
4. One of the commonest poisonings is with paracetamol. This is treated with gastric lavage and replacement of glutathione if poisoning has occurred within 10 hours using methionine 2.5 g via a gastric tube. In addition N acetyl cysteine 150 mg/kg over 15 minutes i.v. followed by 50 mg/kg i.v. in 5% dextrose over four hours and 100 mg/kg i.v. in 5% dextrose over 16 hours is given[2].
5. Treatment with haemoperfusion is recommended in young patients seen early in their illness and attending a unit specialising in this treatment.

FOLLOW-UP

Patients with acute liver disease due to drugs do not require follow-up if they survive.

[1] Zimmerman HJ (1978) Hepatotoxicity. In *The Adverse Effects of Drugs and Other Chemicals on the Liver*. New York: Appleton–Century–Crofts.
[2] Prescott LF *et al.* (1979) *Lancet*, **i**, 59.

Hepatitis

Hepatitis is an acute generalised inflammatory disorder of the liver. Although several drugs, toxins and spirochaetes produce such a disorder in susceptible people the term is generally used to describe a viral inflammation of which the most important are: a) Virus A, incubation period 15–20 days, occurs sporadically or epidemically spread by faeces; b) Virus B, incubation period 7–8 weeks; spread by blood and blood products; c) Virus Non A Non B, three recognisable viruses (May 1986): (i) blood transmitted (post transfusion), (ii) coagulation factor transmitted (Factor VIII and IX), (iii) epidemic water-borne from water supplies.

PROGNOSIS

- The prognosis of Virus A infection is very good. Complete recovery occurs and the mortality is about 0.1%. This is caused by occasional cases who develop acute hepatic necrosis or aplastic anaemia.
- Virus B infection has a much worse prognosis. A mortality of up to 10–20% is recorded, particularly in the elderly and those with an underlying disease which might require blood transfusion and hospitalisation. Coexistent infection with δ agent worsens the short and long term prognosis. Death is from fulminant liver failure. Chronic liver disease and hepatoma are possible long-term sequelae in survivors. In areas of high incidence of hepatoma more than 90% patients have evidence of previous Virus B infections.
- Virus Non A Non B infections with the exception of the water-borne form run a mild apyrexial course. Arthritis and pyrexia are particular features of the water-borne type in which the mortality may be up to 12%. The mortality in the two other types is 1% or less but the risk of chronic liver disease with these two is uncertain, and evidence of persisting biochemical activity occurs in up to 50%.

TREATMENT

1. Prophylaxis

    a) A vaccine against Hepatitis B is available and should be given to those at high risk. Three intramuscular or subcutaneous injections at 0, 1 and 6 months usually produce effective protection, but the immunosuppressed and those with renal disease may need larger doses[1].

    b) Gammaglobulin is used to protect against Virus A infection, e.g. those going to high incidence areas or in an epidemic, whilst high titre antihepatitis B globulin is available for those who have been accidentally exposed by needle prick etc. It must be used within a day or two of exposure.

2. There is no specific treatment for viral hepatitis but isolation and careful disposal of excreta; care with blood samples is essential.

3. In severe cases and in particular where there are cholestatic features corticosteroids (e.g. prednisolone 40 mg daily) will lessen jaundice and produce euphoria but there is a risk of relapse on cessation of therapy, and in fulminant attacks they are not recommended. Further, in Virus B cases there is evidence of increased viral replication with corticosteroids[2].

4. Otherwise the treatment of hepatitis is bed rest and a nutritious diet. Although neither of these has been proven to be beneficial, in an ill patient they would seem to be sensible.

5. Cyanimidol (Catechin), a bioflavin, has been shown to influence favourably the course of Virus B hepatitis but it is not widely used.

6. Drugs which are hepatotoxic and those which accentuate the features of liver cell failure, e.g. sedatives and sodium-retaining drugs, and drugs which cause gastric irritation and bleeding should be avoided. Similarly alcohol should be avoided.

FOLLOW-UP

Virus B cases need six-monthly estimation c

Virus B and e antibody status. Patients and medical attendants must be warned of the risks of transmission. Alcohol is usually withdrawn for 3-6 months. The course of the illness can be checked by LFTs, and HBS Ag which should disappear after 2-3 months. HBe antigen should decline before HBS Ag, but if it remains positive this is a sign of continuing disease.

---

[1] Szmuness W *et al.* (1980) *New Eng. J. Med.*, **303**, 833.
[2] Scullard GH *et al.* (1979) *Gastroenterology*, **77**, 43A.

Pancreatitis

Two forms of the disease are recognised. Acute pancreatitis is an acute generalised inflammation of the pancreas caused by biliary tract disease, alcoholism and more rarely hyperlipoproteinaemia, hypercalcaemia and the action of drugs and toxins. It also occurs postoperatively. Chronic pancreatitis is more commonly related to alcoholism; biliary tract disease is less important. In chronic pancreatitis fibrosis of the gland may be associated with calcification. Dilatation and stricturing of the duct system leads to faulty drainage and stones may form within the ducts. Diabetes may occur, and cancer is a possible sequela.

PROGNOSIS

- The mortality of acute pancreatitis is about 20% from all causes, death being from cardiovascular, pulmonary or septic complications.
- The prognosis in postoperative pancreatitis is poor (40% mortality). Bad signs include urea retention, a low serum calcium and low PaO_2 and raised transaminases (> 250 i.u./l), particularly in a patient over 55 years of age.
- In chronic pancreatitis the course is variable – the seven-year mortality is 50%[1] but in those with an alcoholic cause the 50% seven-year survival may be prolonged to 12.5 years. Death is often due to other alcoholic-related problems like cirrhosis, whilst suicide and malignant diseases, including carcinoma of the pancreas, may occur.

TREATMENT

1. *Acute pancreatitis*

    a) Careful monitoring of fluid balance, tissue oxygenation, blood glucose, calcium.
    b) Limiting pancreatic secretion by nasogastric suction and withholding oral feeding.
    c) Electrolyte and fluid replacement – hypokalaemia and hypocalcaemia are particularly important and must be treated vigorously.
    d) Anoxia is treated with oxygen therapy but endotracheal intubation and mechanical ventilation may be required in progressive cases.
    e) Prophylactic H_2 blockers may prevent gastrointestinal bleeding.
    f) Surgery is limited to diagnostic laparotomy if there is doubt concerning the diagnosis. Even if biliary pathology is present this is best managed after the pancreatitis has subsided. Peritoneal lavage may ameliorate the course of acute pancreatitis but does not prevent late complications like pancreatic abscess which occur in up to 10%.
    g) Pancreatic abscess formation may require antibiotics and surgical drainage.
    h) Nutritional support using parenteral infusion is often required.
    i) Antibiotics are given on clinical suspicion of infection.

2. *Chronic pancreatitis*

    a) A careful search for aetiological factors and correction of these where it is possible. Alcoholism must be vigorously tackled.
    b) Analgesia for abdominal pain (this may require potent drugs and there is a small risk of addiction).
    c) H_2 blockers with pancreatic supplements, e.g. Nutrizym, may lessen steatorrhoea and have been shown to diminish the severity of abdominal pain.
    d) A low fat diet diminishes steatorrhoea resistant to H_2 blockers and pancreatic supplements.
    e) Diabetes may require treatment.
    f) Coeliac axis block may help if pain is intractable and surgery should also then be considered. Pseudocysts are usually treated by anastomosing the cyst cavity to the stomach or small bowel if they do not resolve spontaneously. Identification of duct stenosis by pancreatography may allow a formal longitudinal pancreaticojejunostomy or subtotal distal pancreatectomy.

FOLLOW-UP

Regular surveillance to ensure abstinence from alcohol and control of diabetes.

[1] Worning H (1984) Chronic pancreatitis: pathogenesis, natural history and conservative treatment. In *Clinics in Gastroenterology 13/3*, p. 871. Philadelphia: W.B. Saunders Company.

6

Diseases of the Nervous System and Voluntary Muscle

J.P. Patten

Cerebral Vascular Accidents (CVAs)

CVAs are complications of thromboembolic disease. They may be occlusive (atheroma and thrombus blocking major vessels in the neck or main intracranial branches), embolic occlusions of normal vessels (emboli originating in neck vessels and damaged or fibrillating heart) or haemorrhagic (ruptured microaneurysms or berry aneurysms on major intracranial vessels). A 1% per annum decline in CVAs had been documented from 1940 but since 1970 a 5% annual decrease in CVAs with a major fall in CVAs due to haemorrhage has occurred. Considering that the population is ageing and therefore more CVA prone, this fall is remarkable. It is thought that hypotensive medication, anti-thrombotic and anti-emolic measures have made a major contribution. The indications for and use of such treatment therefore assumes important and still controversial significance. CVA causes 100 000 deaths per annum in GB and 200 000 per annum in USA. The prevalence is 160 per 100 000 population with a peak range 50–70 years. The male to female ratio is 2:1. CVAs in carotid artery territories account for 80–90% cases, vertebral basilar territory 10–20%. The following symptoms occur in completed stroke and transient ischaemic attacks (TIAs) in carotid territory (in order of frequency): hemianaesthesia, hemiparesis, dysphasia, confusion, visual loss, dysarthria and vertigo; in vertebral basilar territory (in order of frequency): vertigo, homonymous visual impairment, falls, dysarthria, hemianaesthesia, hemiparesis, tetraparesis, facial anaesthesia and confusion.

PROGNOSIS

- Varying definitions, different diagnostic criteria and different methods of obtaining trial patients makes for a bewildering variety of prognostic statistics. Included are the generally accepted figures on which treatment strategies are based. The figures are based mainly on carotid artery disease – there is not thought to be any major difference for the prognosis in the vertebral basilar territory, although survival is marginally better (70% v. 60%).
- Mortality rate of first attack: 20% (carotid territory).
- 50% survivors will eventually die of myocardial infarction (MI). Hypertension (70%), ischaemic heart disease (IHD) (30%), peripheral vascular disease (30%), diabetes mellitus (20%), hyperlipidaemia, heavy smoking, oral contraceptives, vasculitis and primary blood disorders play a role in specific cases.
- 90% patients having CVA have no premonitor symptoms[1].
- 50% patients having TIAs have a major stroke within five years (20% within one month, 60% within six months).
- 6% patients with recurrent TIAs have a fatal CVA within one year.

- 30% patients with TIAs die of other causes, mainly ischaemic heart disease.
- At post-mortem up to 15% asymptomatic patients have one or other carotid artery occluded and 40% have severe atheroma.
- Bruits appear in the carotid vessels with increasing age (3.5% at ages 45–54, 7% at ages 67–79), more frequently in patients with hypertension and ischaemic heart disease, and diabetics. The subsequent CVA rate in these patients is twice that of patients without bruits but the CVA usually occurs in another vascular territory and is often non-embolic in type. The incidence of MI is also increased twofold in patients with bruits. Bruits should be regarded as evidence of diffuse vascular disease, not as a disease in their own right[2].
- The outcome of completed CVAs: Good recovery (20%), moderate disability (30%), severe disability (30%), death (20%). Bearing in mind that most survivors will die of ischaemic heart disease, treatment strategies to prevent CVAs are of little use unless similar benefits for the vascular disease elsewhere apply. For this reason surgical treatment of localised carotid artery disease can have only limited application.
- Increasing age does not protect, the risk increases with age.

- Lipid abnormalities are a high risk factor in CVA and IHD below age 55, after this it is less significant.
- Diabetes is a more important factor in women than men – diabetic women lose their relative immunity to IHD and CVA. Detection and strict management of diabetes unfortunately seems to achieve little reduction of neurological complications and strokes.
- Haematocrit:

  a) There is increasing evidence that a high haematocrit, even in upper normal range, carries risk when associated with narrowed atherosclerotic arteries.
  b) Venesection leads to *increased* cerebral blood flow.

- Oral contraceptives carry a risk especially in women over 35 years who smoke.

TREATMENT AND PREVENTION

1. Hypertension

   a) At all levels a higher risk of CVA occurs – there is no safe level.
   b) Sex difference does not matter – women have the same risk of CVA as men.
   c) Systolic blood pressure matters. Even with a normal diastolic pressure, a high systolic pressure results in twice the rate of CVA.
   d) Detection and treatment of high blood pressure has dramatic effects on reducing CVA risk and improving the prognosis in CVAs. Reduction of blood pressure *increases* cerebral blood flow and the approach of not treating high blood pressure for fear of causing CVAs is quite unjustified[3].

2. Cardiac abnormalities

   a) All forms of ischaemic heart disease predispose to CVA and appropriate treatment especially of congestive heart failure is important.
   b) Atrial fibrillation, even without co-existent vascular disease, is dangerous.

There is a five times greater risk of embolic CVA.

3. Anti-platelet therapy: Aspirin alone has proved to be effective (without the addition of sulphinpyrazone and dipiridamole) in reducing the frequency of TIAs and subsequent stroke, although dose and duration of treatment varies. Minimal benefits in females in studies so far reported may reflect the smaller number and known lower risk in females. The dose used is up to 1500 mg/day in most trials. Theoretical considerations suggest 300 mg/day should be adequate and until further trials are reported this seems the safest dose to avoid gastrointestinal problems[4, 5, 6].

4. Anticoagulant therapy

   a) The evidence *against* anticoagulant therapy as treatment after CVA with the exception of atrial fibrillation is impressive.
   b) For strokes in evolution there is no firm evidence of value but recent reports suggest benefit. Since it is a rare situation formal trials are virtually impossible.
   c) The writer uses heparin i.v. 5000 units, four hourly, 48–72 hours in patients with stroke in evolution[7].

5. Transient ischaemic attacks

   a) If aspirin fails to prevent TIAs or they occur in rapid sequence, anticoagulation has to be considered. Unfortunately there is no real evidence of benefit and in older patients the risk of haemorrhagic complications is a definite consideration.
   b) The author's own policy, if aspirin fails, is to start a heparin trial for four days and proceed to anticoagulant therapy if heparin prevents further episodes[8, 9].

6. Emboli from the heart

   a) 50% CVAs in under 40-year-olds are due to fibrillation, 10–15% all TIAs are secondary to emboli from the heart.
   Contd.

b) 90% all emboli leaving the heart go to the brain.
c) 20–30% all patients with cardiac originating emboli are dead within one year.
d) For patients with rheumatic valvular heart disease: 30–75% will suffer a repeat stroke, 30% within two weeks.
e) For those with post myocardial infarction emboli: 25% will have a repeat stroke within two weeks.
f) For those with atrial fibrillation (no valve lesion) there is a 42% recurrence rate, 5% within two weeks.
g) In all embolic situations anticoagulant therapy achieves a 50–75% reduction in repeat embolisation rates. Timing is difficult – a six-week delay to avoid bleeding into the cerebral infarct is recommended but known high two-week embolic recurrence rate makes delay dangerous. The risk of haemorrhage is low if the CT scan is clear and blood pressure controlled.
h) The author's own policy is to start heparin and warfarin as soon as the diagnosis is confirmed, *if* no risk factors for bleeding exist. Heparin is continued for the first 72 hours until the prothrombin time is satisfactory.

7. The author's view of carotid endarterectomy: In spite of little solid evidence of value, endarterectomy in carotid artery disease continues to be performed at an increasing pace. At first performed to remove 'an obstruction to flow', when evidence suggested flow was not an important factor, the operation was continued 'to remove a source of emboli', in spite of other purely medical methods of preventing embolus formation. The risks of preliminary angiography are rarely included in reports, although they are actually greater than the subsequent surgical procedure. Digital subtraction angiography may lessen this risk. Mortality rate of surgery is 3.3%. 7.7% have a CVA in the perioperative period. At two years following surgery 15% of a group of operated patients have had a CVA and 14% of a medically treated group had a CVA. The figures are improved if *only* severely stenosing lesions are considered separately. Whatever the angiographic/operative risks, it still has to be established that localised surgical treatment of a systemic condition benefits the patients in the long term. The evidence that it does is still dubious and given the current combined mortality-morbidity rate of 11% it is difficult to regard surgery as an established primary procedure in embolic cerebrovascular disease. Even if mortality rates are brought down, it still has to be demonstrated that the procedure alters the immediate and long-term prognosis and the benefits of a medical approach to the generalised vascular disease will remain an important factor[10, 11].

8. A multi-centre trial of internal carotid – external carotid by-pass surgery has shown no benefit from this procedure in any group of patients[12, 13]. A similar controlled trial of carotid endarterectomy is urgently needed.

FOLLOW-UP

Continuing supervision of anti-hypertensive therapy is important. Anticoagulant therapy should be monitored in an anticoagulant clinic. Neurological follow-up is only necessary if residual CNS problems or further events occur in spite of recommended therapy.

[1] Whisnant JP (1974) *Stroke*, 5, 68.
[2] Wolf RA (1981) *J. Am. Med. Assoc.*, 245, 1442.
[3] Kannell WB *et al.* (1970) *J. Am. Med. Assoc.*, 214, 301.
[4] Bousser MG *et al.* (1983) *Stroke*, 14, 5.
[5] Fields WS *et al.* (1977) *Stroke*, 8, 301.
[6] Canadian Cooperative Study GP (1978) *New Eng. J. Med.*, 53, 299.
[7] Millikan C (1975) *Med. Clin. North Am.*, 63, 897.
[8] Carter AB (1957) *Q. J. Med.*, 26, 335.
[9] Ebert JA (1973) *J. Am. Med. Assoc.*, 225, 724.
[10] Barne TT *et al.* (1984) *Stroke*, 15, 941.
[11] Fields WS *et al.* (1970) *J. Am. Med. Assoc.*, 211, 1993.
[12] Bypass Study Group (1985) *New Eng. J. Med.*, 313, 1191.
[13] Plum F (1985) *New Eng. J. Med.*, 313, 1221.

Dementia

Dementia is a descriptive term meaning failure of previously normal intelligence. Frequency increases with age, hence it is a growing medical problem. It has been classified as presenile if onset is under 60 years of age. The neuropathological changes are senile plaques, neurofibrillary tangles and loss of neurones and are identical in all age ranges and also found in the brains of 30–40-year-old patients with Down's syndrome. Severe depression may cause *pseudo-dementia* (10% all cases). Approximately 15% suspected cases of dementia are not demented. 50% demented patients have a demonstrable (not necessarily treatable) cause. A full range of haematological, biochemical and endocrine investigations must therefore be performed in each patient. There is a variable presentation depending on the area of brain affected. Frontal lobe damage produces changes in behaviour, emotions and social skills, poor judgement, loss of abstract thought, labile mood, impaired personal hygiene, incontinence, secondary depression (25–30% cases) and psychotic thought disorder. Parieto-temporal lobe damage in the dominant hemisphere causes nominal aphasia, receptive aphasia, dyslexia, loss of constructional skills and sequencing difficulty. The female to male ratio is 3:1[1, 2].

PROGNOSIS

- The average lifespan from diagnosis is 2–5 years.
- Most patients continue in their family setting for 2–3 years and most survive 1–2 years after admission to hospital.

TREATMENT

1. Appropriate treatment of underlying disorder if identified.
2. Withdrawal of drugs that may be causing or aggravating the condition.
3. Recognition and aggressive treatment of co-existent depressive or psychotic features. Electro-convulsive treatment may be indicated[3].
4. Social and environmental adjustments, family care, day care centres and support groups may enable the patient to live in their home and community for long periods, but most eventually need custodial hospital care, by which time most are unaware of their circumstances and often fail to identify relatives who continue to visit them after admission.
5. No measures using vasodilator drugs, cholinesterase inhibitors, polypeptides, choline precursors or vitamin supplements, have been shown to produce indentifiable benefits.
6. There is currently no specific treatment of proven benefit.

FOLLOW-UP

No specific neurological follow-up is necessary. Review if new problems such as epilepsy occur. Psychogeriatric in-patient care often necessary in latter stages.

[1] Marsden CD *et al.* (1972) *Br. Med. J.*, **ii**, 249.
[2] Wells CE (1979) *Am. J. Psychiat.*, **136**, 895.
[3] Yesavage J (1979) *Geriatrics*, **34**, 51.

Epilepsy

The treatment and prognosis of epilepsy depend on the correct identification of the type of attack and confirmation that the attacks *are* epileptic in nature. Pseudo-seizures (non-organic seizures) can account for 25% of 'uncontrollable' epilepsy.

Petit-mal epilepsy[1]

Petit-mal epilepsy is a rare form of epilepsy (2.5%) unique to children 4–12 years old. It is slightly more frequent in females and there may be a genetic factor. It consists of short-lived (5–45 seconds) impairment of awareness, and is associated with 2–3 cps spike wave bursts on EEG in every attack. A brief clonic jerk of eyelids and arms occurs in 71%, and short automatisms, chewing, swallowing and finger fumbling in 88%. The latter features occur particularly in long attacks and the differentiation between these and brief complex partial seizures becomes very difficult.

PROGNOSIS[2]

- In fewer than 2% patients attacks continue into adulthood.
- Nearly all sufferers cease having attacks by 17 years of age.
- If major attacks supervene the prognosis alters and different medication may become more appropriate.

TREATMENT

1. Patients treated with a pure anti-petit-mal therapy have a higher incidence of subsequent major attacks (80%) than those on composite regime who have only a 35% chance of developing other seizure types.
2. Therapy should be withdrawn at 10–14 years of age or after four years complete control.
3. Sodium valproate 20–60 mg/kg in divided doses twice daily, depending on control – drug of choice[3].
4. Ethosuximide 250–1000 mg daily: risk of provoking other types of epilepsy[4].
5. Treatment of petit-mal status

   a) Rebreathe from paper bag.
   b) Diazepam 10 mg i.v. by slow injection.

c) Valproate dosage increased.
d) Ketogenic diet (see neurological texts for details).

Complex partial seizures (psychomotor seizures, temporal lobe attacks)

Complex partial seizures are the commonest type of seizure in adolescence and adulthood. They occur in any age range in either sex. In childhood, they are often incorrectly identified as petit-mal. Almost any intellectual or autonomic function may be affected. The main features are sudden alterations in mood, behaviour, and personality, which may be associated with repetitive semi-purposeful movements and followed by confusion and even denial of the attack. The seizures do not occur at any special times although daydreaming and mealtimes are often cited. Patients eventually recognise the premonitory signs: epigastric distress, perineal numbness, nausea, giddiness, visual, auditory, olfactory or gustatory hallucinations, or *deja-vu* phenomena. In the attack confusion, staring, running in circles, chewing, lip-smacking, clothing removal and aimless fiddling with objects may occur. Attempts to restrain or assist may provoke physical resistance and attacks may proceed to collapse with convulsive movements.

PROGNOSIS

- Attacks may occur several times daily or very infrequently. Associated behavioural disturbance is common, sometimes prior to attack
- 10% patients have cerebral tumours (usually late onset adults).
- Generally the prognosis is poor as it is the hardest type of epilepsy to control completely.
- Associated social/behavioural problem

make it difficult for the sufferer to hold employment.

- The association with occasional grand mal attacks often requires a high dose regime or complex polypharmacy with attendant problems of drug side-effects.

TREATMENT[5] (see dose regimes, p. 102)

1. Carbamazepine is the drug of choice.
2. Phenytoin is effective, but may provoke petit-mal if the diagnosis is wrong.
3. Primidone carries the risk of worsening behavioural upset.
4. Sodium valproate is occasionally successful, and is ideal if petit-mal is also present[6].
5. Benzodiazepines alone are disappointing – clobazam 10 mg bd or nocte is occasionally an effective supplement to other agents.

Grand-mal epilepsy

Grand-mal epilepsy is the second most common form of epilepsy (but accounts for 80% childhood seizures). It affects about 0.8% of the population – up to 3% have had one seizure. Loss of consciousness is the main feature – movement is not essential (akinetic epilepsy). Tonic (sustained) or clonic (jerking) movements commonly occur. Incontinence (<50% cases) is not essential to diagnosis. It mainly occurs in those aged 0-15 years and those over 50 years old when the incidence rises steadily due to vascular disease and neoplasms.

PROGNOSIS

- In the younger age group metabolic and hormonal factors rather than structural disease are the main causes. In the older age range toxic, vascular or neoplastic causes are more likely (approximately 30%).
  Episodes may be diurnal or nocturnal.
- Diurnal attacks tend to occur within 1-2 hours of awakening.
- Nocturnal attacks tend to occur within two hours of onset of sleep or within one hour of wakening – many patients *only* ever convulse nocturnally and are therefore allowed to drive provided they have had three years of nocturnal episodes only.

- Idiopathic epilepsy

  a) Starting before 5 years old: unlikely to remit completely.
  b) Starting between 5 and 15 years old: high chance of remission by age 20 years (approximately 75% will not have repeat episodes when drugs withdrawn after three years of freedom from attacks).
  c) Attacks continuing beyond 20 years need lifelong therapy.

- Attacks due to structural lesions, trauma, tumour, angioma are unlikely to remit and lifelong therapy is necessary.
- Attempts to stop therapy are generally made after 3-4 years of complete control if the risk of recurrence seems low or where an attack will not destroy a career or prevent essential driving.

TREATMENT[7, 8, 9]

1. All anti-convulsant drugs demonstrate about 70% effectiveness against major epilepsy – personal preferences dictate the regime in most cases.
2. Phenytoin 300–500 mg daily in a bd regime is a safe, effective drug. It has numerous but rare side-effects including skin reaction, gum hyperplasia, and macrocytic anaemia as the main problems. Teratogenic problems occur but rarely considering the widespread use of the drug since 1938.
3. Sodium valproate 600–1500 mg daily in bd or tds dosage may cause gastric side-effects, weight gain, hair loss and skin rashes. Tremor can occur. It may possibly be teratogenic.
4. Carbamazepine 300–1200 mg daily in tds dosage may cause severe skin reaction, vertigo, and occasional fluid retention. Bone marrow toxicity is rare, most reported cases being in the elderly. It improves behavioural disturbance in brain-damaged children. It has no known teratogenic potential.
5. Primidone 375–750 mg daily in tds dosage may cause giddiness and vertigo, frequently
   Contd.

severe. Drowsiness even in small dosage is a problem. Many patients cannot tolerate it even with low starting dose and slow increments.

6. Barbiturates and benzodiazepines are no longer regarded as first line drugs.

7. It is important to note that the dose of any medication must be adequate (assessed by clinical results and secondarily by blood level determination). Missed doses, particularly of the short acting drugs, may provoke attacks.

8. Toxic levels of any medication cause drowsiness, ataxia, diplopia, nausea and exacerbation of the epileptic attacks.

9. In occasional patients a full range of agents may be tried before control established. Polypharmacy should be avoided.

Other forms of epilepsy

TREATMENT

1. *Focal motor epilepsy.* Phenytoin/Primidone combined best therapy.

2. *Myoclonic seizures* – 'messy breakfast syndrome'. Clonazepam 0.5–2 mg nocte or methsuximide 300 mg nocte are both extremely effective. Methsuximide available to special order from manufacturers.

3. *Status Epilepticus*

   a) Intravenous diazepam 10 mg bolus, repeated hourly as necessary.
   b) Rectal diazepam 1 mg per year of age plus 1 mg in infants.

   c) Paraldehyde, 0.3 ml/kg in children, 5–10 ml in adults i.m. into buttock only. May be repeated six hourly over 24 hours.
   d) Chlormethiazole 0.8%, 8 mg/ml solution by i.v. infusion. In infancy 5–10 mg/kg/hour. In adults 15–60 drops/minute according to response *must* be given via central venous line.
   e) Maintenance doses of previous regime should be continued or reintroduced by nasogastric tube if necessary.

FOLLOW-UP

As long as attacks continue follow-up at three, six, nine or 12 month intervals is necessary, reconsidering the therapy at each visit. Early follow-up (2–4 weeks) is advisable after any major change in medication to assess response and side-effects. When attacks controlled (over two years since last episode) discharge from hospital follow-up into care of family doctor pending further episodes with strict instructions not to alter or discontine therapy without medical advice.

[1] Penry J et al. (1975) Brain, 98, 427.
[2] Sato S et al. (1973) Neurology (Minneap.), 23, 1135.
[3] Sato S et al. (1982) Neurology (Minneap.), 32, 157.
[4] Coatsworth J J et al. (1972) Antiepileptic Drugs p. 87. New York: Raven Press.
[5] Cereghino J J et al. (1974) Neurology, 24, 401.
[6] Bruni J (1979) Arch. Neurol., 36, 393.
[7] Porter R J et al. (1985) The Epilepsies. Guildford: Butterworth.
[8] Pedley TA et al. (1983) Recent Advances in Epilepsy 1. Edinburgh: Churchill Livingstone.
[9] Pedley TA et al. (1985) Recent Advances in Epilepsy 2. Edinburgh: Churchill Livingstone.

Parkinson's Disease

Parkinson's disease is a syndrome produced by failure of striato-nigral dopaminergic neural systems, consequent upon degeneration of the substantia nigra. It can be a consequence of degenerative, infective metabolic or pharmacological processes. Most cases are idiopathic. The prevalence is 130 per 100 000 and there appear to be no genetic factors (based on twin studies). Usual onset is after 40 years of age – 1% population over 60 is affected. In 50% patients with Parkinson's disease over 70 years, Alzheimer-like changes are present in the cerebral cortex. Early symptoms are non-specific: stiffness, slowness, muscle aching. Tremor is often mild, marked at rest or while walking and is often embarrassing rather than disabling. Rigidity is usually the most dependable physical sign, best detected on passive movement. Bradykinesia is the most disabling feature of the disease. Progressive confusional and dementing state occurs in 20–30% older patients[1, 2].

PROGNOSIS

- Symptoms often start unilaterally and become bilateral in 2–3 years in those patients who are going to run a progressive course.
- A few patients show a rapidly deteriorating course, often indicated by rapidly failing or poor initial response to medication, or confusional side-effects.
- In most a slow decline over a 5–10 year period is the rule with age and problems related to therapy becoming increasingly significant.

TREATMENT

1. Treatment must aim to enable the patient to lead a normal life, to reach retirement age in employment, and to enjoy hobbies. But it must be borne in mind that the long-term problems of therapy, as many of the later complications, are dose/duration related.

2. The anticholinergics (benzhexol (Artane), benztropine (Cogentrin), orphenadrine (Disipal))

   a) The oldest medications in use, best for tremor with little effect on other parameters.
   b) May cause problems with confusion, visual hallucinosis and urinary retention in males.
   c) In the author's view have a limited place in therapy and inadvisable in patients over 60 years.

3. Amantadine hydrochloride (Symmetrel)

   a) The mode of action may be facilitation of dopamine-release or some anticholinergic effect.
   b) It may cause nocturnal hallucinations, oedema and skin rash on legs (livedo reticularis), and epileptic fits in overdose.
   c) The maximum dose is 100 mg bd. It has a good dopamine sparing action but the effect lessens after several months of therapy. The evening dose should not be taken later than 6 pm.

4. Selegiline hydrochloride (Eldepryl)

   a) This is a monamine oxidase B-blocking agent.
   b) It has no tyramine effect, and prevents dopamine breakdown.
   c) It has few side-effects but may potentiate the side-effects of levodopa.
   d) It must be used with a dopamine-containing agent.
   e) Dosage is 5–10 mg daily mane.

5. Levodopa

   a) Available in combination with carbidopa (Sinemet) and benserazide (Madopar) which avoids gastrointestinal and systemic side-effects.
   b) Is very effective but has long-term side-effects. Dyskinesias and on/off phenomena seem related to dose and duration of use.

Contd.

c) Use should be delayed by using other agents if possible; when used the dose should be kept low and cover the active period of the day only – no retiring dose.

d) Dosages are Madopar: 62.5 mg, 125 mg, 250 mg tds; Sinemet Plus: $\frac{1}{2}$–1 tab., tds; Sinemet: 110–275 mg, $\frac{1}{2}$–1 tab., tds. All doses are given with meals to avoid nausea and vomiting. The dose should be reduced if choreiform or athetoid movements intrude. In some patients this will allow parkinsonian symptoms to return, but a permanent dyskinetic state, only blocked by ever higher dosage of causal drug, occurs if allowed to persist. This remains the major unsolved dilemma of treatment.

6. Bromocriptine

a) The only dopamine agonist available for general use.

b) Its role as primary medication still under evaluation.

c) Mainly used in patients developing choreiform movements and on/off effects.

d) May cause severe nausea, vomiting, and postural hypotension.

e) 2.5–5 mg tds is usually the maximum dosage tolerated.

7. At present no safe agent is available to block the involuntary movements produced by medication, such agents are being actively sought.

8. The author's regime

a) Amantadine hydrochloride, 100 mg bd (8 am and 6 pm) for as long as it is effective.

b) The smallest dose of dopamine-containing agent is added to achieve control.

c) Selegiline is used to enhance control but is continued only if effective.

d) Bromocriptine is considered when response fails, dyskinetic movements or on/off symptoms occur, or if dopamine not tolerated.

9. Other useful agents

a) Constipation. Bisacodyl one tab. nocte and one suppository mane.

b) Postural hypotension. Ephedrine hydrochloride 15 mg tds or fludrocortisone 100 μg od.

c) Depression. Imiprimine hydrochloride 10–25 mg tds.

d) Psychotic changes. Thioridazine 25 mg tds is the only agent with a low potential for worsening the parkinsonian features. However withdrawal of anti-parkinsonian drugs is often necessary.

10. The treatment of Parkinson's disease complicating other disorders is particularly difficult, as response to medication is less predictable. Confusional side-effects and postural hypotension are more likely as is progressive failure of medication to benefit patient as disease progresses. These conditions include post-encephalitic, drug-induced, multi-system atrophies, post-traumatic and post-CVA parkinsonian syndromes.

11. Pseudo-parkinsonism (arteriopathic rigidity) does not respond to any anti-parkinsonian medication.

[1] Marsden CD et al. (1981) Movement Disorders: Neurology 2. Guildford: Butterworths.
[2] Jankovic J et al. (1984) Neurol. Clin., 2, 417.

Multiple Sclerosis

Multiple sclerosis (MS) is a syndrome in which episodes of demyelination occur at different times and in different areas of the central nervous system producing widespread and increasing disability. In its classical relapsing form in young adults it is readily diagnosed. Increasingly patients with a progressive course from the onset are being positively identified. This pattern may occur at all ages but particularly in patients over 50 years. It is therefore a spectrum of diseases produced by local plaques of demyelination as both its causal and distinguishing lesion. It is twice as frequent in females as males and has prevalence rates 85 per 100 000 in Europe and GB, 58 per 100 000 in USA and 4 per 100 000 in Japan. The peak age of onset is 20–40 years (older in males), with 5% cases under 15 years and 10% over 50 years.

PROGNOSIS[1]

- The spinal cord is mainly affected, Babinski sign (65%), Lhermitte's phenomena (paraesthesial in limbs on neck flexion) (40%), sensory symptoms (35%), painful dysaesthesias (20%).
- Acute transverse myelitis may be a presenting sign but only 20% cases go on to get MS.
- Cerebellar symptoms occur in 50% cases.
- Cranial nerve problems occur in 42% (diplopia, nystagmus, internuclear ophthalmoplegia).
- Acute retrobulbar neuritis may be a presenting sign but only 20–40% cases subsequently develop MS. It occurs in 25–40% patients with MS.
- Bladder problems occur in 5% as initial symptom but 90% will ultimately get bladder involvement.
- Depression is common, true euphoria quite rare.
- Dementia is rare (5%) as are seizures (1–2%) which usually occur in childhood onset disease.
- Single system symptoms clear most completely.
- Brain stem, optic nerve lesions and sensory symptoms have a good prognosis for recovery.
- Sensory signs, spasticity and weakness have a fairly good prognosis.
- Bowel, bladder and cerebellar dysfunction generally persist.
- 90% will show a relapsing course from onset; 10% will progress without remission from onset.

- After five years' illness 50% will have begun a progressive decline.
- After 10 years, 40% will be leading normal lives, 50% will be quite disabled.
- After 20 years only 35% still leading normal lives.
- Overall 25-year survival is 50%.
- Very severe life-threatening attacks (brain stem, hemispheric lesions) do *not* necessarily carry a poor prognosis.
- Only 5% patients die within five years of onset, no predictive features – initial symptoms are often mild.
- High temperature may exacerbate or cause new symptoms – patients should avoid very hot baths or holidays in hot climates.
- Pregnancy carries 5% relapse risk in puerperium.
- Trauma, including surgical procedures, occasionally provokes relapse – insufficient risk to preclude necessary surgery.

TREATMENT[2]

1. ACTH in acute attacks may improve recovery, but over 60% acute attacks improve spontaneously. Trials show no benefit from long-term use.
2. There is no evidence that oral steroids (prednisolone or dexamethasone) influence acute attacks and some evidence that in long-term use the prognosis is worsened (although this may reflect the cases selected for treatment).

Contd.

3. Acute severe, life-threatening attacks or episodes with poor anticipated recovery (cerebellar, bladder, bowel or motor symptoms) should be treated with ACTH. The author's regime is a 10-day course of ACTH of 80, 60, 40, 20, 10 units each for two days. A positive response is indicated by clear improvement on day 5 or 6 of the course.

4. For attacks with high recovery rates (retrobulbar neuritis, brain stem attacks or sensory symptoms) ACTH should be withheld unless very severe or no recovery within four weeks of onset.

5. Long-term immunosuppression (cyclophosphamide, antilymphocytic serum, whole body radiation and cyclosporin A) has been used or is under evaluation. The benefits of such treatment should be measured against the hazards of the therapy.

6. Azathioprine has few side-effects and is ideal for long-term therapy. Dosage is 2 mg/kg daily, average 150–200 mg daily. Latest trials show benefit in intermittent progressive disease but no effect on single attack or chronic deteriorating type of disease. Haematological monitoring monthly is essential.

7. Plasmapheresis, interferon and epsilon aminocaproic acid have been tried with no proven benefit.

8. Dietary measures: in spite of 30 years' enthusiasm and many trials there is no convincing evidence of any benefit from dietary modification or supplementation on the course of MS.

9. Hyperbaric oxygen is currently under investigation, although the theoretical basis for its use is far from clear. It is hazardous in unskilled hands. No convincing evidence of benefit has been shown from published studies.

10. Treatment of specific problems

a) Spasticity. Diazepam 2–10 mg tds is the best antispastic agent, although it may produce 'jelly' legs if too effective. Baclofen 5–20 mg tds is also effective. Dantrolene sodium not very effective in MS.

b) Retention of urine. Bethanechol chloride (Myotonine) 10–30 mg tds; Propantheline 15–30 mg tds; Phenoxybenzamine hydrochloride (Dibenyline) 10 mg bd can all be useful.

c) Urinary incontinence. Emepronium bromide (Cetiprin) 100–200 mg tds, Flavoxate hydrochloride (Urispas) 200 mg tds can be used with urological advice following cystometrography. If drugs fail, intermittent self-catheterisation, chronic catheterisation or urinary diversion procedures may need to be considered.

d) Trigeminal neuralgia, spinothalamic pain and painful paraesthesiae may respond to phenytoin 100 mg tds or carbamezipine 100–200 mg tds.

e) Cerebellar symptoms are unresponsive to medication but may improve with stereotactic surgery.

f) Impotence can be helped only by mechanical aids or implanted prosthesis.

g) Constipation. Bisacodyl 5–10 mg nocte Bisacodyl suppositories 10 mg on wakening.

FOLLOW-UP

In the early stages regular follow-up alarms rather than reassures patients and in general discharge until next attack is in order. In established disease six monthly review can be helpful for the patient's morale, but the author prefers to see patients when specific problems occur. Severely disabled patients and their relatives benefit from short holiday admissions once or twice a year when the disease progress and new problems can be identified and perhaps helped.

[1] Reder T (1983) *Med. Clin. North Am.*, **1**, 573.
[2] Mathews WB (1984) *Rec. Adv. Clin. Neurol.*, **4**, 17

Migraine

Migraine is a syndrome of severe recurrent headaches which may be unilateral, frontal or orbital, generalised or localised (neuralgic migraine), particularly in the eye, nose or ear. All types may be associated with a variety of neurological phenomena thought to be related to cerebral vasospasm. A wide range of emotional and physical concomitants of uncertain aetiology also occurs and migraine should be regarded as an important differential diagnostic consideration in a variety of neurological conditions, such as transient ischaemic attacks, epilepsy, meningitis, acute confusional states, vertigo, unexplained vomiting, and any severe headache, since migraine in its worst form is regarded as the most severe headache that can be experienced. It affects females to males in the ratio 60:40, and is period-related in 60% and relieved by pregnancy in 64% females. The peak range of onset is 15–45 years. The first attack occurs by 10 years of age in 25% patients, but they may occur at any age[1]. There is a positive family history in 46%.

PROGNOSIS

- Visual phenomena occur in 30% cases.
- Pain may be unilateral (60%), bilateral (40%) or *always* on the same side (20%).
- 90% patients feel nauseated (10% actually vomit).
- Photophobia occurs in 80% patients, diarrhoea in 20% and brainstem symptoms in 25%.
- Average frequency is 1–4 attacks per month.
- 75% attacks last less than 24 hours.

TREATMENT

1. Prophylactic therapy (all drugs probably act by anti-5HT effect)[2]

   a) Propranolol 10–20 mg tds (avoid in asthmatics)[3, 4].

   b) Pizotifen 1.5 mg nocte (may cause drowsiness, marked appetite increase especially in females).

   c) Cyproheptadine 2–4 mg nocte (may cause appetite increase, drowsiness)[5].

   d) Methysergide maleate 1–2 mg tds (patient may feel unwell, suffer thigh pain, and there is a risk of retroperitoneal fibrosis in prolonged high dose – but still the most effective agent and well worth a trial in intractable cases).

   e) Clonidine 50–75 μg bd (can cause depression, and variably effective).

2. Alteration of life style (easy to advise, usually impossible to achieve!).

3. Anti-anxiety and anti-depressant therapy where indicated.

4. Ergotamine in acute attack has limited success, often causes vomiting and diarrhoea, and high doses can cause rebound headache. In patients with isolated headache with identifiable prodrome, 2 mg repeated once only at 60 minutes can be tried on a few occasions and recommended if effective.

5. Although many formulations of aspirin/anti-nausea agents are available, severe migraine sufferers do not respond to simple analgesics, however administered, and the writer finds them of limited value.

FOLLOW-UP

Continue effective regime until pain-free for three weeks. Resume therapy if headaches recur. Reconsider diagnosis wherever atypical features occur.

[1] Heyck H (1969) *Headache*, **2**, 1.
[2] Fozard J (1975) *J. Pharm. Pharmacol.*, **27**, 297.
[3] Diamond S et al. (1976) *Headache*, **16**, 24.
[4] Weber RB et al. (1971) *Neurology*, **21**, 404.
[5] Lance J et al. (1970) *Br. Med. J.*, **ii**, 327.

Cluster Headache

Cluster headache affects males almost exclusively, females tend to have localised neuralgias (lower teeth and face – Sluder's headache). Most patients are aged 35–45 years (range 17–70 years). The headaches are mainly nocturnal (alarm clock headache) at the same time each night, and are unilateral and *always* on the same side. The pain is located to the eye and nostril with lacrimation, nasal discharge and conjunctival infection[1].

PROGNOSIS

- Attacks have sudden onset and offset, lasting 10–90 minutes, and are excruciatingly severe, occurring 2–3 times each night and occasionally in the day.
- There is a tendency for symptoms to occur annually at distinct seasons, e.g. autumn/spring.
- Individual attacks last 5–16 weeks (can be continual).
- Yearly recurrences throughout middle age should be anticipated.

TREATMENT

1. Methysergide maleate 1–3 mg tds is the traditional therapy supplemented by ergotamine suppositories 2 mg nocte for seven days.

2. Lithium carbonate 250–400 mg tds can be dramatically curative often within hours of first dose and is the author's recommended regime supplemented if necesssary with methysergide 1–2 mg nocte[2].

3. Treatment should continue for three weeks after pain subsides.

FOLLOW-UP

Discharge when attack subsides. Give starter supply of medication for use in next attack. See after seven days on treatment in next attack to confirm success and lack of side-effects.

---

[1] Graham JR (1972) *Headache*, **11**, 175.
[2] Kudrow L (1977) *Headache*, **17**, 15.

Trigeminal Neuralgia

Trigeminal neuralgia is a condition dominated by severe needle-like episodes of burning facial pain lasting 15–30 seconds usually in the region between the 1st–2nd or 2nd–3rd divisions of the 5th cranial nerve. It is one of the most painful conditions known, and is of uncertain aetiology. It occurs in the elderly and therefore affects females more than males (3:2). Age of onset is usually 50–60 years old, although it can occur as young as the teens, in which case multiple sclerosis must be considered. It is more common on the right side (6:4), is rarely bilateral (1–2%), and is very rare at night. 60% occur in the lower jaw to ear distribution (triggered by eating, yawning, biting); 30% occur in the upper lip, nose and orbit (triggered by light touch, hot or cold fluids, draughts).

PROGNOSIS

- Initially attacks last from days to weeks, then remit – sometimes for years.
- Attacks almost always recur and may then last longer and be less likely to remit.

TREATMENT[1, 2]

1. Carbamazepine is the drug of choice 100–200 mg 3–6 hourly, best taken one hour before meals as eating is often provocative. 600–1200 mg is the maximum daily dose depending on age and effectiveness.
2. Phenytoin 100 mg tds was the previous best agent and remains effective with less risk of giddiness in the elderly. If supplemented with carbamazepine 100 mg taken one hour before meals 3–4 times per day this is often a good combination with minimal side-effects.
3. An effective long-term alternative is to use phenytoin 100 mg tds continually, with carbamazepine added in exacerbations.
4. Non-narcotic and narcotic pain killers are completely ineffectual and should never be used.
5. Alcohol nerve block, radiofrequency nerve lesions and partial root section via a craniotomy have to be considered in intractable cases. Patients need to be warned that surgical division will cause numbness of the face, and that analgesia of the cornea may require the cornea to be protected with goggles.

FOLLOW-UP

Follow closely while initiating treatment for effectiveness and side-effects. Weekly follow-up may be necessary. Discharge when attack over with starter supply of medication for next episode. When regular attacks established implement 3 under *Treatment* above and follow-up three monthly.

[1] Loesser JD (1978) *J. Am. Med. Assoc.*, **239**, 1153.
[2] Dalessio J (1977) *Clinical Neurosurgery* vol. 24, p. 579. Baltimore: Williams and Wilkins.

Post Herpetic Neuralgia in the Trigeminal Distribution

Post herpetic neuralgia in the trigeminal distribution is a severe burning pain often triggered by light touch, occurring in the area previously affected by shingles. It occurs in 30% patients with an herpetic eruption in the ophthalmic division. Severe pain initially, that fails to ease as the rash erupts, provides a strong clue to the likely development of this syndrome.

PROGNOSIS

- Over the first two years some spontaneous improvement may occur but if not the neuralgia may persist indefinitely.

TREATMENT

1. Phenytoin 100 mg tds plus imipramine 10–25 mg tds is some help especially where triggering by touch is a major feature.

2. All pain killers are totally ineffectual.
3. Acupuncture, transcutaneous nerve stimulation and nerve blocks have no proven value.

FOLLOW-UP

If treatment fails there is nothing that can be done. Patients often request review every few months in the hope that new treatment will be available.

Atypical Facial Pain

Atypical facial pain is a classic facial pain syndrome usually seen in young middle-aged females. Once established and untreated the pain may persist indefinitely and symptoms of 20 years standing or more are not uncommon. Onset is often after some major life crisis although dental care has been given in the previous month in 30% cases. Initial pain is in upper teeth often leading to multiple tooth extractions without benefit. Later pain spreads to a cheek when sinus disease could be suspected. It may extend to the opposite cheek and has been described as terrible, awful, *continual*, 24 hours per day. Often there is an increasing belief by patient that widespread malevolent disease is responsible, even when symptoms have been present for 30 years[1].

PROGNOSIS

- Untreated the pain will not recover.

TREATMENT

1. Controlled trials and experience show that treatment with antidepressants/tranquillisers in combination is effective[2].
2. The author's treatment is chlordiazepoxide 5 mg tds combined with amitriptyline 10–25 mg tds.

FOLLOW-UP

Treatment is usually effective over 6–10 week Review at six weeks and again two weeks aft cessation of treatment. Resume if necessary.

[1] Lesse S (1956) *J. Nerv. Ment. Dis.*, **124**, 346.
[2] Lascelles RG (1966) *Br. J. Psychiat.*, **112**, 651.

Benign Hemifacial Spasm

Benign hemifacial spasm is non-stop twitching of facial muscles, usually starting round the eye, eventually spreading to the entire half face. It usually affects elderly females – probably due to arteriosclerotic vessels irritating the VII cranial nerve. Cholesteatoma is the commonest surgical cause.

PROGNOSIS

- Untreated the condition continues and may worsen. The area involved may increase.

TREATMENT

1. It usually responds well to carbamazepine 100–200 mg tds.

2. Surgical exploration and decompression worth considering in younger patients.

FOLLOW-UP

Frequency of follow-up consultations will depend on patient's symptoms and response to medication.

Spasmodic Torticollis

Spasmodic torticollis is the most frequent naturally occurring form of dyskinesia. There is jerking spasm in one sternomastoid and the opposite trapezius which results in a rotated attitude of the head.

PROGNOSIS

- The likely prognosis is persistence for the rest of life.

TREATMENT[1]

. Extreme effort or gently placing a finger on the chin may control movements briefly.

. Diazepam up to 30 mg tds may help some, and may reduce pain from the muscle spasms.

3. Benzhexol (Artane) in high dose (up to 60 mg daily) occasionally helps.
4. Tetrabenazine (Nitoman) or chlorpromazine (Largactil) may have some success in doses of 12.5–25 mg tds for each.
5. Haloperidol 4 mg daily has been successful but there is a high risk of later side-effects[2].

---

[1] Shaw KM *et al.* (1972) *Lancet,* **i,** 1339.
[2] Gilbert G J (1972) *Arch. Neurol.,* **27,** 503.

Motor Neurone Disease

Motor neurone disease is a fatal disease of unknown aetiology due to progressive death of ventral horn cells, motor cranial nerve cells and the cortico-spinal and cortico-bulbar fibres. This produces a wide array of upper (UMN) and lower (LMN) motor neurone lesions in various combinations. The prevalence is 1.4 per 100 000. It is familial in 5% cases. The mean age of onset is 52 years, mean age of death 62 years. In the sporadic form the male to female ratio is 2:1, in the familial form 1:1. All races are affected – there is a particularly high incidence in Guam and Japan. There are a number of different clinical types. The lesions are mixed in amyotrophic lateral sclerosis (ALS) (52% cases) (UMN in legs, LMN in arms). They are mainly LMN in progressive muscle atrophy (PMA) (28% cases). Arms are affected in 40% cases, legs in 25%, cranial nerves in 25%, and mixed in 10%. The progressive bulbar palsy type accounts for 20% cases and has either UMN or LMN lesions.

PROGNOSIS

- 20% patients survive five years. The PMA type starting in the legs has the best prognosis.
- 80% patients succumb within three years. The bulbar palsy type is worst.
- 10% patients develop dementia – some also autonomic neuropathy with parkinsonian features (Shy Drager syndrome). Some show early dementia and rapid course (Creutzfeld–Jakob syndrome).

TREATMENT

1. No known treatment affects the course of the disease.
2. Small transient improvement in muscle strength can be achieved in PMA type with neostigmine (Prostigmin) 15–30 mg before meals.
3. With severe spasticity some minimal benefit may be derived from diazepam 2–10 mg tds, or baclofen 5–20 mg tds.
4. Muscle cramps may respond to procainamide 250–500 mg tds.
5. Mechanical and electronic aids can be useful.
6. Some patients benefit from crico-pharyngeal myotomy in their final weeks when severe swallowing difficulty exists, but only if the tongue is still mobile and can protrude between the teeth.
7. Fine bore nasal tube feeding in patients with pure bulbar problems can be useful.
8. Assisted respiration is almost never indicated.

FOLLOW-UP

Follow-up can only document the progression of the disease but some help at all stages of the disorder is possible and makes follow-up until death a worthwhile exercise.

Myasthenia Gravis

Myasthenia gravis is a disorder of impaired neuro-muscular transmission due to end plate antibodies preventing access to acetylcholine receptors. The prevalence is 1 per 10 000. There are two distinct groups – females 20–30 years of age, males 50–70 years of age. In the females proximal muscle fatigue develops first followed by ocular symptoms. In the males there is early bulbar/ocular involvement, and proximal muscle problems later. There is a strong association with other auto-immune disorders – 10% have thyrotoxicosis, others have myxoedema, pernicious anaemia, polymyositis, myositis, rheumatoid arthritis, systemic lupus erythematosus, or diabetes mellitus. There is a transient neonatal form in children born to myasthenic mothers. If positive, a response to 10 mg i.v. edrophonium (Tensilon) is diagnostic. The correct performance of the Tensilon test is imperative: inject 2 mg i.v. and wait 30 seconds. If there are no untoward effects inject a further 3 mg and wait one minute. A response is usually apparent. Only give the other 5 mg as a bolus injection if no response or side-effects are noted. Obviously weak muscle groups should be observed for improvement (i.e. ptosis, diplopia, speech, swallowing and arm strength)[1].

PROGNOSIS[2]

- Before treatment was available 30% died within three years, after 10 years; 13% were in incomplete remission, 57% had persistent disease.
- A stormy course in the first three years suggests a poor prognosis.
- Eventual prognosis with modern management is still uncertain.

TREATMENT

1. Anticholinergics – used since 1935 – achieve partial control of symptoms but have no effect on prognosis. Dosages include neostigmine (Prostigmin) 15–30 mg four hourly, and pyridostigmine (Mestinon) 60–120 mg six hourly to control symptoms.
2. Thymectomy is indicated in females under 50 years old. Unless a thymoma is found 25–50% remit but response may take years and relapse later. A thymic tumour should be removed but this often has no effect on the myasthenia[3].
3. Corticosteroids are now standard treatment, initially prednisolone 5–20 mg tds to establish control. They are especially effective in the elderly male group (90% will show good response).
4. Immunosuppression – azathioprine 25–50 mg tds with steroids – is now the treatment of choice, with thymectomy if indicated. The response may not be apparent for some months[4].
5. Ptosis. Ephedrine hydrochloride 25–50 mg tds may help.
6. Oral atropine has been used to control gastrointestinal symptoms produced by the anticholinergics. It can be hazardous because of the block of warning symptoms of a cholinergic crisis due to overdosage which can be as hazardous as the disease itself.
7. The long-term use of modest doses of anticholinergics is usually necessary in patients on combination therapy with steroids and azathioprine.

FOLLOW-UP

Myasthenia is a difficult disease to manage and expert follow-up is essential, including haematological monitoring and prevention of steroid side-effects. In general, three monthly follow-up with immediate clinic access in emergencies is advisable.

[1] Compston DAS et al. (1980) Brain, 103, 579.
[2] Engel AG et al. (1973) Neurology (NY), 23, 1273.
[3] Bartococcini E et al. (1980) J. Neurol., 249, 9.
[4] Mertens HG et al. (1981) Am. Acad. Sci., 377, 691.

Muscle Disorders

Diseases of muscle include those due to metabolic or toxic damage, those due to inherited disorders – the muscular dystrophies, and inflammatory disease. Only those disorders that can be treated are discussed in this section. In many instances correct identification and treatment of the underlying disease resolves the muscle problem.

Familial hypokalaemic periodic paralysis

Inheritance is autosomal dominant. The male to female ratio is 4:1. The usual age at onset is 10–20 years. Paralysis occurs on waking in the morning after provocation, e.g. a heavy carbohydrate meal or exertion.

PROGNOSIS

- Attacks generally last 12–24 hours but occasionally several days.
- Attacks tend to decrease with age.
- Some patients develop permanent limb girdle weakness.

TREATMENT

1. For an acute attack, 5 g KCl should be given orally two hourly up to 15 g total dose.
2. Prophylaxis

   a) Avoid provocative factors, e.g. violent exercise or heavy carbohydrate meals.
   b) Acetazolamide (Diamox) 125–150 mg daily; spironolactone 100–200 mg daily; KCl 5 g orally on retiring to bed.

Familial hyperkalaemic paralysis

Inheritance is autosomal dominant. The male to female ratio is 1:1. Attacks often begin in early childhood and are not as severe as hypokalaemic attacks. Fasting is an important provocative factor and exercise at onset of attack may delay paralysis.

PROGNOSIS

- Attacks last 10–60 minutes.
- Attacks may occur in the day or on retiring.
- Proximal myopathy may develop as a long-term complication.

TREATMENT

1. Oral glucose may abort a mild attack at the onset.
2. 100 g glucose orally and insulin 20 units subcutaneously are necessary for a severe attack. Calcium gluconate 0.5–2 g i.v. is also effective.
3. As prophylaxis acetazolamide (Diamox) 125–250 mg daily can be helpful and hypoglycaemia should be avoided by frequent small meals.

Dystrophia myotonica

Inheritance is autosomal dominant, and a variable expression is common. The prevalence is 3–5 per 100 000 with a male to female ratio of 1:1. The usual age of onset is 10–20 years.

PROGNOSIS

- Myotonia in forearm flexors is a common early feature.
- Wasting and weakness occur in extensors arms and legs.
- 66% patients have disordered cardiac conduction.
- 90% have anterior and posterior subcapsular cataracts.
- Infertility and menstrual irregularities are common.
- The rate of progress of the disease varies. Patients with diffuse disease generally become chairbound after 20–30 years.

TREATMENT

1. Avoidance of cold may reduce myotonia.
2. Gentle exercise improves the condition.
3. Procainamide 250–1000 mg daily, quinidine sulphate 300 mg four hourly prn, phenytoin 100 mg qds may reduce myotonia but may also depress cardiac conduction and are not well tolerated. Phenytoin is probably safest for long-term use.

FOLLOW-UP

Yearly review is helpful to monitor the progress of the disease and advise the patient about prognosis.

Polymyositis (if associated with a skin rash – dermatomyositis)

Polymyositis may occur at any age and is an inflammatory muscle disorder characterised by progressive proximal muscle weakness.

PROGNOSIS

- The prognosis in pure polymyositis ranges from acute cases dying after a few months' illness to chronic, relapsing cases living for many years.
- Dysphagia is an early and serious problem in 30% cases.
- Cranial nerve territory involvement is rare.
- Skin rash occurs over cheeks, nose and nail beds.
- Children always have skin rash and never have malignancy.
- Malignant disease occurs in 8% overall – 20% in patients over 50 years. The risk rises to 60% in men over 40 years age with dermatomyositis.

TREATMENT

1. Spontaneous improvement has been documented.
2. Steroid treatment is effective in 70% cases. Prednisolone 5–20 mg tds is the usual dose required.
3. Azathioprine 25–50 mg tds may be necessary with incomplete response to steroids or as a steroid-sparing alternative if more than 10 mg tds prednisolone is necessary for disease control. Treatment can be tapered after three years but many patients relapse and need continuing treatment.

FOLLOW-UP

Routine follow-up for steroid/immunosuppression management. Six monthly review to search for underlying malignancy.

Peripheral Nerve Disorders

Peripheral nerve disorders may consist of damage to single nerve trunks (entrapment neuropathies) or diffuse nerve damage caused by a wide variety of toxic, metabolic, infective or deficiency disorders on an acquired or inborn basis. Only disorders amenable to treatment will be discussed.

Carpal tunnel syndrome (CTS)

Carpal tunnel syndrome is an entrapment of the median nerve in the carpal tunnel at the wrist. The female to male ratio is 3:1. Characteristically nocturnal pain occurs in the median innervated fingers although it may occur during the day when the hands are elevated, i.e. when typing, knitting, etc. It is rapidly eased by clenching and relaxing the hand. Acromegaly, myxoedema, amyloidosis, rheumatoid arthritis, polyarteritis nodosa, diabetes mellitus, myelomatosis and pregnancy predispose.

PROGNOSIS

- In pregnancy CTS responds to diuretics, and clears on delivery.
- In other instances symptoms will continue unless treated.

TREATMENT

1. Night splinting with cock-up splint is effective and diagnostic.
2. Diuretics relieve symptoms in pregnancy and menstrual related cases.
3. Local steroid injections are temporarily effective.
4. Surgical decompression offers the best chance of permanent relief.

Ulnar nerve compression

The ulnar nerve may be damaged at any point on its course but particularly at the elbow by anatomical abnormality, and at elbow and wrist by external trauma. It is most frequent in males due to the greater risk of repeated trauma, e.g. occupational trauma, resting on elbows, hitting heel of hand. Symptoms include pain and paraesthesiae in ring and little finger, insidious development of weakness of intrinsic muscles of hand. Lesion at wrist will usually only affect motor function. Acute onset can occur while bedbound, after overdose, during anaesthesia. All medical conditions above, except pregnancy, may predispose.

PROGNOSIS

- Acute lesions due to trauma may recover fully provided the nerve fibres have not been severed.
- Chronic lesions, whatever the cause, are unlikely to recover spontaneously.

TREATMENT

1. Surgical transposition to the front of the humerus if the nerve is damaged at the elbow
2. Surgical decompression if the deep branch is damaged at wrist.

Radial nerve palsy

Radial nerve palsy is caused by trauma in axilla by crutch or chair (Saturday night palsy), damage in the mid-arm by midshaft humeral fractures, or damage within the supinator muscle by twisting forearm strain. It causes weakness of finger and wrist extension and minimal numbness over the dorsum of the thumb and index finger.

PROGNOSIS

- All palsies recover well over 3–6 months even if trapped in mid-humeral fracture callus, unless the nerve is transected.

TREATMENT

1. Damage within the supinator may require surgical decompression.

2. The need for surgery is relatively rare.
3. Contracture must be prevented while recovery takes place.

Peroneal nerve palsy

Peroneal nerve palsy is usually due to external pressure at the neck of the fibula. Marked weight loss, bed rest or anaesthesia all predispose. It causes foot drop and weakness of toe extension, and minimal sensory loss over the dorsal aspect of the foot.

PROGNOSIS

- Recovery is usually spontaneous if the aetiology is identifiable.

TREATMENT

1. A splint should be worn until recovery is assured.
2. If the palsy is not recovering within three months exploration is advisable.

Diabetic neuropathy

Overt neuropathy occurs in 5–10% diabetics. Nerve conduction studies reveal mild disease in 40–60%. 50% maturity onset diabetics present with neuropathy. Painful peripheral paraesthesiae are the main symptom. Mononeuritis multiplex may occur (nerve trunk infarcts), and diabetic amyotrophy due to upper lumbar root infarction (usually in recent onset disease with rapid weight loss).

PROGNOSIS

Generalised neuropathy progresses insidiously.
Mononeuritis multiplex and amyotrophy recover over months.

TREATMENT

Tight diabetic control may have slight beneficial effect.
Local pressure avoidance is important.

3. Trials of myo-inositinol, sorbitol and aldose reductase inhibitors are still in progress.

Alcoholic neuropathy

Alcoholic neuropathy is usually due to heavy alcohol intake combined with poor nutrition. Presentation is often with muscle tenderness or painful paraesthesiae in the feet. It can produce ascending motor weakness if untreated.

PROGNOSIS

- The prognosis is poor unless total abstinence is practised.
- The recovery period following severe motor involvement may take years.

TREATMENT

1. Abstention from alcohol is essential.
2. A balanced diet should be achieved as soon as possible.
3. Vitamin B_1 replacement therapy (vitamin B compound strong, six tabs. daily) and other vitamins (e.g. vitamin B_{12}) as indicated by the patient's general state.

Guillain–Barre syndrome

The Guillain-Barre syndrome is an acute or chronic, progressive or relapsing neuropathy which accounts for 30–40% of all acute neuropathy in adults. The incidence is 1 per 100 000 per year. Presentation is usually with ascending motor paralysis which may become total. Painful paraesthesiae are common, but sensory loss is minimal. 60% cases have prior respiratory or intestinal virus disease[1, 2].

PROGNOSIS[3]

- 50% develop respiratory insufficiency.
- 50% progress for two weeks with peak disability at four weeks in 90%.
- The recovery rate is variable, often a similar time scale to onset.
- The plateau phase is unpredictable and may last days to weeks.

Contd.

- 15% remain permanently disabled by their attack.

TREATMENT

1. Careful respiratory monitoring is essential.
2. Respiration should be assisted as soon as indicated.
3. General nursing, as necessary, for unconscious or paralysed patients. Bulbar paralysis may necessitate a stomach tube to ensure adequate fluid and calorie intake.
4. Plasmapheresis is claimed to help but variable prognosis makes isolated case reports difficult to assess. No full-scale trial has yet been reported[4].
5. There is conflicting evidence about the use of ACTH, including some authors' suggestions that it is harmful. The author uses a 10-day course of ACTH in all patients seen in the acutely progressive phase (exactly as for *Multiple sclerosis*, see p. 107).
6. In cases becoming chronic, immunosuppression may be of benefit although no full-scale trials have been reported so far. Azathioprine 25–50 mg tds[5].

Polyneuritis due to malignancy

This is a rare condition given the prevalence of malignant disease. It usually presents as a predominantly sensory neuropathy. It may precede discovery of malignancy by months or years and may complicate any form of malignancy but bronchial and ovarian carcinomas predominate.

PROGNOSIS

- Variable, not necessarily remitting if the malignancy is treated. By contrast it may remit in the presence of persisting malignancy.

TREATMENT

Cytotoxic therapy, where appropriate, may be indicated but further nerve damage due to medication is then a problem.

Facial nerve palsy (Bell's palsy)

Bell's palsy is one of the commonest neurological conditions. It may occur at any age, but most frequently from 20–40 years old. It is often painful around the ear at onset, and complete paralysis of the facial nerve occurs by 48 hours in 75% cases. Altered taste and hearing sensation occurs only in severe cases. Nearly all patients complain of sensory symptoms (i.e. numbness of the face) but objective signs are usually absent.

PROGNOSIS

- 80% recover fully over 3–6 weeks. Incomplete palsies are more likely to recover fully.
- 15% make a delayed recovery over 3–6 months, often complicated by the development of synkinetic movements.
- 5% fail to make significant recovery.
- The palsy can be recurrent in some patients.

TREATMENT

1. Protection of the exposed cornea is essential
2. Prednisolone 50 mg daily for five days or ACTH over a similar period have been recommended but there is increasing doubt as to the value.
3. Surgical decompression in acute stage is not justified – the claimed success rate being the same as the natural history.
4. Exclusion of underlying hypertension, diabetes and sarcoidosis is worthwhile.
5. Cosmetic surgery may sometimes be required.

---

[1] Eiben RM et al. (1963) Med. Clin. North Am., 47, 1371.
[2] Eisen A et al. (1974) Arch. Neurol., 30, 438.
[3] Löffel NB et al. (1977) J. Neurol. Sci., 33, 71.
[4] Gross MLP et al. (1982) J. Neurol. Neurosurg. Psych., 45, 675.
[5] Hughes RAC et al. (1981) Ann. Neurol., 9, 125.

7

Diseases of the Skin

S. K. Goolamali

Acne Vulgaris

Acne is a disease of the sebaceous glands which is exacerbated or precipitated by puberty. Increased sebum production is an invariable feature but other factors which also play a part in the pathogenesis of acne include bacteria in the pilosebaceous duct, sebaceous lipid composition and obstruction of the sebaceous duct. The comedone is the hallmark of acne and forms in response to sebum components. Many acne lesions occur without comedones and some patients with severe acne have few or no comedones. Acne lesions include papules, pustules, nodules and cysts. Although the frequency of acne is greatest at adolescence one study[1] showed that 42% 8–10 year-old-girls and 36% boys of a similar age had comedonal acne.

PROGNOSIS

- There is general agreement that acne is more common and severe in late teenage boys than in girls. Approximately 3–4% boys and 0.5% girls have very severe acne[2].
- The age at which acne begins does not influence the risk of subsequent scarring.
- For both sexes the greater the duration of acne the greater the risk of scar formation.

TREATMENT

1. Topical

   a) Obsessional or very frequent washing of the face or other acne-bearing sites is not recommended though cleansing of the skin to keep within the bounds of social acceptability is helpful.
   b) Topical preparations usually contain antibacterial or exfoliating agents. There is little evidence that antiseptics, sulphur, salicylic acid or corticosteroids help acne. Topical antibiotics, e.g. neomycin and chloramphenicol, have been used with benefit but are recognised sensitisers and are best avoided.
   c) Benzoyl peroxide is useful because it produces exfoliation and is also bacteriostatic. 5% gel or lotion is tried initially though the strength may be varied between 2.5% and 10% according to the clinical response.
   d) Tretinoin modifies the abnormal keratinisation in the pilosebaceous duct. Formulated in alcoholic solution (Retin-A) it is particularly useful in the treatment of open ('blackhead') and closed ('whitehead') comedones. In papular acne the benefits are not so marked and in pustular or cystic acne it is of minimal help.

2. Systemic therapy (indicated in moderate and severe forms of acne)

   a) Tetracycline is the drug of first choice. Its absorption is affected by food, it is best taken between meals. Antacids containing aluminium and magnesium, iron supplements and milk interfere with its absorption. The dose is normally 250 mg twice daily given for a minimum of three months. Improvement is usually seen after two months but patients need to be warned that the drug may be required for very much longer.
   b) The more lipid soluble tetracyclines, minocycline and doxycycline are less affected by food or milk and may be successful where tetracycline has failed.
   c) Trimethoprim[3] and co-trimoxazole[4] are other anti-acne drugs and indicated when acne is non-responsive to the tetracyclines. The dose for acne is half the normal antibiotic dose and it is given for a minimum of three months.
   d) Erythromycin is also an effective anti-acne drug but as it is also widely used for systemic infections it is prudent to choose tetracycline.
   e) Anti-androgens, e.g. cyproterone acetate inhibit the binding and retention of testosterone and dihydrotestosterone (DHT within the target cell and also suppress gonadotrophin secretion[5]. As endogenous androgen is the main stimulus to sebum output in acne the use of anti-androgen

appears logical in acne. However it is contraindicated in both males and females, and the effects of long-term use are not known. One product containing 2 mg cyproterone acetate and 50 μg ethinyloestradiol (Diane) has been marketed both as a contra-acne and a contraceptive drug.

f) Isotretinoin is a vitamin A analogue which markedly reduces sebum production. It is indicated for the treatment of severe, antibiotic-resistant nodulo-cystic acne. Careful patient selection is essential and female patients who receive the drug are advised that strict contraception is essential during therapy and for two months after cessation of therapy. The oral contraceptive pill does not interact with isotretinoin. Dosage varies between 0.1-1.0 mg/kg/day. The recommended treatment time is 16 weeks. Facial lesions improve in 80–90% patients whilst truncal lesions in approximately 60%. Side-effects include dry lips, angular cheilitis and facial dermatitis. Teratogenicity, elevation of serum triglycerides, liver function abnormalities, pancreatitis and pseudotumour cerebri are other well-recognised unwanted side-effects. Isotretinoin 0.5 mg/kg/day has proved more effective than Diane for antibiotic-resistant acne in women.

g) Miscellaneous
   i) Dietary restriction is unnecessary.
   ii) Ultraviolet therapy helps only temporarily.
   iii) Intralesional steroids are helpful with acne cysts and keloids.
   iv) Zyderm is a bovine collagen useful for depressed acne scars but very expensive.
   v) Dermabrasion is helpful in selected patients with predominantly superficial acne scars but is not indicated in pigmented skin as often postoperatively it may heal with variegated pigmentation.

FOLLOW-UP

Patients with acne should be reviewed in the first instance after two months of treatment and then after a further two months. The decision to reduce dosage or alter therapy should be made at the second return visit when improvement or otherwise is usually apparent.

[1] Burton JL et al. (1971) Br. J. Derm., 85, 119.
[2] Kligman AM (1974) J. Investigative Derm., 62, 268.
[3] Gibson JR et al. (1982) Br. J. Derm., 107, 221.
[4] Nordin K et al. (1978) Dermatologica, 157, 245.
[5] Neumann G (1977) Horm. Metab. Res., 9, 1.

Atopic Dermatitis

Atopic dermatitis or eczema is a chronic relapsing skin disease which commonly begins in childhood. There is often a personal or family history of allergic rhinitis or asthma. One study[1] showed that 60% patients developed atopic dermatitis in the first year of life and 85% under the age of five years. The prevalence of the disease has been variously estimated as 3% among children under the age of five years[2] and 7–24 cases per 1000 of the population[3].

PROGNOSIS

- Follow-up studies suggest that approximately 40% patients show clearing of the disease.
- Patients with severe disease are twice as likely to have persistent disease[4].
- Atopic dermatitis-like disease may occur in unrelated conditions such as phenylketonuria and the Wiskott–Aldrich syndrome. In these cases the prognosis of the skin disease relies on the progress of the underlying systemic disorder.
- Patients with atopic dermatitis show an increased susceptibility to virus infections particularly herpes simplex, warts and molluscum contagiosum.
- 30-50% cases of eczema subsequently develop asthma or allergic rhinitis.
- Serum IgE, reaginic antibody, is inevitably increased in atopic eczema but there is little correlation between titres of IgE and severity of eczema.

TREATMENT

1. The natural history of the disease, as far as is known, should be carefully explained to the parents emphasising in particular that the condition waxes and wanes and although there is no cure very adequate control can be achieved in most patients with simple topical measures.
2. The basic principle of therapy is to suppress or prevent pruritus. Extremes of temperature should be avoided. Excess heat may provoke miliaria. Wool next to the skin commonly triggers off itching.
3. The child should be bathed regularly and the use of soap decreased. Many children will tolerate a superfatted soap provided it is not left on the skin for too long. After bathing an emollient such as aqueous cream, ung

emulsificans or related preparation should be applied liberally to the skin.

4. Some evidence suggests that atopic eczema may be lessened in infants with a family history of atopy by strict avoidance of allergens, especially cow's milk, up to the age of six months[5]. Two good studies however have shown no advantage of soya milk or breast feeding in the prevention of allergy[6,7]. One other study[8] claims that the control of atopic dermatitis may be enhanced by certain food avoidance but again in most patients exacerbations cannot be related to a specific 'food-allergen' cause.
5. Topical therapy

   a) Acute patches of eczema should be treated with a topical steroid cream to which an antibiotic is added if there is evidence of secondary infection. The use of a systemic antibiotic will depend on the severity and extent of infection.

   b) The strength of steroid initially for acute eczema may be of Group 3 or the strong variety (betamethasone, beclomethasone dipropionate, fluocinonide) applied only for a week or 10 days. As soon as is practicable the strength is reduced to the Group 2 (clobetasone butyrate, fluran drenolone) and Group 1 (hydrocortisone varieties.

   c) In infants the aim should always be to use as weak a steroid as possible for as short a time as the clinical situation allows.

   d) The face, intertriginous areas such as the axillae, submammary region and the perianal skin should be treated with a weak steroid and preferably hydrocortisone.

6. Chronic lichenified lesions especially on the lower limbs may be usefully treated with a

occlusive bandage impregnated with corticosteroid or tar.

7. Oral antihistamines reduce nocturnal itching by virtue of their central action and are best employed only for a few days when acute exacerbations occur.

8. Occasionally short-term systemic corticosteroid therapy (10–14 days) may be necessary in erythroderma induced by eczema. Long-term corticosteroid therapy has virtually no place in the management of atopic eczema.

9. Oral 8-methoxypsoralen with high intensity long wave ultraviolet light is sometimes indicated in adults with generalised eczema recalcitrant to routine measures. The success with this treatment modality is variable.

FOLLOW-UP

Children with severe atopic dermatitis need frequent review until the acute phase has subsided. In practice, review once a week for a fortnight and then once a fortnight for a month is often required. Once the condition is under reasonable control monthly review or assessment at longer intervals is arranged according to the needs of the child and the parents. In general children require more frequent review than adults.

[1] Rajka G (1975) *Atopic Dermatitis*. London: W.B. Saunders Company.
[2] Walker RB *et al.* (1956) *Br. J. Derm.*, **68**, 182.
[3] Johnson ML (1977) National Center for Health Statistics, United States, No 4, Jan 26.
[4] Roth HL *et al.* (1964) *Arch. Derm.*, **89**, 209.
[5] Matthew DJ *et al.* (1977) *Lancet*, **i**, 321.
[6] Kjellman NI *et al.* (1979) *Clin. Allergy*, **9**, 347.
[7] Halpern SR *et al.* (1973) *J. Allergy Clin. Immun.*, **51**, 139.
[8] Atherton DJ *et al.* (1978) *Lancet*, **i**, 401.

Psoriasis

Approximately 2% of the population is affected by psoriasis. Its cause is unknown but it is considered to have a polygenic mode of inheritance. Twin studies provide evidence that psoriasis is hereditary but the mode of inheritance remains speculative since it is difficult to distinguish between multifactorial inheritance and two alleles at a single locus with empiric data alone. There is a family history in 30% patients[1] and recently it has been found that the HLA-C antigen, Cw6, is the most frequent HLA antigen to be detected in psoriasis patients[2]. Individuals with HLA-B17 also have a five times greater chance of developing psoriasis. The disease is characterised by silvery scales overlying well-defined erythematous patches, commonly over the scalp, elbows, knees and sacrum. Psoriatic epidermis proliferates some seven times more rapidly than normal epithelium[3], and since this increased rate of epidermal cell replacement is considered by most to be fundamental in the pathogenesis of psoriasis most treatments are designed to reduce the rate of epidermal turnover.

PROGNOSIS

- The prognosis is unpredictable for the most part.
- Guttate psoriasis carries a better prognosis and has longer remissions after treatment[4].
- An early onset and family history appear to worsen the prognosis[5].
- Infections with beta-haemolytic streptococci cause relapse of the acute guttate type of psoriasis in children.
- Pregnancy appears to improve psoriasis more commonly than worsen it.
- Remissions of psoriasis lasting one year or more were reported in approximately 40% of 5355 patients[6].
- The incidence of polyarthritis in psoriasis was estimated in one series as occurring in 7% patients[7]. There is a significantly greater frequency of HLA-B27 in patients with psoriatic arthritis[8].

TREATMENT

1. Nearly all patients respond well to topical therapy. Dithranol or anthralin remains the most effective. Dithranol is usually applied daily as a paste combined with tar baths and ultraviolet B (UVB) (sunburn range 290–320 nm) (the 'Ingram' regime[9]). For hospital-treated patients the dithranol is combined with Lassar's paste as it confines the action of the dithranol to the involved skin. However, ointments or creams containing dithranol are less messy and equally effective and may be preferred for domiciliary use.

2. Coal tar may also be used either alone or in combination with tar baths and UVB (the 'Goekerman' regime[10]).

3. In selecting the starting concentration of dithranol or tar attention must be paid to the patient's skin colouring and the type of psoriasis to be treated. Small children and adults who burn easily on exposure to sunlight are susceptible to the irritant action of dithranol or tar and in these a low starting concentration of the agent should be prescribed.

4. The preparations are applied until the psoriasis lesions are no longer palpable.

5. Topical corticosteroid therapy may occasionally be appropriate for chronic plaque psoriasis, especially if the lesions are localised and treatment with tar or allied products has been unhelpful.

6. 1% hydrocortisone cream or ointment is permissible on the face (where dithranol is contraindicated) and on the flexures and genitalia. Potent fluorinated steroids are best avoided. Steroid scalp applications are useful with severe scalp psoriasis but whenever possible non-steroid preparations should be tried. Topical steroids lose effectiveness with time, seldom produce long remissions and the lesions of psoriasis often 'rebound' on withdrawal of the steroid.

7. Antimetabolites: These limit the synthesis of DNA in epidermal cells and therefore decrease the turnover time of psoriatic epidermis. Methotrexate is the most successful and best tried. The indication for this therapy is severe recalcitrant psoriasis unresponsive to routine topical measures. 75% respond and

best results occur with palmar and plantar psoriasis and in psoriatic arthritis[11]. Methotrexate is hepatotoxic and liver biopsy should be performed before and every two years whilst on therapy. 3–5% develop cirrhosis on methotrexate.

8. Psoralen + UVA (PUVA) was first reported as successful anti-psoriatic therapy in 1974[12]. Indications are as for antimetabolite treatment. 85% show partial or total clearing of the disease. Treatment is 2–3 times weekly until clearing and then maintenance once weekly or longer. In one study[13] the mean time to clearance in patients with chronic plaque psoriasis was about 34 days. The advantages of PUVA are that it is an outpatient therapy, it is cosmetically very acceptable – most patients substitute a tan for their psoriasis – and it obviates the use of preparations which may be messy or stain the skin. Potential disadvantages include premature cataract formation, skin ageing and early skin cancer.

9. Oral retinoids are synthetic derivatives of vitamin A and its metabolite vitamin A acid. The aromatic form etretinate is the most effective[14]. The drug is especially good for pustular and erythrodermic psoriasis. It may be used in combination with PUVA when neither treatment modality used alone is sufficiently helpful. Side-effects include angular cheilitis, conjunctivitis and alopecia. Increased plasma triglycerides occur but may be controlled with a low fat diet.

FOLLOW-UP

Review of patients with psoriasis is guided by the treatment used. For those receiving topical therapy, usually dithranol, review fortnightly until the maximum tolerated concentration of dithranol is reached. Subsequently, follow-up at monthly intervals for three months and if all is progressing satisfactorily after this period review at longer intervals may be arranged. Patients receiving PUVA are reviewed weekly until maximum improvement or clearance of the psoriasis is obtained. Further review is then arranged at monthly intervals during maintenance therapy. At three monthly intervals a full blood count, renal and liver function tests are performed.

[1] Abele DC (1963) *Arch. Derm.*, **88**, 38.
[2] McMichael A J *et al.* (1978) *Br. J. Derm.*, **98**, 287.
[3] Weinstein GD *et al.* (1968) *J. Investigative Derm.*, **50**, 254.
[4] Durham GA *et al.* (1974) *Br. J. Derm.*, **91**, 7.
[5] Church RE (1958) *Br. J. Derm.*, **70**, 139.
[6] Farber EM *et al.* (1974) *Dermatologica*, **148**, 1.
[7] Ingram JT (1954) *Br. Med. J.*, **ii**, 823.
[8] Svejgaard A *et al.* (1974) *Br. J. Derm.*, **91**, 145.
[9] Farber EM *et al.* (1970) *Arch. Derm.*, **101**, 381.
[10] Goekerman WH (1925) *Northwest Med.*, **24**, 2.
[11] Black RL *et al.* (1964) *J. Am. Med. Assoc.*, **189**, 743.
[12] Parrrish JA *et al* (1974) *New Eng. J. Med.*, **291**, 1207.
[13] Rogers S *et al.* (1979) *Lancet*, **i**, 455.
[14] Goerz G *et al.* (1978) *Dermatologica*, **157**, 38.

Dermatophyte Infections

Tinea capitis

Tinea capitis or scalp ringworm may be caused by fungal infection within the hairshaft (endothrix infection) or where the spores are both within and around the hairshaft (ectothrix infection). The clinical appearances vary between diffuse alopecia, diffuse scaling and thinning of the hair (favus) or a boggy, oedematous inflammation (kerion). Hairs infected with a Microsporum species will fluoresce green with Wood's light (long-wave ultraviolet light). Samples of hair should always be examined for fungus.

TREATMENT

1. The scalp should be shampooed each night with a mild shampoo and an antifungal lotion or cream applied.
2. Griseofulvin is the treatment of choice and should be continued for three months.
3. A kerion will require griseofulvin, often an antibiotic for secondary bacterial infection, and a short course of oral prednisolone to clear the infection and inflammation as quickly as possible and prevent permanent scarring.

FOLLOW-UP

Further examination of hair from the previously infected sites is necessary to ensure that the fungus has been completely eradicated.

Tinea corporis

Tinea corporis is a superficial fungal infection of the skin which may present as dry, scaly lesions or an acute eczema-like eruption often annular in configuration. Scales from the edge of the lesion should be examined for fungus.

TREATMENT

1. Benzoic acid ointment (Whitfield's ointment) should be applied twice daily to the affected areas for at least four weeks. It is inexpensive but messy.
2. Clotrimazole, an imidazole derivative, is an effective topical agent. It is aesthetically more acceptable but there is little evidence that for dermatophyte infections any topical preparation is significantly superior to Whitfield's ointment.

Tinea unguium

Tinea unguium is a fungal infection of the fingernails or toenails. The nails become thickened and friable and are often discoloured. It is important to ensure that fungus is present and sensitive to griseofulvin.

TREATMENT

The only satisfactory treatment for nail plate infection due to one of the trichophytons is griseofulvin. Patients should be warned that prolonged treatment is necessary: for fingernails six months (or occasionally longer) of griseofulvin; for toenails 12–24 months. Relapse after apparent cure is not infrequent. Courses of griseofulvin after the first course are not as effective.

Tinea pedis

Tinea pedis or athlete's foot usually begins in the web between the fourth and fifth toes and extends to adjacent toe webs and the plantar and dorsal aspects of the foot. It is particularly common in the shoe-wearing peoples of the world emphasising the influence shoes have in creating a warm hospitable environment for dermatophytes and candida.

TREATMENT

1. Griseofulvin (provided the organism is sensitive to the drug) for 4–6 weeks for long

standing infections. This is usually allied with Whitfield's ointment or clotrimazole cream applied to the affected skin.

2. Candida is treated with Nystatin or one of the imidazole anti-fungal preparations which are effective against both dermatophyte and candida infection.

FOLLOW-UP

Further examination of skin, hair or nails, as appropriate, from the previously infected site is necessary to ensure that the causative organism has been completely eradicated.

Alopecia

Hair growth is normally expressed in three different follicular phases – anagen or growth phase, catagen when the follicle regresses and telogen or the resting phase. Approximately 85% scalp hairs are in anagen and hair grows at the rate of 0.35 mm per day. The duration of the hair cycle determines the different lengths of scalp, axillary or eyebrow hair. Alopecia may result from a structural weakness of the hair; a loss of hair follicles as in scarring alopecia or from follicular dysfunction.

PROGNOSIS

- In drug-induced alopecias with cytotoxic drugs (cyclophosphamide, actinomycin), anti-coagulants, anti-thyroid drugs, allopurinol, oral contraceptives or synthetic vitamin A related retinoids, hair returns as a rule on cessation of therapy.
- Alopecia areata
  a) In a study of 736 patients[1] 89% were less than 50 years of age with an average age of 32 years. 54% of the children (16 years or younger) and 24% of the adults developed total loss of terminal hair (alopecia totalis) implying a worse prognosis for children. 21% children and 30% adults with alopecia totalis showed no regrowth.
  b) Nail changes occur in 10% and are thought to indicate a poor prognosis.

TREATMENT

1. Spontaneous regrowth is common.
2. Topical corticosteroids are ineffective perhaps because adequate concentrations at the hair follicle are not achieved.
3. Intralesional triamcinolone acetonide or hexacetonide via Pan-jet induces hair regrowth. In one study[2] 60% patients had responded 12 weeks after intralesional triamcinolone given weekly for three weeks.
4. Photochemotherapy has also been found useful – in one study of 41 patients, 73% responded[3].
5. Dinitrochlorobenzene (DNCB) used as a contact allergen on areas of alopecia areata has been found successful[4,5]. Positive Ames test (carcinogenic in laboratory animals) demands caution with this treatment modality. The new contact sensitiser diphencyprone may be safer and equally effective[6].

6. Minoxidil, a vasodilator used as an antihypertensive, has been reported as inducing hair growth in alopecia areata[7]. Most other workers have not found it an effective treatment[8].
7. Male pattern baldness (androgen-dependent dominantly transmitted hair loss): Antiandrogen, cyproterone acetate is not effective in reversing process. Hair transplantation with hair plugs obtained from non-androgen sensitive areas over the occiput will grow normally when inserted into the bald areas.
8. Female pattern alopecia (akin to male pattern baldness): Treatment with cyproterone acetate in a reversed sequential pattern with oestrogen may be helpful. 100 mg cyproterone acetate is given on days 5–14 of the menstrual cycle and 30 μg ethinyl-oestradiol from days 5–25.

FOLLOW-UP

In alopecia areata patients should be reviewed three months after receiving intralesional triamcinolone therapy. Further review is guided by the response to treatment but once there has been sufficient regrowth of hair three monthly assessments are justified until doctor and patient are satisfied that there are no new patches of hair loss.

[1] Muller SA et al. (1963) Arch. Derm., 88, 290.
[2] Abell E et al. (1973) Br. J. Derm., 88, 55.
[3] Lassus A et al. (1980) Dermatologica, 161, 298.
[4] Breuillard F et al. (1978) Lancet, ii, 1304.
[5] Hehir ME et al. (1979) Clin. Experimental Derm., 4, 385.
[6] Happle R et al. (1983) Acta Dermato-Venereologica (Stockholm), 63, 49.
[7] Fenton DA et al. (1983) Br. Med. J., 287, 1015.
[8] Vestey JP et al. (1985) Br. J. Derm., 113, Suppl. 29, 35.

Pityriasis Versicolor

Tinea or pityriasis versicolor is an extremely common superficial yeast infection which occurs predominantly in young adults. The causative organism has reliably been shown to be the yeast *Pityrosporum orbiculare* which converts to the pathogenic form *Malassezia furfur* in tinea versicolor. In adults, widespread infection may be associated with uncontrolled diabetes mellitus or undiagnosed Cushing's syndrome. A potassium hydroxide preparation of the skin scraping will confirm the diagnosis and show the characteristic short hyphae and large spores ('spaghetti and meat-balls') of *M. furfur*. Wood's light examination of affected skin often reveals a yellowish fluorescence and helps to delineate the extent of infection.

PROGNOSIS

- Untreated, the condition gradually becomes more widespread and produces a mottling of the skin.

TREATMENT

1. Many different treatments are recommended – possibly because of the lack of a truly effective measure which would both clear the condition and prevent recurrence.
2. Benzoic acid compound (Whitfield's ointment) is effective and inexpensive, but patient compliance is reduced because the preparation is messy.
3. Clotrimazole cream 1% is also effective and more aesthetically acceptable but expensive when compared with Whitfield's ointment. It is applied twice daily for at least six weeks.
4. Griseofulvin is ineffective in tinea versicolor.
5. Ketoconazole clears tinea versicolor but is potentially hepatotoxic. The effect of ketoconazole on the liver ranges from asymptomatic transient abnormalities of the liver enzymes to potentially fatal acute hepatic necrosis[1].
6. Selenium sulphide shampoo, available in cream-shampoo form is also useful and best results are obtained if the preparation is applied on three separate occasions a few days apart. It should be applied to the affected patches and the surrounding skin at bedtime and washed off in the morning.

FOLLOW-UP

Review after six weeks of therapy and finally at three months.

---

[1] Lewis JH *et al.* (1984) *Gastroenterology*, **86**, 503.

Scabies

Scabies is an infection caused by the ubiquitous mite *Sarcoptes scabiei*. Typically it presents as nocturnal itching. The adult female mite is commonly seen in the scabies burrow, usually found on the hands (finger webs and sides of digits) and the wrists.

PROGNOSIS

- Untreated the patient continues to scratch. With appropriate treatment the disease is cured.

TREATMENT[1]

1. Gammabenzene hexachloride (GBHC) is effective and easy to use. The lotion is applied to the entire skin surface except for the head and neck, and left on for 12 hours. Recent reviews suggest that application may be made to dry, cool skin to reduce percutaneous absorption which bathing in a hot bath prior to lotion application may induce. One application is usually sufficient.
2. 25% benzyl benzoate application is another good scabeticide though a little less pleasant to use than GBHC.
3. Crotamiton cream is a weak scabeticide but very useful in controlling the itch which inevitably stays for a week or more, in spite of adequate scabies therapy.
4. Intimate articles of clothing need routine laundering and ironing only. Outer garments and furniture do not need to be discarded.

FOLLOW-UP

All members of the household and sexual contacts of infected patients should be followed-up and treated, even if they are asymptomatic. The patient should be seen two weeks after therapy.

[1] Orkin M *et al.* (1976) *J. Am. Med. Assoc.*, **236**, 1136.

Pediculosis

There are three types of lice infection of importance to man, pediculosis capitis, pediculosis corporis and pediculosis pubis. All live on blood sucked from the host into whom they inject saliva which in turn causes sensitisation and irritation. The head louse measures 3 mm and is intermediate in size between the body louse, the largest, and the pubic louse, the smallest. In all cases the lice appear to prefer blood from the female – the human male hormone is thought to interfere with the metabolism of the lice. Fever tends to rid the host of lice and the pediculi always disappear with the death of the host!

PROGNOSIS

- Untreated the patient continues to scratch. With appropriate treatment the disease is cured.

TREATMENT

1. *Pediculosis capitis*

    a) Carbaryl lotion 0.5% is rubbed gently into the hair and allowed to dry naturally. Twelve hours later the scalp is shampooed with non-medicated shampoo and combed thoroughly whilst wet. The treatment may be repeated a week later.

    b) Gammabenzene hexachloride (GBHC) preparations are effective against head lice and also possess an ovicidal action[1]. Resistant strains have emerged and respond to malathion.

    c) Malathion preparations. These are probably the treatment of choice for resistant infections with the so-called 'super-louse'. Chlorine inactivates the lotion and patients should not go to swimming baths for a week after treatment.

2. *Pediculosis corporis:* 1% gammabenzene hexachloride (GBHC) lotion is applied to the body except the face and neck and washed off after 12 hours. One application is usually sufficient. Clothes are also treated with GBHC then sent for laundering.

3. *Pediculosis pubis:* Treatment is as for head lice.

FOLLOW-UP

The patient should be seen two weeks after therapy.

---

[1] Gardner J (1958) *J. Paediatrics*, **52,** 448.

Warts

Warts are epidermal tumours caused by infection by the Papova group of viruses. The virus may be found in the surface layer of the wart so spread of infection can occur if infected debris comes into contact with abraded skin (indirect contact). Infection may also occur as a result of direct contact or auto-inoculation as might occur with nail biting or shaving.

PROGNOSIS

- 20% warts, especially in children, disappear spontaneously within six months. It is argued that as common warts (verruca vulgaris) resolve spontaneously sooner or later, treatment in very young children should be deferred and the warts simply covered with collodion, plaster or a clear nail varnish to prevent spread. However, in most, warts are socially unacceptable or painful and require treatment.

TREATMENT

1. Patients should be advised that no certain or quick cure exists for warts and no matter which treatment is chosen the time for cure can extend to three months or longer.
2. Wart paints. Many are available. Most contain salicylic acid. One formula containing salicylic acid and lactic acid in flexible collodion (Salactol, Duofilm) is useful. It is important that the paint is applied to the lesion itself, that surrounding skin is protected with soft paraffin and the surface of the wart is abraded with a pumice stone or manicure emery board prior to paint application. In one study[1], 67% hand warts had cleared by 12 weeks. Plantar and anogenital warts may be treated with compound podophyllin paint containing podophyllum resin 15%. With genital warts the paint is left on for a maximum of six hours and then washed off with ordinary soap and water. Applications are made once weekly, though for plantar verrucae two or three times a week is acceptable. Pregnancy is a contraindication to the use of podophyllin preparations as fetal abnormalities may occur as a result of absorption of podophyllin which is cytotoxic and antimitotic.
3. Cryotherapy: Liquid nitrogen ($-196°C$) has substituted CO_2 snow as the treatment of choice for warts apparently resistant to paint therapy and for lesions on the face. The warts are frozen until a halo appears around the base of the lesion – 5 to 20 seconds depending on the size of the lesion. One series[2] showed that 69% responded to light frequent applications of liquid nitrogen.
4. Surgery: In selected patients only, as for example those with large warts on the face or groins, curettage and electrodesiccation under local anaesthetic may be the treatment of choice.

FOLLOW-UP

Patients prescribed paints for their hand and foot lesions may be reviewed three months after the therapy. Those who receive liquid nitrogen treatment are best reviewed within three weeks and patients with anogenital warts should be reviewed once a week and investigations completed to exclude other sexually transmitted disease.

[1] Bunney MH (1974) *Prescribers' J.*, **14**(6), 11.
[2] Barr A *et al.* (1969) *Trans. St. John's Hosp. Derm Soc.*, **55**, 69.

Basal Cell Carcinoma (BCC)

Basal cell carcinoma is a slow-growing tumour which normally arises from the epidermis although some develop from hair follicles[1]. Sun-exposed areas of the body are more likely to develop BCC than sun-protected areas[2]. BCC may arise in scarring whether induced by burns[3], trauma, vaccination or even chickenpox[4]. Naevi, such as naevus sebaceus[5] and junctional naevi, may also form BCC.

PROGNOSIS

- After therapy high recurrence rates are frequently quoted for lesions over the nasolabial fold[6], medial canthus, postauricular area and scalp[7].
- BCCs rarely metastasise even when present for several years.
- Metastasis (estimated at one in a thousand) usually occurs to the regional lymph nodes (68%) whilst distant metastases to bone, lungs and liver occur in fewer than 20%[8].

TREATMENT

1. Curettage and electrodesiccation: Probably the most frequent technique used by dermatologists. Useful for (a) BCCs 1.5 cm or less in size with well-defined borders, and (b) BCC in areas with little mobile tissue, e.g. over ears, nose and temples. Low risk outpatient technique. Wound heals by secondary intention.

2. Surgical excision with or without graft: Useful where primary closure after excision of adequate margin is possible. Quick healing. Indicated for BCC of the morphoeic variety and 'recurrent' tumours.

3. Radiotherapy: Especially useful for BCCs over ears, eyelids, nose and lips and for large tumours in elderly patients. Scars from radiation therapy tend to worsen in appearance in time. Radiation should be avoided if possible in patients under 50 years of age.

4. Mohs' chemosurgery: First described by Frederic Mohs in 1936. Useful for almost all types of BCC but the technique is time consuming and requires multiple patient visits over a period of 2–7 days. Healing by secondary intention. Requires special equipment and training for surgeon and histopathologist.

5. Cryosurgery: Best used for BCCs which show well-defined borders. Liquid nitrogen is the cryogen of choice. Requires local anaesthetic. Particularly useful for tumour in areas where keloids likely to form, e.g. sternum. Healing by secondary intention.

6. 5-Fluorouracil: May be useful for early superficial BCC. Nodular BCCs do not respond. Excellent for actinic keratoses and makes obscure BCCs more apparent and amenable to one of the treatment modalities above.

FOLLOW-UP

Patients should be reviewed six monthly in the first year and then annually until five years post-therapy. Review may be more frequent if lesions were large, multiple or showed atypical (basi-squamous) histology.

[1] Zachheim HS (1963) *J. Investigative Derm.*, **40**, 283.
[2] Scotto J (1974) *Cancer*, **34**, 1333.
[3] Connolly JG (1960) *J. Can. Med. Assoc.*, **83**, 1433.
[4] Hendricks WM (1980) *Arch. Derm.*, **116**, 1304.
[5] Fergin PE (1981) *Clin. Experimental Derm.*, **6**, 111.
[6] Mora RG (1978) *J. Derm. Surg. Oncology*, **4**, 315.
[7] Gormley DE (1978) *Arch. Derm.*, **114**, 782.
[8] Costanza ME *et al.* (1974) *Cancer*, **34**, 230.

Malignant Melanoma

Primary cutaneous malignant melanoma is commonly classified into lentigo malignant melanoma, superficial spreading melanoma, acral lentiginous melanoma and nodular melanoma[1].

PROGNOSIS

- Breslow[2] determined that melanoma thickness measured precisely from the granular layer of the epidermis to the deepest invasive part of the tumour by ocular micrometry correlated closely with five-year survival.
- It is also generally accepted that thickness for thickness there is no prognostic difference between nodular melanoma and superficial spreading melanoma[3].
- The Melanoma Clinical Cooperative Group[4] concluded that prognosis worsens with increasing tumour thickness in a stepwise rather than linear fashion. The melanoma thickness categories were classified as less than 0.85 mm invasion, 0.86–1.69 mm, 1.70–3.60 mm and greater than 3.60 mm invasion.
- Ulceration of a melanoma is a bad prognostic sign. Although the incidence of ulceration increases with increasing thickness, the prognosis is worse for patients with ulcerated melanomas in lesions with similar thickness[5].
- Women with melanoma have a better prognosis than men[6].
- In most series patients younger than 50 years of age have a better prognosis than those above 50 years.
- Patients with melanomas on the upper back, upper arms, neck and shoulder (BANS) areas have a significantly worse prognosis than those with lesions over other body areas[7].
- Evidence of a pre-existing naevus in association with the malignant melanoma is associated with a better prognosis[8].

TREATMENT

1. Surgery

   a) Studies suggest that the margin of excision of the malignant melanoma, provided there is complete removal of the tumour, has no significant effect on subsequent survival. In many centres the extent of excision is correlated with the depth of tumour. Tumours 1 mm or less in thickness are only locally excised. Lesions deeper receive 3 cm excision and graft.

   b) Controversy relates to prophylactic node dissection. In general the view appears to be that patients with a poor prognosis as assessed by Breslow thickness may benefit from lymph node dissection.

   c) If there are clinically enlarged nodes full dissection of the appropriate nodes is necessary.

   d) If only one lymph node in a drainage site shows metastatic tumour histologically the prognosis appears no worse than if no lymph nodes were involved. If two or more lymph nodes are involved the prognosis worsens.

2. Chemotherapy: The response of patients with advanced malignant melanoma to all forms of chemotherapy whether given singly or in combination is poor. Some regression of tumour is seen in approximately 20% patients and the duration of response is usually measured in weeks rather than in months. The two single agents used most commonly are dimethyl triazeno imidazole carboxamide (DTIC) and vindesine, a semi synthetic vinca alkaloid. Combination therapy includes bleomycin, vincristine, lomustine and DTIC (BOLD), and vindesine in combination with bleomycin, lomustine and DTIC.

3. Radiotherapy: Melanoma is mostly regarded as radioresistant. However large fraction radiotherapy is occasionally useful for individual cutaneous nodules. Radiotherapy may also be useful for relieving pain from bone metastases, and for cerebral metastases when given in combination with dexamethasone which reduces cerebral oedema.

4. Hormonal therapy: Antioestrogen tamoxifen is of some benefit in postmenopausal women with advanced malignant melanoma.
5. BCG, acting as a non-specific immune stimulator, is of little benefit in advanced malignant melanoma.

FOLLOW-UP

Patients should be reviewed every three months in the first year after treatment for melanoma restricted to the skin. The frequency of review would need to be increased in patients with deep lesions or those with evidence of metastasis to nodes or beyond.

[1] Clark WH Jr et al. (1969) Cancer Res., 29, 705.
[2] Breslow A (1970) Ann. Surg., 172, 902.
[3] Schmoeckel C et al. (1978) Arch. Derm., 114, 871.
[4] Day CL Jr et al. (1981) New Eng. J. Med., 305, 1155.
[5] Balch CM et al. (1980) Cancer, 45, 3012.
[6] Shaw HM et al. (1980) Cancer, 46, 2731.
[7] Day CL et al. (1981) Surgery, 89, 599.
[8] Friedman RJ et al. (1983) Arch. Derm., 119, 455.

Vitiligo

Vitiligo is an acquired pigmentary disorder and results from destruction of melanocytes in the skin and eyes. Three major theories exist to explain the development of vitiligo. The auto-destructive theory suggests that melanocytes synthesising melanin at an accelerated rate are more susceptible to destruction and this would explain why patients with Addison's disease who are hyperpigmented develop vitiligo. The immune theory is based on the association of auto-immune diseases with vitiligo and finally the neural hypothesis relies on the fact that melanocytes and nerve cells are both of ectodermal origin and many patients develop vitiligo in a dermatomal distribution.

PROGNOSIS

- Commonly associated with thyroid disease[1] (15%) in particular thyrotoxicosis[2] and Hashimoto's thyroiditis and diabetes mellitus (5%). In most patients the disease is slowly progressive. Spontaneous repigmentation is uncommon as is total depigmentation of the entire skin surface.
- Patients with vitiligo have a high incidence (40%) of subclinical retinal pigmentary disease.
- The onset of vitiligo in a patient with a past history of malignant melanoma is an ominous sign that metastases have occurred.

TREATMENT

1. 8-methoxypsoralen, a furocoumarin from the fruits of the Ammi majus plant, was introduced in 1947 by Fahmy and El Mofty to Western medicine, for treatment of vitiligo. Patients take the drug on a weight-related basis and are then exposed to sunlight two hours later or longwave (PUVA) ultraviolet light produced artificially. The improvement obtained appears to vary with the age of the patient, the duration of the vitiligo and the length of treatment. In one series[3] 70% patients showed marked improvement within one year of PUVA therapy. Others have seen improvement in 15-25% patients only.
2. Localised areas of vitiligo may respond to topical therapy with a neat fluorinated steroid such as 0.05% clobetasol propionate cream or 0.1% betamethasone valerate cream applied sparingly twice daily for 6-8 weeks.
3. Intralesional injections with triamcinolone acetonide via Pan-jet (needleless injector) may produce some improvement.
4. Cosmetic treatment with staining lotion, e.g. dihydroxyacetone solution, or with cosmetic masking agents are useful psychological props and should not be overlooked.

FOLLOW-UP

With PUVA therapy monthly review is satisfactory. Patients should be photographed prior to and at the end of treatment to assess repigmentation.

[1] Cunliffe WJ et al. (1968) Br. J. Derm., 80, 135.
[2] Ochi Y et al. (1969) Ann. Int. Med., 71, 935.
[3] Parrish JA et al. (1976) Arch. Derm., 112, 1531.

Lichen Planus

Lichen planus (LP) is an inflammatory dermatosis characterised by pruritic, polygonal lesions which heal with pigmentation. Mucous membrane lesions are common. The disease occurs most frequently between 30 and 60 years of age and in a 10-year study of 200 patients[1] 60% affected were males and 40% females. Its incidence is estimated at approximately 0.15–1% of all skin conditions seen by dermatologists[2,3]. Its aetiology is unknown though it may have an immune basis. An LP-like eruption as a form of graft versus host reaction may follow bone marrow transplantation[4].

PROGNOSIS

- It may develop rapidly into an acute generalised eruption.
- Mucous membrane lesions occur in 7 out of 10 patients.
- 15–25% patients who present with oral LP never have skin lesions[5].
- 1 out of 4 male patients with LP has genital lesions.
- Chronic erosive or atrophic oral lichen planus may predispose to an oral squamous cell carcinoma though the risk is considered low[6].
- Nails are affected in 10% patients[7].
- Acute or subacute LP can be expected to clear in the vast majority (95%) within 24 months. 45% clear within nine months. 60% within 12 months and 90% within 21 months[1].
- Relapse or recurrence is reported in about 15% patients.

TREATMENT

. Lichen planus will improve without treatment.
. Pruritus is lessened with oral antihistamines and topical corticosteroids.
. Acute widespread LP may require a short tapered 2–4 week course of systemic corticosteroids.
. Oral lesions require a potent corticosteroid, e.g. adcortyl in orabase.
. Hypertrophic LP often responds to intra-lesional triamcinolone acetonide or hexacetonide or steroid cream under polythene occlusion.
6. Oral griseofulvin has been claimed to be beneficial[8].
7. Oral etretinate may be useful in some patients with LP[9].

FOLLOW-UP

When treatment with systemic steroids is required patients should be reviewed once weekly for two weeks and then once a fortnight for a month. If there has been sufficient improvement, further review after another month and then at three-monthly intervals until the disease shows no signs of recrudescence. With intralesional triamcinolone therapy, as for hypertrophic lichen planus, review at two-monthly intervals is usually satisfactory.

[1] Samman PD (1961) Trans. St. John's Hosp. Derm. Soc., **46**, 36.
[2] Calnan C et al. (1957) Trans. St. John's Hosp. Derm. Soc., **39**, 56.
[3] Schmidt H (1961) Acta Dermato-Venereologica, **41**, 164.
[4] Saurat JH et al. (1975) Br. J. Derm., **92**, 675.
[5] Arndt KA (1979) In Dermatology in General Medicine 2nd edn. p. 655. Maidenhead: McGraw-Hill Book Co.
[6] Dusek JJ et al. (1982) J. Oral Maxillo-facial Surg., **40**, 240.
[7] Norton LA (1980) J. Am. Acad. Derm., **2**, 451.
[8] Sehgal VN et al. (1972) Br. J. Derm., **87**, 383.
[9] Mahrle G et al. (1982) Arch. Derm., **118**, 97.

Fixed Drug Eruption

The term fixed drug eruption was introduced by Brocq[1] when he described three patients in whom an erythematous pigmented eruption developed after ingesting antipyrine. It usually presents as a solitary erythematous macule which forms into an oedematous plaque. Pruritus is often associated and the lesion heals with mild scaling and pigmentation.

PROGNOSIS

- With repeated attacks existing lesions increase in size and new lesions appear elsewhere on the skin. The lesions, which later may present as vesicles or bullae, appear anywhere on the body though the lips, hands and glans penis are commonly affected. The length of time from re-exposure to a drug and onset of symptoms varies between $\frac{1}{2}$ hour and 8 hours[2]. The condition is not life threatening.

TREATMENT

1. Identify the causative drug. In a recent review of the literature[3] 68 drugs had been reported as causing a fixed drug eruption. Common offenders include barbiturates, sulphonamides, phenolphthalein, oxyphenbutazone, chlordiazepoxide and quinine. Phenolphthalein is found in some proprietary purgatives and quinine in tonic water. It is not uncommon for patients to forget when they last took a drug if at all, and then the only way of identifying the offending agent is by testing in turn with the drugs known to cause a fixed eruption.

2. For pruritus associated with the eruption a medium potency steroid (Metosyn, Synalar) applied to the affected area three times a day for a few days together with an oral antihistamine is helpful.

FOLLOW-UP

No specific follow-up required although patients must be warned to avoid the causative drug.

[1] Brocq L (1894) *Annales de Dermatologie et d Syphiligraphie (Paris)* 5 (Series 3), 308.
[2] Stubb S (1976) *Acta Dermato-Venereologica*, **56**, 1.
[3] Korkij W *et al.* (1984) *Arch. Derm.*, **120**, 520.

Erythema Multiforme

Erythema multiforme is an acute, usually self-limiting, disease characterised by target or iris-shaped lesions and occasionally associated with mucosal involvement – the Stevens–Johnson syndrome. It is considered to be a hypersensitivity reaction, commonly to a drug or to an underlying virus or bacterial infection. The commonest associations are with preceding herpes simplex or Mycoplasma infection. The most common drugs causing erythema multiforme are sulphonamides, phenytoin, barbiturates, phenylbutazone, sulphonylureas, penicillin and salicylates.

PROGNOSIS

- In erythema multiforme without mucosal lesions (EM minor) new lesions usually appear for 3–5 days though occasionally they may form over 1–2 weeks. The duration from onset to healing is usually two weeks.
- Stevens–Johnson syndrome (EM major) takes very much longer to heal, reflecting the more serious nature of the disease. In most the condition resolves within six weeks[1].
- In EM minor recovery is complete and complications are rare. In EM major visual impairment may occur as a result of keratitis or conjunctival scarring[2,3]. A permanent visual defect may occur in some 10% patients with ocular disease[1].
- Pneumonia or upper airways disease may complicate 30% cases of EM major.
- With herpes simplex associated disease EM minor usually occurs – primarily in young adults and tending, like the herpes lesions, to be recurrent. Both Type 1 and 2 herpes viruses have been associated with EM.

TREATMENT

1. EM *minor* usually clears with symptomatic treatment only.

2. For *EM major* prednisolone 30 mg as a single morning dose tailed off over 14 days is often indicated. Bullae are punctured with a sterile needle and a fluorinated steroid cream applied three times daily for 7–10 days as necessary.
3. Secondary infection is common and if streptococcal or other bacterial infection is thought, on laboratory evidence, to have triggered the disease it should be treated with appropriate antibiotics.
4. Mucous membrane lesions require a topical steroid preparation and usually respond well to 0.1% triamcinolone in sodium carboxymethyl cellulose (Orabase).

FOLLOW-UP

With EM minor review two and six weeks after the onset of the illness. With EM major weekly review for the first month, then two weekly for the next month.

[1] Ashby DW (1951) *Lancet*, i, 1091.
[2] Patz A (1950) *Arch. Ophthalmology*, 43, 244.
[3] Howard GM (1963) *Am. J. Ophthalmology*, 55, 893.

Dermatitis Herpetiformis

Dermatitis herpetiformis (DH) is a chronic papulo-vesicular, extremely pruritic dermatosis which occurs most commonly in the 20–40 years age group. Patients with the disease have an associated asymptomatic gluten (wheat protein) sensitive enteropathy of the small intestinal mucosa[1,2]. Jejunal biopsy shows a variable flattening of intestinal villi and increased numbers of lymphocytes between epithelial cells similar to coeliac disease. Granular deposits of IgA occur in dermal papillae, demonstrated by immunofluorescent techniques, in perilesional and uninvolved skin.

PROGNOSIS

- The disease runs a long course of exacerbations and remissions. 40% have active lesions after 10 years.
- Overt symptoms of malabsorption are unusual in dermatitis herpetiformis although abnormalities of intestinal function may be demonstrated.

TREATMENT

1. Dapsone (diaminodiphenylsulphone) is the treatment of choice. Tests for glucose-6-phosphate dehydrogenase deficiency should be completed prior to administration. Side-effects of dapsone include haemolysis, methaemoglobinaemia, and rarely agranulocytosis.
2. Sulphapyridine is also beneficial but less effective than dapsone.
3. Gluten-sensitive enteropathy improves with gluten-free diet and after 5–6 months of the restrictive diet it may be possible to reduce the dose of dapsone and in some patients discontinue the drug.
4. Iodide should be eliminated from the diet as it is known to exacerbate DH.

FOLLOW-UP

Review one week after commencing therapy, then after a fortnight. If progress satisfactory, monthly for three months and finally three-monthly intervals in the first year.

[1] Marks J et al. (1966) Lancet, ii, 1280.
[2] Katz SI et al. (1978) J. Investigative Derm., 70, 63.

Pemphigoid

Pemphigoid is a chronic bullous disorder which occurs predominantly in the elderly. 80% patients are over 60 years old at the onset of the disease which is characterised by the formation of tense, subepidermal blisters with a predilection for the flexor aspects of the arms, the axillae and the thighs. Clinically there are two types of blisters – those which develop on inflamed skin and those which arise on normal-looking skin. The inflammation in both occurs at the basement membrane zone of the skin where dermo-epidermal separation occurs and where immunoglobulins (IgG) and complement are deposited. Using standard indirect immunofluorescent techniques anti-basement membrane zone (anti-BMZ) antibodies are detected in the sera of 70–80% patients[1].

PROGNOSIS

- Prior to steroid therapy a third of patients died of the disease. With steroid therapy the mortality has been significantly lowered. In one series[2] 30 of 68 patients (44%) went into remission such that treatment could be discontinued. In only 3% could death be attributed to the complications of treatment.
- Controversy exists regarding the association of pemphigoid with malignancy. Recent work[3] suggests that there may be a true increase in malignancy in those patients with negative indirect immunofluorescent findings, i.e. absence of anti-BMZ antibody.
- There is no correlation between the severity of pemphigoid and the titres of anti-basement membrane zone antibodies.

TREATMENT

1. Prednisolone 60–90 mg as a single morning dose together with azathioprine 100–150 mg daily in divided doses. The latter acts as a 'steroid-sparing' drug. The dose of steroid is gradually reduced once new blisters have stopped forming but the reduction needs to be slow or there is a recurrence of the disease necessitating much larger increases in steroid dosage.
2. Blisters often rupture leaving large denuded areas of skin which become sore and are readily infected. Topical therapy with a steroid-antibiotic cream for 10–14 days is both symptomatically and therapeutically rewarding.
3. Oral lesions require steroid cream, 0.1% triamcinolone acetonide in orabase applied thinly 2–4 times daily.
4. It is often possible to tail off systemic therapy within a year or two and many patients remain in remission for several years.

FOLLOW-UP

Patients with pemphigoid are usually hospitalised for investigations and treatment. Once the blisters have stopped forming and the skin has healed it is justifiable to continue treatment as an out-patient. A suggested review programme is two weekly for 6 weeks, three weekly for 9 weeks, monthly for 6 months, two monthly for 6 months and three monthly for 6 months. Full blood count, renal and liver function tests should be completed weekly in the first three months of treatment when steroid-sparing drugs such as azathioprine are given in conjunction with prednisolone. Subsequently monthly laboratory assessments are usually sufficient.

[1] Jordon RE et al. (1967) J. Am. Med. Assoc., 200, 1967.
[2] Stevenson CJ (1960) Br. J. Derm., 72, 11.
[3] Hodge L et al. (1981) Br. J. Derm., 105, 65.

Pemphigus Vulgaris

Pemphigus vulgaris is an auto-immune, non-infectious, non-familial blistering disorder. It commonly occurs in the 40–60 years age group and more frequently in Jews[1]: Histologically there is acantholysis in the epidermis and direct and indirect immunofluorescence studies show the presence of immunoglobulin in the intercellular substance (ICS) of the epidermis and anti-ICS antibody in the serum[2].

PROGNOSIS

- Without treatment it is inexorably fatal.
- One study[3] showed that 12% pemphigus patients developed an internal malignancy.
- Thymoma[4] or myasthenia gravis may be found in patients with pemphigus.
- Most studies show a drop in serum anti-ICS antibody titre with successful therapy[5,6].
- Systemic corticosteroids have lowered the mortality to approximately 25%, though the prognosis appears less favourable in Jews than in other races.

TREATMENT

1. Systemic corticosteroids and immunosuppressive drugs are the mainstay of treatment. Prednisolone 90–120 mg as a single morning dose until new blisters stop forming.
2. Azathioprine 100–150 mg daily is added to the systemic steroid as a steroid-sparing drug.
3. Other steroid-sparing drugs include cyclophosphamide[7], methotrexate and dapsone.
4. Oral lesions are managed as for bullous pemphigoid (see p. 143).

FOLLOW-UP

See *Pemphigoid* (p. 143).

[1] Rosenberg FR et al. (1972) Arch. Derm., 112, 962.
[2] Ahmed AR et al. (1980) Ann. Int. Med., 92, 396.
[3] Krain LS et al. (1974) Cancer, 33, 1091.
[4] Stillman MA et al. (1972) Acta Dermato-Venereologica, 52, 393.
[5] Weissman V et al. (1978) J. Investigative Derm., 71 107.
[6] O'Loughlin S et al. (1978) Arch. Derm., 114, 1769.
[7] Fellner MJ et al. (1978) Arch. Derm., 114, 889.

Dermatomyositis

Dermatomyositis is a disorder characterised by musculocutaneous signs and symptoms. It may occur in childhood, usually before the age of 10 and in adults commonly after the age of 40. It affects females twice as often as males. The myopathy is predominantly proximal but may also involve the tongue and pharangeal muscles. Impaired gastrointestinal motility is a common feature. The rash, typically a heliotrope erythema associated with oedema, begins around the eyes but may spread, especially on exposure to sunlight, to the rest of the face, the neck, the axillae and the exposed skin of the arms. The degree of muscle involvement does not correspond with the severity of the skin signs.

PROGNOSIS

- Variable. Children may be left with gross disability with contractures of the limbs and calcinosis.
- 75% children followed-up for 5-15 years survived.
- Calcinosis is associated with a good prognosis.
- In adults, the mean duration of dermatomyositis in men was two years and in women five years[1].
- Dermatomyositis is associated with internal malignancy in adults. The reported incidence of cancer varies between 6% and 25% patients, with an incidence of 50% in patients over the age of 40[2,3,4].
- In women the commonly associated cancers are those of the breast, ovaries, cervix and uterus whilst in men the neoplasm is usually that of the lung, stomach, colon or prostate. In Chinese patients dermatomyositis has been associated with nasopharangeal carcinoma in 75% cases.

TREATMENT

1. Rest is essential in the acute phase.
2. An underlying carcinoma must be excluded.
3. Prednisolone 60-90 mg daily is the treatment of choice with the dose reduced as the symptoms improve.
4. Azathioprine is given concurrently with the systemic steroid as a steroid-sparing agent.
5. Children with minimal myopathy may respond to indomethacin without steroids.
6. Physiotherapy is important in prevention of contractures, particularly in children.

FOLLOW-UP

With children physiotherapy is one of the mainstays of treatment and review is gauged by the severity of muscle involvement. In the adult form the underlying malignancy determines the frequency of review.

[1] Degos R et al. (1971) Trans. St. John's Hosp. Derm. Soc., 57, 98.
[2] Barnes BE (1976) Ann. Int. Med., 84, 68.
[3] Scaling ST et al. (1979) Obstet. Gynec., 54, 474.
[4] Talbott JH (1977) Sem. Arth. Rheum., 6, 305.
[5] De Vere R et al. (1975) Brain, 98, 637.

8
Diseases of the Blood and Lymphoreticular System

N. C. Allan

Iron Deficiency Anaemia

This anaemia is due to failure of haemoglobin synthesis caused by a lack of adequate iron available to the erythropoietic precursors. It results in small (microcytic) under-haemoglobinised (hypochromic) red cells. It is the commonest type of anaemia, and accounts for over 90% of all anaemias. About 3% men, 20% women during the reproductive years and up to 90% pregnant women, if not given prophylaxis, may be deficient.

PROGNOSIS

- Prognosis is that of the underlying disorder, since in almost all cases this type of anaemia is secondary to other problems which either prevent adequate absorption of iron, result in excessive loss of iron, usually through bleeding, or make it unavailable (see *Anaemia of chronic disorders*, p. 155).
- Nearly 100% patients respond to iron therapy if adequate iron is given other than in association with chronic disease.
- Relapse occurs unless the cause is removed or treatment given continuously. If the cause is not removed, treatment may be required continuously.

TREATMENT

1. The cause should be removed or corrected.
2. Ferrous sulphate 200 mg tds orally (minimum of 100 mg elemental iron per day). Treatment should be continued until the haemoglobin is normal. Then the dose may be reduced to 200 mg daily and continued for up to one year to establish body stores. Single daily doses are best taken last thing at night.
3. Delayed release iron preparations should be avoided.
4. 30% patients have unpleasant side-effects and may require alternative iron preparation, e.g. ferrous gluconate, fumarate, glycine sulphate, succinate.
5. Liquid iron (ferrous sulphate mixture) is available for children or adults unable to swallow tablets.
6. Less than 5% patients genuinely require parenteral iron[1]. If required, oral iron should be avoided for over 24 hours before starting.
7. Intramuscular iron: iron sorbitol (Jectofer) 2 ml (50 mg/ml) daily may be given for 10 doses on alternate days. The course should be started with a test dose.
8. Intravenous iron may be given as iron dextran 50 mg iron per ml (Imferon) in slow infusion diluted in normal saline (500 ml) over 6–8 hours. Close observation is required in the first 15 minutes of transfusion. It should not be given if serum iron is normal or iron binding capacity is low. Antihistamine and steroids should be available to cover reactions.
9. Blood transfusion: red cell concentrate should be given only if absolutely essential, i.e. when oral or parenteral iron may prove too slow (500 ml blood = 250 mg iron).

FOLLOW-UP

A monthly blood count until remission: then at six months and one year. More frequent surveillance may be required depending on underlying cause.

---

[1] Callander STE (1982) *Clin. Haemat.*, **11**, 327.

Pernicious Anaemia

This is a disorder caused by failure to absorb vitamin B_{12} due to a lack of intrinsic factor production in the stomach. In turn, this is due to an auto-immune destruction of gastric parietal cells. Deficiency of vitamin B_{12} causes a failure in DNA synthesis in all dividing cell systems in the body, most obvious in the haemopoietic precursors. The effect is a maturation arrest in the bone marrow and progressive failure of erythrocyte, leukocyte and platelet production. About 2% cases present with evidence of neurological damage to the posterior and lateral columns of the spinal cord, and peripheral neuropathy (sub-acute combined degeneration of the cord).

PROGNOSIS

- Without treatment, death is inevitable although temporary remissions may occur. Survival varies from 12 months to 3 years.
- With treatment, the prognosis is excellent. The patient's haematological problems are corrected and remain in remission as long as treatment is continued.

If treatment is discontinued, relapse will usually occur within 2–5 years.

In sub-acute combined degeneration of the cord, symptoms and signs due to peripheral neuropathy usually respond well to treatment. Long tract signs tend to respond less well with only partial recovery.

There is a three-fold increase in the incidence of gastric carcinoma.

TREATMENT

An intramuscular injection of hydroxocobalamin 1 mg should be given weekly for six weeks. Thereafter a dose should be given every three months for life if there are no neurological problems. If there are neurological signs, monthly injections are required for life. During the recovery phase from anaemia, potassium supplements may be required.

2. Iron deficiency commonly emerges during the recovery phase. Oral iron therapy may then be given.
3. If there is a history of poor diet, folic acid 5 mg daily may be required. Folic acid should never be given without vitamin B_{12} unless vitamin B_{12} deficiency has been excluded.
4. Oral vitamin B_{12} preparations are not recommended except for patients allergic to injected material.
5. Liver extract preparations are satisfactory, but add nothing and are considerably more expensive.
6. Blood transfusion should be used only if really necessary. It is almost never required in patients under 50 years. It is required mainly for elderly patients with a haemoglobin of 5 g/dl or less[1].

FOLLOW-UP

A full blood count should be performed annually. A watch should be kept for the development of iron deficiency. Annual barium meal examinations are not generally recommended, but should be done if any gastric symptoms arise.

---

[1] Chanarin I (1976) *Clin. Haemat.*, 5, 747.

Hereditary Spherocytosis (HS)

This is a chronic haemolytic disorder due to an inherited Mendelian dominant intrinsic red cell abnormality which causes sphering of the red cells and, as a result, excessive destruction in the spleen. The exact nature of the defect is unknown, but it is associated with a leaky cell membrane and excessive sodium pump activity[1]. The severity of the disease is very variable, even within a family. Both sexes are affected equally.

PROGNOSIS

- Without treatment prognosis varies from early death from aplastic crises and much morbidity, to little or no effect on life expectancy and very little morbidity.
- Following splenectomy, most patients are effectively cured, although still retaining the abnormal red cells.

TREATMENT

1. Splenectomy is the definitive treatment as it produces a clinical cure in virtually all cases. However, it should be postponed until early adult life if possible and followed by penicillin V prophylaxis for at least five years. Pneumococcal vaccination before splenectomy may enhance resistance to this organism. Splenectomy at an earlier age may be necessary if the disease is severe.

2. Folic acid 5 mg daily may be required in cases with very active haemolysis.
3. Cholecystectomy may be required for complicating gall bladder disease, usually due to pigment stones.
4. Blood transfusions should be used only if absolutely essential.
5. Iron therapy is contraindicated unless frank deficiency is demonstrated.

FOLLOW-UP

Before splenectomy in young patients, follow up should be six monthly unless the disease is very severe when more frequent visits may be required. After splenectomy, annual review for five years until penicillin withdrawn, after which the patient should be discharged.

---

[1] Becker PS et al. (1985) Clin. Haemat., **14**, 15.

Sickle Cell Anaemia

This is a hereditary, moderately severe, chronic haemolytic anaemia due to the homozygous inheritance of abnormal β globin genes which code for the production of abnormal β globin chains and hence the abnormal haemoglobin, *Haemoglobin S*. Under hypoxic conditions, this haemoglobin forms pseudocrystals (tactoids) which distort red cells into elongated sickle cells. This causes excessive red cell destruction (haemolysis) and recurrent episodes of microvascular obstruction with infarction of tissues. The disorder manifests in the third to fourth month of life, causes marrow hyperplasia and distortion of bones, particularly facial, early in life and is a lifelong problem. The patient suffers from episodic exacerbation of haemolysis (haemolytic or sequestration crises) and painful infarction crises, often in the bones. Aplastic crises may also occur. The majority of sufferers are of black African stock, although the disorder is also seen in the Mediterranean area, the Middle East, India and South America. The highest incidence is in Central Africa and its original distribution correlates well with that of falciparum malaria perhaps because heterozygous carriers are more resistant to *P. falciparum* than normal individuals.

PROGNOSIS

- Prognosis is dependent on social and other environmental conditions.
- In poor social and medical circumstances the majority die before the age of two from anaemia and intercurrent infection exacerbated by malnutrition and folate deficiency.
- Under optimal social conditions and good medical care, survival into middle age is possible.
- The severity of the manifestations tends to ameliorate with age after puberty. Autosplenectomy often occurs as a result of repeated splenic infarctions.
- Relatively few women achieve successful pregnancy unless under optimal social and medical conditions.

TREATMENT[1]

1. The patient requires a good standard of nutrition and general care.
2. Folic acid 5 mg daily should be given.
3. Antimalarial prophylaxis should be given for life in malarial areas.
4. Anything promoting dehydration should be avoided and adequate fluid intake maintained.
5. Infections should be treated early and vigorously. Prophylactic penicillin may be offered to young patients who show evidence of autosplenectomy.
6. Infarction crises require rehydration and pain relief avoiding addictive analgesics if possible, but their use should not be withheld if really necessary. Broad spectrum antibiotic therapy may be required.
7. Haemolytic crises may require transfusion but this should be avoided if possible.
8. Transfusion with red cell concentrate or exchange transfusion may be given before surgery to reduce the risks of sickling. The use of diuretics should be avoided. Long-term transfusion therapy is not generally recommended.
9. Bloodless field surgery should not be practised.
10. Antisickling agents such as urea, cyanate, carbamyl phosphate and carbon monoxide are not recommended.

FOLLOW-UP

Regular visits, preferably to a specialist clinic, are the ideal with the possibility of attending if and when crises occur. Lifelong surveillance is required.

---

[1] Davies SC *et al.* (1984) *Br. J. Hosp. Med.*, **31**, 440.

Homozygous β Thalassaemia

This is an inherited disorder due to the homozygous inheritance of genes incapable of adequate β globin chain synthesis. The majority of patients have inherited two β+ thalassaemia genes capable of limited β chain synthesis of between 5% and 30% normal. Others with two β⁰ genes have virtually no β chain synthesis and are the most profoundly affected. The clinical result is severe chronic anaemia due to production failure and increased destruction of misshapen red cells, excessive iron absorption, retardation of development and bone changes.

PROGNOSIS

- Without transfusion support survival is limited and death occurs after 2–5 years in many cases.
- With transfusion maintaining the haematocrit above 27%, iron overload problems appear at about puberty and few patients survive beyond the age of 20.
- With supertransfusion (haematocrit above 35%) and use of neocytes the onset of iron overload toxicity may be delayed and survival extended[1,2].
- Allogeneic bone marrow transplantation is the only treatment that offers the possibility of cure, but is available only to children with compatible sibling donors.

TREATMENT

1. Bone marrow transplantation from histocompatible sibling donor if possible.
2. Supertransfusion to maintain haematocrit above 35%. This reduces gut iron absorption. The use of selectively harvested young red cells (neocytes) extends the donor cell survival.
3. Desferrioxamine (DF) therapy[3,4] is usually given subcutaneously by infusion over 12 hours, five days per week. Daily doses for longer periods (up to 22 hours) can be given to adults if tolerated. The dose for children under six years should be 0.25–1 g daily. Patients over six years should be given 2–4 g daily.
4. Ascorbic acid (vitamin C) supplement given parenterally enhances iron mobilisation and loss during desferrioxamine (DF) therapy, but should be given only during DF therapy otherwise it may exacerbate iron toxicity.
5. Splenectomy may be required to remove a large organ, improve red cell survival and remove a mass of storage iron. It should be postponed as long as possible.
6. Folic acid 5 mg daily.

FOLLOW-UP

Follow-up will be dictated by transfusion requirements in cases not able to have allogeneic transplantation.

[1] Propper RD et al. (1980) Blood, 55, 55.
[2] Corash L et al. (1981) Blood, 57, 599.
[3] Ley TJ et al. (1982) Clin. Haemat., II, 437.
[4] Pippard MJ et al. (1983) Br. J. Haemat., 54, 503.

Auto-immune Haemolytic Anaemia (AIHA)

This is a haemolytic disorder caused by the production of antibodies against red cell antigens by the body's own immune system. Two types are found: a) those associated with 'warm' (thermal optimum 37°C) antibodies, usually IgG in type and Rhesus if showing specificity; and b) 'cold' (thermal optimum 4°C) antibodies usually IgM in type and anti-I in specificity. Complement is involved in both types but more importantly in the 'cold' type of disease. 'Warm' type AIHA is often idiopathic, but may be secondary to viral infections, lymphoproliferative disorders, other auto-immune disorders, drug therapy and occurs across a wide age spectrum. 'Cold' AIHA (often called cold haemagglutinin disease or CHAD) occurs mainly in the elderly, is often idiopathic but may be associated with malignancy, usually lymphoma, and infection.

PROGNOSIS

- If secondary to other disease, the outlook may be that of the primary disease unless the haemolytic disease is severe and unresponsive to treatment.
- With 'warm' type AIHA, approximately 20% patients may achieve long-term, disease free remission. About 10% have severe disease which progresses despite treatment. The remainder show a varied response to treatment and may survive for years.
- With 'cold' type AIHA, the disease is usually chronic and slowly progressive and compatible with years of life.

TREATMENT[1]

1. 'Warm' type AIHA

   a) Corticosteroids, usually prednisolone 60 mg per day orally as enteric coated tablets is the first line treatment and should be continued for 3-6 weeks in which time response should be evident if it is to occur. Thereafter, the steroids are gradually reduced and if possible stopped. If a dose greater than 15 mg per day is required to control disease, splenectomy is necessary.

   b) Splenectomy. About 50% patients who have 'failed' on steroids respond.

   c) Immunosuppression. Azathioprine 150 mg daily or cyclophosphamide 150 mg daily with or without prednisolone for six months. Used for patients who have failed on above treatments or cannot have them. About half of the patients respond.

   d) Blood transfusion. Often difficult or impossible to use unless the auto-antibody shows specificity and antigen free blood can be obtained. May be forced to use 'least incompatible' blood covered by high doses of corticosteroid if anaemia is life threatening.

   e) Folic acid 5 mg daily during periods of active haemolysis should be prescribed.

   f) Intravenous immunoglobulin G may be beneficial but requires further evaluation.

   g) Thymectomy is of doubtful value.

2. 'Cold' type AIHA

   a) The patient must be kept warm, especially in cold weather. Electric blankets and heated gloves may help.

   b) Immunosuppressive therapy may help in some cases especially if secondary to other disease.

   c) Blood transfusion is often required. Washed red cells should be used to avoid giving complement.

   d) Corticosteroids and splenectomy are of less value and risk promoting more problems than they cure.

   e) Folic acid 5 mg daily is worth prescribing.

   f) Plasmapheresis reduces antibody levels but is required frequently. Elderly patients do not tolerate it well.

Contd.

3. All types of AIHA secondary to other disease may respond to the treatment of the underlying disease.

FOLLOW-UP

Regular clinic visits 3–6 monthly for patients in remission. More frequent visits required for patients with active disease.

---

[1] Flaherty T *et al.* (1979) *Br. J. Hosp. Med.*, **22**, 334.

Anaemia of Chronic Disorders

This is a common chronic anaemia, usually normocytic normochromic, but quite often showing hypochromia and less often microcytosis. It is associated with disturbances in the handling of body iron to the detriment of red cell production. The anaemia is caused mainly by a failure of red cell production, but a variable reduction in red cell life span may also contribute.

PROGNOSIS

- The anaemia and its severity is symptomatic of the underlying disorder, and generally reflects the activity of that disease. The anaemia will improve if the underlying disease remits.
- It will relapse or recur despite therapeutic efforts if the underlying disease is active.
- It is a cause of morbidity, not mortality.

TREATMENT

1. Unless the anaemia is causing morbidity in its own right, it may be best not treated. Patients tolerate mild anaemia well.
2. Treatment directed to the underlying disorder is the most important measure.
3. Oral iron therapy may produce improvement. Ferrous sulphate 200 mg tds may be given. Response is slow and treatment should be continued for four months before abandoning it. The benefit disappears if it is stopped.
4. Parenteral iron therapy is better avoided as body iron stores are already replete if not overloaded.
5. Blood transfusion of red cell concentrate should be used only if essential. The benefit is usually transient. It adds to iron overload.
6. Cobaltous chloride; 100–300 mg daily may produce response, but side-effects such as anorexia and other gastrointestinal symptoms usually discourage its use. The effect is transient without lasting benefit. It is not recommended.
7. Corticosteroids will improve the anaemia mainly by inducing remission in the underlying disease. They should not be used merely for the anaemia unless it is severe.
8. Androgenic steroids (e.g. oxymetholone 50 mg daily) are of little benefit and may be hepatotoxic.

FOLLOW-UP

Follow-up is generally dictated by the underlying disease. Blood counts should be monitored approximately every three months.

Idiopathic Thrombocytic Purpura

This is a syndrome in which the diagnosis is reached by exclusion of known causes of secondary thrombocytopenia together with the demonstration of normal or increased numbers of megakaryocytes in the bone marrow. In many cases an immune cause for excessive destruction of platelets may be demonstrated. The disorder may present as an acute and, in young children, evanescent problem. In adults it tends to be chronic and follow an intercurrent illness. Two-thirds of cases occur in patients under 21, and it is more common in females than males, with a ratio of 3:1.

PROGNOSIS

- In very young children the prognosis is excellent, and over 90% remit without treatment.
- Older children and adults usually become or are chronic.
- 90% show a response to prednisolone but 50% relapse and require splenectomy. Of these, 50-60% respond to splenectomy with lasting remission, although relapse occurs years later in a few.
- If the platelet count peak exceeds $400 \times 10^9/l$ after splenectomy, the outlook is probably good. If it does not, relapse is likely.
- About 25% patients are left with chronic long-standing thrombocytopenia. Few respond to immuno-suppressive therapy.
- The severity of the disorder in chronic refractory disease fluctuates spontaneously.

TREATMENT

1. In young children (2-6 years) management should be conservative unless bleeding is severe. Splenectomy should be avoided if possible.

2. In older children and adults up to 60 years:

   a) Corticosteroids: prednisolone 1 mg/kg body weight daily for 3-4 weeks thereafter tailing off gradually over a further 3-4 weeks. Restart if relapse occurs. If fails – splenectomy is indicated.

   b) Splenectomy for failed corticosteroid therapy. Delay should be avoided. It is preceded with pneumococcal vaccination and followed by prophylactic penicillin V for five years.

   c) Intravenous immunoglobulin G 0.4 g/kg/day for five days. Expensive: may induce lasting remission, but benefit often evanescent. Useful for inducing temporary remission to cover splenectomy[1].

   d) Immunosuppressive therapy
      i) Vincristine (up to 2 mg)/vinblastine (up to 10 mg) – may also stimulate platelet production.
      ii) Cyclophosphamide 50-200 mg daily orally.
      iii) Azathioprine 100 mg daily.
      iv) Note that ii) and iii) require blood count monitoring.

   e) Platelet infusion. Unsatisfactory – very temporary benefit if any. Used only for life-threatening situations.

3. For patients over 60 years the above treatments may be used, but generally in more elderly patients more problems may be caused by the treatment than the disorder. It is often best not to treat unless bleeding is really troublesome. Patients can survive for years with moderately severe thrombocytopenia.

FOLLOW-UP

In children, none is required if spontaneous remission occurs. If not, follow-up is as for adults. In adults regular surveillance is required indefinitely if patient is not in remission. If patient in remission, six monthly follow up is required for five years.

[1] Newland AC et al. (1983) Lancet, i, 84.

Haemophilia

This is a hereditary sex-linked disorder found almost exclusively in males. It is characterised by increased susceptibility to bleeding, particularly into tissues, joints, muscles and viscera, and, in severe cases, not necessarily initiated by known trauma. It is due to a lack of functionally active factor VIII which is an essential component of the intrinsic system in the coagulation cascade. Either the gene on the X-chromosome which codes for the coagulant fraction of the factor VIII molecule is defective or deleted. Prevalence is 1 per 10000 of the population. Approximately 50% cases are severe (less than 2% factor VIIIc), 25% are moderate (2–5% factor VIIIc) and 25% are mild (5–30% factor VIIIc). Between 5 and 21% patients develop inhibitors to factor VIII.

PROGNOSIS

- Severe cases: Adequately treated patients should now have a near normal life expectancy but there is always a risk of lethal bleeding, e.g. intracranial and sublingual bleeds.
- Moderate: patients have a normal life expectancy.
- Mild: patients have a normal life expectancy.
- The presence of inhibitors exacerbates the problem, making therapy more difficult.

TREATMENT

1. Replacement therapy with factor VIII[1]:
   a) *Materials available*
      (1) Heat-treated human factor VIII concentrate best material. Suitable for home therapy.
      (2) Cryoprecipitate useful. Not suitable for home therapy.
      (3) Porcine AGH antigenic. Reserve for severe problems where human concentrate inadequate. Useful for 7–10 days only.
   b) *Usage of factor VIII concentrate*
      (1) Minor spontaneous bleeding—8–10 u/kg body weight.
      (2) Severe bleeds; minor surgery—20–40 u/kg body weight.
      (3) Major surgery—80-100 u/kg body weight. Repeat every 4–5 hours with coagulation monitoring.

2. For mild cases DDAVP may stimulate factor VIII production and obviate the need for factor replacement (0.3 μg/kg in 50 ml saline over 30 minutes). Should be used with anti-fibrinolytics[2].

3. For surface bleeding: e.g. tooth extraction – tranexamic acid 0.5 g i.v. plus factor VIII concentrate in severe cases.

4. Supportive measures:
   a) Prevention of deformity and contracture and restoration of function.
   b) Pain relief.

5. Early treatment: most haemophiliacs can cope with home therapy.

6. Prophylaxis: regular administration is used only for the most severe cases as it is costly.

7. Inhibitors present: bleeds require intensive factor VIII concentrate therapy to overwhelm inhibitor. Porcine material is often used. Exchange transfusion and immunosuppressive therapy may also have a place[1].

8. Ancillary methods: topical thrombin, Russell's viper venom. Pressure to bleeding site. Human factor VIII paste, where the bleeding point is accessible.

9. There should be social and educational supervision to ensure adequate education and suitable occupation.

FOLLOW-UP

Patients should attend a special haemophilia centre regularly and as necessary with bleeds. The majority of patients eventually become HTLV III positive, especially if commercial blood products have been used. This carries the risk that some may develop and transmit AIDS.

[1] Rizza CR (1981) *Haemostasis and Thrombosis*, p. 371. Edinburgh: Churchill Livingstone.
[2] Mariani G et al. (1984) *Clin. Lab. Haemat.*, 6, 229.

Polycythaemia Vera

This is a chronic, excessive and inappropriate production of red cells, generally regarded as a neoplastic disorder. It is associated with a high haemoglobin, raised red cell mass, normal plasma volume, increased white cell and platelet counts, and a tendency to the problems of hyperviscosity and thrombosis. The mean age is 60 years and the range is 15–90 years. The male to female ratio is 1.4:1.

PROGNOSIS

- If it is untreated, 50% patients will be dead within 18 months[1].
- If it is treated, the outlook is relatively good with a mean survival in excess of 12 years.
- 50% patients progress slowly to a refractory 'spent' phase with a failure of red cell production.
- 25% patients progress to a myelofibrosis type of disease.
- 15% patients develop an acute leukaemic transformation, usually myeloblastic.
- The remainder succumb to other complications or disorders.

TREATMENT

1. At diagnosis venesection should be performed up to 500 ml on alternate days, depending on the patient's tolerance, until haematocrit is less than 45%. The volume and frequency should be less in elderly patients. The median survival on venesection alone is 3–5 years.
2. Radioactive phosphorus (^{32}P dibasic sodium salt) 5 mCi i.v. The effect is seen in about 6–12 weeks. Further doses up to a total of 15 mCi in one year may be used. This should usually be repeated in about 12–18 months and thereafter as necessary until the disease is refractory. Ideal for elderly patients[2].
3. Chemotherapy: busulphan should be given 2–4 mg daily until the red cell proliferation is controlled. Control may depend more on the white cell and platelet count. The dose should be reduced or stopped as indicated by the counts. Care is needed since an overdose may produce busulphan aplasia. Melphelan 2 mg daily is given along the same lines as busulphan. Chlorambucil should be avoided, as it has been shown to promote the development of acute leukaemic transformation.
4. The refractory phase may require blood transfusion support.
5. The patient should be monitored for folate deficiency and given 5 mg folic acid weekly if it is required.
6. Venesection produces iron deficiency. Treatment is unnecessary if the patient is asymptomatic. If there are side-effects, e.g. sore mouth, angular stomatitis, 200 mg of ferrous sulphate weekly is often enough to eliminate symptoms.

FOLLOW-UP

There should be regular three monthly blood counts and clinical scrutiny, more often if patient is on chemotherapy, depending on the stability of the control. After ^{32}P with very stable disease, six monthly review is adequate.

---

[1] Gilbert HS (1975) *Clin. Haemat.*, **4**, 263.
[2] Loeb V Jr (1975) *Clin. Haemat.*, **4**, 441.

Acute Lymphoblastic Leukaemia

This is due to a monoclonal defect in maturation of primitive lymphoid elements which overgrow the bone marrow and spill in increasing numbers into the peripheral blood. There is decreasing production of red cells, white cells and platelets, which gives rise to anaemia, susceptibility to infection and bleeding. A peak incidence is seen in children under the age of five. The incidence rises again in adults. About 70% are the common type (cALL), 27% T-cell, 1% B-cell and 2% Null cell.

PROGNOSIS

- Good prognostic features at diagnosis are:

  a) Age 2-5.
  b) Female sex (in children).
  c) Low total white cell count – less than $5 \times 10^9/l$.
  d) Absence of thrombocytopenia – more than $150 \times 10^9/l$.
  e) cALL type disease.
  f) Lymphadenopathy – none.

- Survival disease-free for patients with these good prognostic features is greater than 90% at five years. The majority are probably cured.
- Bad prognostic features are:

  a) Age. The prognosis worsens with increasing age in the adult and in infants less than one year old.
  b) Male sex (less significant in adults)[1].
  c) High total white cell count – greater than $200 \times 10^9/l$.
  d) Thrombocytopenia.
  e) Evidence of CNS involvement.
  f) B-cell (worst). T-cell is better than B-cell. L3 Burkitt type is very bad.

- In adults, the response to treatment is less good, but lasting remission can be achieved in about 30% patients. Relapse on treatment means a very grave outlook. Relapse off treatment – a second remission can be induced, but long-term freedom from disease is unlikely unless there is bone marrow transplantation.

TREATMENT

1. Remission induction. There are many regimes but they are mostly based on weekly vincristine 1.4 mg/m² i.v. (max 2 mg) with high dose prednisolone daily (40 mg/m²) and the addition of other drugs such as anthracyclines, l-asparaginase, cyclophosphamide. Good remission is usually established within the first six weeks[2,3,4].
2. Remission consolidation. Further chemotherapy with drugs such as 6-mercaptopurine, intrathecal methotrexate and cranial irradiation (24 cGy) as CNS prophylaxis.
3. Remission maintenance. This is usually a three month cycle of varying combinations of the above drugs given to eliminate residual disease. Treatment should be stopped after 2-3 years of maintenance.
4. Bone marrow transplantation is usually offered in second remission. 50% long-term survival claimed[5].

FOLLOW-UP

Long-term regular surveillance is required with regular blood counts and bone marrow. In the first year, six-weekly visits with marrow examination every three months. Thereafter the frequency can be diminished until after five years when an annual visit may suffice.

[1] Baccarani M et al. (1978) Br. Med. J., ii, 1646.
[2] Lister TA et al. (1978) Br. Med. J., i, 199.
[3] Willemze R et al. (1980) Scand. J. Haem., 24, 421.
[4] Kirshner J. et al. (1984) Butterworth Int. Med. Rev., 8, 190.
[5] Blacklock HA et al. (1984) Exp. Haemat., 12 Suppl. 15, 29.

Acute Myeloblastic Leukaemia

This is usually a rapidly progressive condition due to a defect in maturation of primitive myeloid (granulocytic, monocytic, erythrocytic and megakaryocytic) elements which accumulate in the marrow, overgrowing the normal elements. In turn, this causes production failure of red cells, white cells and platelets giving rise to problems of anaemia, infection and bleeding respectively. It occurs at all ages but the incidence rises sharply in old age[1]. Seven varieties are recognised by the French, American, British (FAB) classification: 1 – Myeloblastic, undifferentiated; 2 – Myeloblastic, differentiating; 3 – Hypergranular or hypogranular promyelocytic; 4 – Myelomonocytic; 5 – Monocytic; 6 – Erythroblastic; 7 – Megakaryoblastic.

PROGNOSIS

- Without treatment half the patients die in the first five weeks; 99% are dead within one year.
- With adequate treatment the results depend on intensity of treatment and adequacy of supportive care. The overall median survival at all ages is 12 months. There is a five year survival of about 20%. The remission rates for patients under the age of 60 is over 70%. Over the age of 60 it is less than 50%. There is a five year survival for patients obtaining remission of about 30%.
- For patients receiving allogeneic bone marrow transplantation, the survival curve plateaus at 40%.
- For autologous bone marrow transplantation in first remission there is a 70% survival at three years.
- There is no significant difference in prognosis for the various FAB types if age is taken into consideration.

TREATMENT

1. Curative intent. This requires aggressive ablation of disease. There are many regimes. The majority use three drugs: anthracycline, cytosine arabinoside and 6-thioguanine. These are given intensively for 2–5 pulses[2].
2. Consolidation and maintenance therapy. The value is not fully established. Late intensification is of value. The benefit of immuno-therapy is marginal. CNS prophylaxis is not usually given.
3. Palliative therapy

    a) Supportive therapy only with transfusion etc.
    b) Non-aggressive therapy with cytotoxic agents such as 6-mercaptopurine, cytosine arabinoside.

4. Bone marrow transplantation (available to only 10% patients). This requires patient to be aged less than 40, have a histocompatible sibling donor and a good first remission. The best results are seen in younger patients. Graft versus host disease is an increasing problem as age increases.
5. Autologous bone marrow transplantation early in first remission either with:

    a) Intensive chemotherapy and rescue with autograft done twice in succession; or
    b) Once with preparation with cyclophosphamide and total body irradiation as for allogeneic transplantation.

FOLLOW-UP

Long-term regular surveillance is required with peripheral blood and bone marrow monitoring.

[1] Boros L et al. (1984) Butterworth Int. Med. Rev., 8 104.
[2] Lister TA et al. (1984) Butterworth Int. Med. Rev. 8, 136.

Chronic Myeloid Leukaemia

Chronic myeloid leukaemia is a monoclonal neoplastic disorder affecting the pluripotent haemopoietic stem cells in the marrow and characterised by an uncontrolled proliferation of myeloid cells. In the majority of cases this involves the neutrophil precursors predominantly, but rarely the eosinophil or basophil precursors dominate. The Philadelphia chromosome (Ph[1] (9q+, 22q−)) is present in 90% cases and usually affects all cells analysed. About 10% cases are Ph[1] negative. 85% cases are over 30 years of age. The male to female ratio is Ph[1] positive 1.3:1; Ph[1] negative 2:1.

PROGNOSIS

- Ph[1] positive cases have a median survival of 40 months. For Ph[1] negative cases it is 16 months unless the patient presents with a platelet count greater than $260 \times 10^9/l$ when the prognosis is similar to Ph[1] positive cases.
- Poor prognostic findings at diagnosis include:

  a) Haemoglobin less than $10\,g/dl$.
  b) Platelet count less than $150 \times 10^9/l$ or greater than $1000 \times 10^9/l$.
  c) More than 5% blast cells in blood.
  d) Splenomegaly greater than $10\,cm$ below the costal margin.
  e) Absence of Ph[1] chromosome with platelet count less than $250 \times 10^9/l$.

- Bone marrow transplantation: syngeneic has a 65% survival, recurrence of leukaemia occurs in the others[1]. It is too early to be sure about allogeneic, but results are encouraging. The majority of patients who survive disease-free at one year are possibly cured.
- Autografting in accelerated phase or blast crisis brings about a disappointingly brief re-establishment of chronic phase in the majority of patients.

TREATMENT

1. Bone marrow transplantation is the only hope of cure. Patients under 40 are screened for the availability of a compatible sibling donor. Syngeneic transplant if there is an identical twin available[1].
2. Chemotherapy. The following regimes are available:

   a) Busulphan $4\,mg$ daily until white cell count is approximately $20 \times 10^9/l$. Treatment should be stopped and restarted with a smaller dose to maintain counts around $10 \times 10^9/l$ by dosage adjustment. The number of days per week the dose is given should be varied.
   b) Busulphan $2\,mg$ plus 6-thioguanine $80\,mg$ daily five days per week until the white cell count is approximately $10 \times 10^9/l$, then dose should be reduced gently to maintain counts as above. White cell count reduction is very rapid, but should plateau in the normal range[2].
   c) Hydroxyurea $0.5-2\,g$ daily. Control is as for busulphan. This is useful in the accelerated phase.
   d) Dibromomannitol $250-750\,mg$ daily. Control is as for busulphan. There is no advantage over busulphan.
   e) Aggressive combination therapy. This is of doubtful advantage as there is much morbidity.
   f) Interferon 2.5 mega units daily – early results suggest that this can induce control of disease and reduction in Ph[1] positivity[3].

3. Leukapheresis – this is useful to reduce hyperviscosity from very high white cell counts.
4. Allopurinol therapy – 300 mg daily during initial treatment to control urate production and avoid secondary gout.
5. Splenic irradiation – this is superseded by chemotherapy. It may be used for intractable splenomegaly, and also as primary treatment.
6. Splenectomy – mainly used for physical problems of excessively large spleens.

Contd.

FOLLOW-UP

Monthly blood counts should be done while on chemotherapy and three-monthly if not on specific therapy.

[1] Goldman JM *et al.* (1984) *Butterworth Int. Med. Rev.*, 8, 239.
[2] Allan NC *et al.* (1978) *Lancet*, ii, 523.
[3] Freireich EJ *et al.* (1984) *Cancer*, 54, 2741.

Chronic Lymphocytic Leukaemia

This is a chronic progressive monoclonal proliferation of lymphocytes with a persistent blood lymphocytosis above $10 \times 10^9/l$. About 98.5% patients have B-cell, 1.5% T-cell type of disease[1]. It is associated with lymphadenopathy, hepatosplenomegaly, bone marrow overgrowth by lymphocytes eventually leading to marrow failure, and progressive reduction in immune competence due to reduction in immunoglobulin levels. The majority of patients are over 50 years and men are affected almost twice as often as women. It is rare among Chinese.

PROGNOSIS

- Binet prognostic groupings[2]:

  a) Group A (55%): <3 involved sites; haemoglobin >10 g/dl; platelet count >$100 \times 10^9/l$. Good prognosis; median survival >10 years.
  b) Group B (30%): ≥3 involved sites; haemoglobin and platelets as Group A. Intermediate prognosis; median survival seven years.
  c) Group C (15%): haemoglobin <10 g/dl; platelets <$100 \times 10^9/l$. Poor prognosis; median survival two years.

- Bone marrow histology is the best single parameter of prognosis[3].

TREATMENT[4]

1. Group A: often no treatment is required. May be observed for years.
2. Groups B and C: chlorambucil 0.05–0.15 mg/ kg body weight daily indefinitely or 0.5 mg/ kg body weight daily, four days per month.
3. If bone marrow rescue is required, the above treatment should be preceded by predniso-lone 40 mg/m² daily for 2–4 weeks, and continued for a further four weeks after chlorambucil is started. If an intermittent chlorambucil regime is employed, it should be combined with intermittent steroids.

4. Radiotherapy (as an alternative therapy)

   a) Splenic irradiation 100 cGy weekly for 10 courses is effective. Best if splenomegaly is present.
   b) Total body irradiation 15 cGy two times per week for five weeks is effective.
   c) Radioactive phosphorus is generally unsatisfactory.

5. Intensive combination chemotherapy – reserve for later stages of disease.
6. Leukapheresis can reduce counts but not organomegaly. Useful for very high white cell counts.
7. Interferon – role not clearly defined.
8. Gammaglobulin – for recurrent infection, sometimes of benefit.
9. Specific immunotherapy with idiotypic antibody – transient benefit: not yet fully evaluated.

FOLLOW-UP

The patient should be followed-up regularly, monthly to six monthly depending on need.

[1] Catovsky D (1984) *Butterworth Int. Med. Rev.*, **8**, 266.
[2] Binet JL et al. (1981) *Cancer*, **48**, 198.
[3] Rozman C et al. (1984) *Blood*, **64**, 642.
[4] Galton DAG (1984) *Butterworth Int. Med. Rev.*, **8**, 299.

Hodgkin's Lymphoma

This is a neoplastic disorder affecting the lymphoid tissue and characterised by progressive lymphadenopathy, organomegaly and histologically by the Reed–Sternberg cell. Four histological types are recognised; lymphocyte predominant (LP), nodular sclerosing (NS), mixed cellularity (MC) and lymphocyte depleted (LD). The disease has a peak incidence in young adults and a second peak may be observed between 50 and 70 years. It affects males more frequently than females. The nodular sclerosing variety is the most common and occurs particularly in young women.

PROGNOSIS

- Depends on clinical stage at diagnosis.

  a) Stage I: five-year survival 94%.
  b) Stage II: five-year survival 91%; if B symptoms 79%.
  c) Stage III: five-year survival 77%; if B symptoms 56%.
  d) Stage IV: five-year survival 70%; if B symptoms 41%.

- Each stage is divided into A, those with no systemic symptoms, and B, those with one or more of the following:

  a) Weight loss exceeding 10% body weight in previous six months.
  b) Drenching night sweats.
  c) Fevers.

- Histological type five-year survival:

  a) Lymphocyte predominant 65%.
  b) Nodular sclerosing 55%.
  c) Mixed cellularity 30%.
  d) Lymphocyte depleted 20%.

TREATMENT

1. Radiotherapy: 35–40 cGy in divided doses over 4–5 weeks. The use is now largely restricted to stage IA and stage IIA with less than three sites involved. Also for residual disease after chemotherapy (combined modality) and debulking tumour in emergencies.

2. Combination chemotherapy for all stages with B symptoms, and stage IIA with three or more sites involved, stage IIIA and IVA.

   a) The original regime was MOPP[1]: mustine HCl 6 mg/m^2 i.v. days 1 and 8; vincristine 1.4 mg/m^2 i.v. days 1 and 8; procarbazine 100 mg/m^2 orally for 14 days; prednisolone 40 mg/m^2 orally for 14 days; six cycles of 28 days.
   b) Two variants are MVPP[2] where vinblastine replaces vincristine and ChLVPP[3] where chlorambucil replaces mustine.
   c) Two alternative regimes are ABVD[4]: adriamycin, bleomycin, vinblastine, DTIC, and EVAP: etoposide, vinblastine, adriamycin, prednisolone.
   d) Many other regimes are being evaluated.

3. Emergency therapy, e.g. if there is pressure on a vital structure. Patient is given a large single dose of mustine HCl or radiotherapy.

FOLLOW-UP

After treatment is finished, follow-up is three monthly in first year; four monthly in second year; six monthly during years 3–5; and annually thereafter.

---

[1] De Vita VT et al. (1970) Ann. Int. Med., 73, 881.
[2] McElwain TJ et al. (1973) Nat. Cancer Inst. Monograph, 36, 395.
[3] McElwain TJ et al. (1977) Br. J. Cancer, 36, 276.
[4] Bonadonna G et al. (1977) Cancer Treatment Rep., 61, 769.

Non-Hodgkin's Lymphoma

This is a diverse, difficult to classify group of monoclonal neoplastic disorders of the lymphoid system. The great majority are B-cell in type, a minority T-cell and are distinguished from Hodgkin's lymphoma by the absence of Reed–Sternberg cells, clinical presentation and disease progression. They are divided broadly into two groups depending on the histological architecture of the biopsy material: a) nodular (follicular); and b) diffuse. In both groups the lymphoid cells show varying degrees of differentiation allowing further subclassification. The disease may arise in the lymphoid system (nodal) or outside (extranodal), e.g. stomach, thyroid etc. The majority of patients are stage III or IV at diagnosis. Nodular disease occurs mainly in the age group 30–60 years; diffuse disease occurs at all ages. These diseases merge with the lymphoid leukaemias and may become leukaemic.

PROGNOSIS

- Cases fall roughly into two main groups, those with a good prognosis and those with intermediate or poor prognosis.

    a) Group A: Good prognosis – nodular histology (except those with lymphoblast cells, i.e. histiocytic in the Rappaport classification) and diffuse well-differentiated lymphocytic histology. Median survival 7–10 years.

    b) Group B: Intermediate or poor prognosis – 'diffuse' histology except those with well-differentiated lymphocytic cells. Median survival 2–3 years.

- There is a subset among group B of large cell lymphomas (Rappaport diffuse histiocytic[1]) who show up to 60% long-term remission with aggressive combination chemotherapy and may be cured.
- Group A are incurable unless by bone marrow transplantation.

TREATMENT

1. If patient is asymptomatic prognosis is good: observation only is needed.
2. Chemotherapy: the treatment of choice for the majority of patients unless they are proven to be stage I or limited stage II.

    a) Group A: single agent therapy chlorambucil 2–5 mg daily. No proven advantage for combination chemotherapy.

    b) Group B: CHOP (cyclophosphamide, adriamycin, vincristine, prednisolone: 21 day cycle for 6–12 pulses); BACOP[2] (bleomycine, adriamycin, cyclophosphamide, vincristine, prednisolone); MBACOP[3] (with methotrexate).

3. Radiotherapy: stage I and II disease, and local problems, e.g. disease involving spinal cord. Total body irradiation for good prognosis disease is effective. Total nodal irradiation – very damaging to bone marrow reserves.
4. Combined modality (chemotherapy plus radiotherapy) is useful when bulk disease is present.
5. Interferon: value not yet established.
6. Supportive therapy: blood transfusion for anaemia, antibiotics for infection and platelets for thrombocytopenic bleeding.
7. Aggressive therapy requires specialist centre care.

FOLLOW-UP

Patient should have regular 1–6 monthly surveillance for life. Patients in long-term remission may require only annual visits to clinic.

---

[1] Rappaport H (1966) *Atlas of Tumour Pathology*, Section III, p. 97. Washington DC: Armed Forces Institute of Pathology.
[2] Schien PS *et al.* (1976) *Ann. Int. Med.*, 85, 417.
[3] Scarin A *et al.* (1980) *ASCO Abstracts*, c, 568.

Myeloma

Myeloma is a neoplastic clonal proliferation of immuno incompetent plasma cells usually capable of producing abnormal immunoglobulins or light chains, but with poor immune function. Overgrowth of the marrow displaces normal haemopoietic tissue and stimulates osteoclast activity causing both osteoporosis, locally destructive bone lesions and increased calcium mobilisation. Immunoglobulin production is excessive and monoclonal (M protein). Excessive light chain production causes renal tubular damage. Immune incompetence renders patients susceptible to infection. Males are slightly more commonly affected than females. 98% patients are over 35 years. The incidence peaks about 60 years of age. Approximately 50% are IgG, 20% IgA, 20% Bence-Jones. IgM, IgD and IgE are rare. 1% are nonsecretory and 2% have plasma cell leukaemia.

PROGNOSIS

- The prognosis depends on:

  a) How far the disease is advanced at diagnosis. The earlier the better.
  b) The rate of disease progression. The slower the progression the better the prognosis.

- Response to treatment: rapid response usually means rapid relapse; slow response is better. 20% show little or no response but this is not always bad.
- Type of immunoglobulin class: IgG has a better prognosis than IgA, which is better than Bence-Jones which is better than nonsecretory. Kappa light chain is better than Lambda.
- Irreversible renal failure at diagnosis means a poor prognosis.
- If it is untreated, the median survival is seven months.
- If it is treated, the median survival is 28 months[1]. Some patients survive for many years.

TREATMENT

1. Alkylating agents

   a) Melphalan $7 \, mg/m^2$ daily or $0.25 \, mg/kg$ for four days every 3–6 weeks under blood count control until the drop in paraprotein level remains static for six months. Melphalan may be combined with prednisolone $40 \, mg/m^2$ daily.
   b) Cyclophosphamide $250 \, mg/m^2/day$ for four days orally as for melphalan. There is no advantage. More hair loss. Given as weekly i.v. dose of $300 \, mg/m^2$ it is useful, especially when there are problems of treatment-induced cytopenia.
   c) Vincristine – does not have a proven value as an addition to the above drugs.
   d) High dose melphalan[2] $140 \, mg/m^2$ i.v. stat with hyperhydration following priming with cyclophosphamide $300 \, mg/m^2$ i.v. seven days before. It is used in patients up to 60 years of age. It is best in the young. It requires intensive care and support and further evaluation.
   e) Combination chemotherapy – this is recommended mainly for relapsed or very aggressive disease. VAD (vincristine, adriamycin, dexamethasone) regime[3] – success may be due mainly to high dose dexamethasone.
   f) Radiotherapy is best reserved for treating local painful lesions, space occupying lesions and fractures, for which it is the most effective management.

2. Hypercalcaemia – requires high fluid intake prednisolone $60 \, mg/day$; calcitonin; phosphates; mithramycin $0.25 \, mg/kg$ body weigh – beware thrombocytopenia.
3. Renal failure – requires high fluid intake dialysis. The myeloma should be treated Alkalinisation of urine may be of some value.
4. Hyperuricaemia – allopurinol $300 \, mg$ daily high fluid intake.
5. Hyperviscosity – plasmapheresis will contain the problem until specific therapy take effect.

FOLLOW-UP

Lifelong six weekly visits for surveillance are required, more frequent when treated intensively. In particular, the level of paraprotein band in the plasma and light chains in the urine should be monitored. β microglobulin estima-tions are also useful in gauging the activity of disease.

[1] Durie BGM et al. (1982) Clin. Haemat., 11, 181.
[2] McElwain TJ et al. (1983) Lancet, ii, 822.
[3] Barlogie B et al. (1984) New Eng. J. Med., 310, 21.

Idiopathic Myelofibrosis

This is a myeloproliferative disorder characterised by excessive proliferation of haemopoietic elements in the bone marrow together with progressive fibrosis of the marrow space which displaces the haemopoietic tissue. The fibrosis is believed to be reactive and the primary defect in the haemopoietic cells. Primitive erythrocyte and leucocyte precursors appear in the blood (leucoerythroblastic) and tissues, particularly the liver and spleen (myeloid metaplasia). Characteristic mis-shapen red cells (tear drop poikilocytes) are seen. Massive hepatosplenomegaly is characteristic although occasionally absent. The male to female ratio is 1:1. Prevalence is 2 per 100 000. Median age 60, range 30–80.

PROGNOSIS

- Very variable: some may live for decades. The median survival is about 5–6 years[1].
- Good prognostic signs at diagnosis are:

  a) Absence of anaemia.
  b) Platelets more than 100×10^9/l.
  c) Absence of hepatosplenomegaly.

- The degree of splenomegaly bears no relationship to prognosis.

TREATMENT

1. If patient is asymptomatic, only observation is necessary.
2. Exclude folate deficiency. 5 mg folic acid weekly should be adequate.
3. Check for hyperuricaemia. Allopurinol 300 mg daily should be given if it is present. A good fluid intake should be advised.
4. Anabolic steroids: oxymetholone 50–150 mg daily, starting with a small dose and building up. Liver function (especially alamine transaminase) should be maintained. It takes months for the full effect to be seen. Results are unpredictable but can be very good.
5. Corticosteroids: prednisolone may curtail fibrosis and improve the patient's wellbeing. Should be combined with a small dose of anabolic steroids. It is not suitable for long-term therapy.
6. Blood transfusion and filtered red cell concentrate should be used, but only if essential. Enough should be given to maintain the quality of life.
7. Splenectomy[2]: this is recommended for discomfort and high transfusion requirement. Should be performed before spleen becomes too large.
8. Bone marrow transplantation: this should be considered for a patient under 40 years with a histocompatible sibling donor.
9. Thrombocytopenic bleeding: platelet cover and corticosteroids should be given. Infection requires antibiotic therapy.
10. Hypermetabolic symptoms: beta blockade is often helpful.
11. Chemotherapy: caution is necessary as patients are often very sensitive. Busulphan is best avoided unless platelet count is high. Hydroxyurea 500 mg daily with blood count monitoring; increase the dose if necessary.
12. Splenic irradiation: this may be tried for reduction of spleen size when splenectomy is not possible.

FOLLOW-UP

There should be regular surveillance 1–6 monthly depending on need lifelong.

---

[1] Ward HP et al. (1971) Medicine, 50, 357.
[2] Benbassa J et al. (1979) Br. J. Haemat., 42, 207.

9
Diseases of Joints and Connective Tissue

G. R. V. Hughes

Rheumatoid Arthritis

Rheumatoid arthritis (RA) is a common multi-system disorder of unknown aetiology characterised by a symmetrical erosive polyarthritis and variable heart, lung, eye and nervous system involvement.

PROGNOSIS

- 20-30% patients have an intermittent course, with recurrent remissions and relatively mild disease[1].
- 10% have long clinical remissions, lasting for several years, with or without later flares[2].
- About 65% pursue a course of remissions and exacerbations and moderate to severe disease.
- An acute explosive onset of disease may have a better prognosis than disease with an insidious onset.
- Female sex, nodules, high titres of rheumatoid factor, eosinophilia and marked thrombocytosis are all associated with a poorer prognosis; slow onset in the elderly tends to indicate a relatively benign course[3].
- Palindromic onset of disease is associated with a relatively good prognosis[4]. 25% patients with palindromic rheumatism develop RA.
- Extra-articular involvement includes lung disease (typically interstitial fibrosis, pleural disease or nodules), cardiac disease (pericardial effusion or myocarditis), systemic vasculitis, Felty's syndrome and amyloidosis[5]. Systemic involvement may lead to death, most commonly from vasculitis.

TREATMENT

1. Non-steroidal drugs (e.g. ibuprofen, indomethacin, naproxen) provide a mainstay of symptomatic therapy, although side-effects (usually gastrointestinal) often limit their use.
2. The same is true of aspirin (4-6 g daily), which though effective has a high incidence of gastric toxicity.
3. Intramuscular gold (sodium aurothiomalate, Myocrisin) is used as a disease-modifier in disease which is uncontrolled by 1 and 2:

a) A commonly used regime starts with a 10 mg test dose, followed by 50 mg weekly for 12 weeks and then 50 mg monthly.
b) Attempts at 'tailoring' of dosage may be tried and are often successful.
c) Remission, total or partial, occurs in 40-60%, after 6-12 weeks.
d) The gold is withdrawn if there is no response after 1 g.
e) Side-effects occur in 25-30%. Rash and/or oral ulceration is the commonest side-effect. It is usually mild but can occasionally give a severe desquamating dermatitis. Marrow suppression (especially thrombocytopenia) and proteinuria are much less common but also require withdrawal from gold permanently.
f) Regular monitoring of urine for proteinuria and full blood count is essential. A rising eosinophil count may herald an allergic reaction.

4. D-Penicillamine tablets. The starting dose is 125 mg daily, increasing 2-4 weekly to a total dose of 500-750 mg in a single daily dose. Used as an alternative to gold it has a similar success rate and range of side effects. Response may take 12 weeks or longer.
5. Anti-malarials (e.g. hydroxychloroquine 200 mg daily) may act as disease-modifiers. The risk of ocular toxicity is minimal at this dose.
6. Immunosuppressives. Azathioprine has anti-inflammatory as well as immunosuppressive effects. It is most often used in conjunction with steroids as a steroid-sparing agent. It may be used if gold and penicillamine have failed. Due to its toxicity cyclophosphamide is rarely used.
7. Corticosteroids are reserved for progressive disease, progressive rheumatoid vasculitis

scleritis, iritis, pericarditis, pleuritis and Felty's syndrome. Steroids should only be used in younger age groups if other second line treatment has failed. Prednisolone 7.5 mg given once daily in the morning minimises the long-term risks of steroid therapy. A dosage of 5–7.5 mg may produce a very good clinical response in the elderly. The evidence for 'pulse' high dose i.v. steroids suggests benefit is short lived and side-effects are not uncommon.

8. The usefulness of plasmapheresis is still unclear.

9. Intra-articular steroids (e.g. methylprednisolone) are often helpful in providing temporary or long-lasting relief in one or two particularly troublesome joints.

10. Yttrium synovectomy is occasionally used for recurrent uncontrolled synovitis of the knee.

11. Surgery may play an important role in advanced disease. Operations include tendon repair, removal of metatarsal heads, wrist fusion and total hip and knee replacements.

12. Bed rest may help articular symptoms but good physiotherapy is important at all stages. Mobility and muscle power should be maintained; hydrotherapy, if available, is particularly useful. Splints (especially for the wrists at night) help to rest joints and prevent contractures. A cervical collar, unless fitted with a brace to chest and skull, is of no useful mechanical support in protection of atlanto-axial subluxation, but serves as a warning to patient and others to take care when handling, e.g. for an anaesthetic. Palliative physiotherapy (e.g. wax baths) may provide some symptomatic relief.

13. Home aids (e.g. special cutlery, tap handles, rails, raised toilet seat, etc.) and occupational therapy are important adjuncts to medical treatment.

FOLLOW-UP

Frequency of follow-up is dependent on the severity of symptoms, disability and medication. Those on gold and penicillamine should have monthly blood counts (including eosinophil counts) and urine tests for proteinuria. Those receiving immunosuppressive therapy also require monthly blood counts.

[1] Short CL (1968) *Med. Clin. North Am.*, 52, 549.
[2] Short CL *et al.* (1948) *New Eng. J. Med.*, 238, 142.
[3] Corrigan AB *et al.* (1974) *Br. Med. J.*, i, 444.
[4] Mattingley S (1966) *Ann. Rheum. Dis.*, 25, 307.
[5] Cobb S *et al.* (1953) *New Eng. J. Med.*, 249, 553.

Juvenile Chronic Arthritis

Juvenile chronic arthritis (JCA) describes a group of conditions presenting in children under 16 years old in whom inflammatory arthritis affecting four or more joints is present for at least three months, or synovial biopsy findings resemble those of adult rheumatoid arthritis. Many children go on to develop a recognisable adult rheumatic disease such as rheumatoid arthritis, ankylosing spondylitis or psoriatic arthritis. The incidence of JCA is approximately one child per 10 000 per year[1].

PROGNOSIS

- Pauciarticular onset usually affects girls under five years old, commonly with one to four large joints affected. Up to 50% develop chronic iridocyclitis; positive ANF is a strong risk factor for this complication. A pauciarticular onset may also occur in older boys of tissue type HLA-B27.
- Polyarticular onset, rheumatoid factor negative: this group, usually young girls, tends to develop a widespread polyarthritis of rheumatoid type, but only mild systemic features.
- Seropositive polyarticular onset ('juvenile rheumatoid arthritis') carries a poorer long-term prognosis than other types of JCA.
- Overall prognosis for all groups: for the majority this is good or excellent. Approximately 10% enter adult life with severe disability.
- Levels of IgM rheumatoid factor are of prognostic value in children with arthritis. Most children ultimately developing a clinical disease pattern similar to adult rheumatoid arthritis are persistently IgM RF positive early in the disease[2].
- Death occurs in 2–4% and is usually due to renal failure or amyloidosis[3].

TREATMENT

1. Salicylates (80–90 mg/kg per day) suppress fever and inflammation in the majority.
2. Other non-steroidal anti-inflammatory drugs (e.g. ibuprofen) are increasingly used as an alternative to aspirin.
3. Gold or D-penicillamine may be used in patients unresponsive to conservative ther-

apy. Both result in overall improvement in about 60% cases[4] (see p. 170 for toxicity monitoring).
4. Corticosteroids are used for life-threatening or uncontrollable disease. They do not alter the prognosis. Gradual reduction of dose whenever possible is important, particularly in view of growth retardation.
5. Intra-articular steroids are used for one or two isolated 'hot' joints.
6. Systemic and/or local steroids should be given for chronic uveitis.
7. Immunosuppressives are occasionally used for life-threatening disease.
8. Bed rest with splints at night, combined with physiotherapy to retain muscle strength and mobility and hydrotherapy are useful.
9. Surgery, e.g. synovectomy, is advised when medical treatment fails. Joints are replaced after cessation of growth if necessary.

FOLLOW-UP

Frequent follow-up is mandatory to ensure early treatment of any newly-involved joints or of any deformities which may occur. Patients on gold and penicillamine should have blood counts and urine tested monthly.

[1] Sullivan DB et al. (1975) Arth. Rheum., 18, 251.
[2] Ansell BM (1976) In Modern Topics in Rheumatology (Hughes GR ed.). London: William Heinemann Medical Books.
[3] Bywaters EGL (1977) Arth. Rheum., 20, 256.
[4] Ansell BM (1981) In Arthritis in Childhood (Moore TD ed.) pp. 127–30. Ross Laboratories: Columbus

Osteoarthritis

Osteoarthritis (OA) is the commonest articular cause of rheumatic complaints. It consists of a limited or widespread arthropathy, and may affect most axial and peripheral joints. It is characterised by cartilage loss and bony regeneration. It may be idiopathic, or secondary to mechanical injury, inflammation or other local damage. There is no visceral involvement. The ESR and Hb are normal and rheumatoid factor test is negative.

PROGNOSIS

- Symptoms, chiefly of pain, limitation of function and disuse stiffness, are variable depending on joint involvement.
- Primary generalised OA (occurring chiefly in middle-aged women) tends to run a mild course.
- Hand function is well preserved.
- Patients with diffuse idiopathic skeletal hyperostosis (DISH)[1] have chronic moderate symptoms, usually back pain.
- Major disability occurs in a small percentage overall. OA knee carries a worse prognosis than OA hip. Time between onset of hip pain and development of a high level of disability averages 8–10 years.
- For most patients OA is slowly progressive. Some develop intermittent acute flare-ups of the disease.

TREATMENT

1. Non-steroidal anti-inflammatory drugs (e.g. ibuprofen, indomethacin, naproxen) are the mainstay of treatment. Simple analgesics are also frequently used with symptomatic benefit.
2. Intra-articular steroid injection for an acute flare-up in one or two involved joints will give temporary or long-lasting symptomatic relief.
3. Weight loss is recommended in obese patients with involvement of spine or lower limb joints.
4. Physiotherapy should involve exercises to maintain muscle power and joint mobility.
5. Aids, e.g. spinal support, walking stick etc. may be required.
6. Any activity likely to exacerbate affected joint should be restricted or stopped altogether, if practical.
7. Surgery. Total hip or knee replacement for severely affected joints.

FOLLOW-UP

Follow-up is dependent on the severity of symptoms and disability.

---

[1] Forestier J et al. (1950) *Ann. Rheum. Dis.*, 9, 320.

Septic Arthritis

In this form of arthritis a joint is infected by pyogenic bacteria. A high index of suspicion should be maintained for sepsis in any acute arthritis, especially if it is a monarthritis. Most infections are due to haematological dissemination of organisms rather than following local trauma or arthrocentesis. The commonest organism causing septic arthritis is *Staphylococcus aureus*, but many others may be implicated including *Neisseria gonorrhoeae*, *Streptococcus pyogenes*, *Streptococcus faecalis*, *Escherischia coli*, *Haemophilus influenzae* and *pseudomonas*. It is commoner in the very young, the elderly, those with a joint prosthesis and those with reduced host resistance, e.g. diabetics and rheumatoid arthritics.

PROGNOSIS

- Untreated, septic destruction of the joint, osteomyelitis, ankylosis, septicaemia and death results.
- With early diagnosis and effective treatment the prognosis is good.
- The prognosis worsens with increasing time from onset of infection to institution of effective treatment[1].
- More virulent organisms will cause greater cartilage damage, and the prognosis is also worse in the presence of osteomyelitis.
- There is a poor prognosis in infections of the infantile hip. There are long-term complications including femoral shortening, femoral head and neck deformity and recurrent dislocation.

TREATMENT

1. Parenteral antibiotics on a 'best-guess' basis initially (e.g. amoxycillin and flucloxacillin). Once culture sensitivities are available, change to appropriate antibiotics if necessary. This therapy continues for two weeks and if the joint is responding, the oral route may be used for a further four weeks[2].
2. There is no indication for intra-articular steroids. Indeed, they may cause a postinfectious synovitis, which occurs after the acute arthritis has been controlled, and which appears as a recrudescence of the disease.
3. Daily aspiration of the joint through a widebore needle to dryness is important as the presence of pus causes enzymatic destruction of cartilage.
4. Surgical drainage of joint is only indicated in the case of the hip which is inaccessible to routine aspiration, or if the infected effusion is loculated.
5. Rest and immobilisation, which may include splinting, is necessary.
6. Physiotherapy in recovery phase to regain range of movement and power, and to minimise deformity.
7. Analgesics: patients may require narcotic analgesia for the first 48 hours followed by simple analgesics.

FOLLOW-UP

No long-term follow-up is required unless joint destruction has occurred.

---

[1] Goldenberg DL *et al.* (1976) *Am. J. Med.*, **60**, 369.
[2] Newman JH (1976) *Ann. Rheum. Dis.*, **35**, 198.

Reactive Arthritis

Reactive arthritis comprises a group of conditions in which a seronegative, mainly large joint polyarthritis occurs secondary to a bacterial or other infection. Reiter's disease is the commonest example: it may follow an episode of gastroenteritis or urethritis, and is largely confined to men. Agents causing reactive arthritis include chlamydia, salmonella, shigella and Yersinia.

PROGNOSIS

- The prognosis is difficult to assess in the individual patient.
- The disease may be persistent or recurrent in 60–70% patients[1,2].
- A small proportion of patients develop progressive iridocyclitis[3].
- Cardiac conduction defects or aortic regurgitation are detectable in 1%.
- The HLA-B27 antigen occurs in 80–90% patients and may predispose a patient to develop sacroiliitis, which occurs in 20–30% cases.
- 1% develop neurological complications.

TREATMENT

1. Eradication of precipitating infection, if this is persistent. (Efficacy at this stage is disputed.)
2. Non-steroidal anti-inflammatory agents (e.g. indomethacin) are the chief form of therapy. They provide symptomatic relief only.
3. Azathioprine or methotrexate may be tried in severe cases[4,5].
4. Joints should be rested and occasionally intra-articular steroids are indicated.

FOLLOW-UP

Long-term follow-up is unnecessary unless symptoms persist. In the case of Reiter's disease patients should be warned to avoid multiple sexual contacts because of the risk of reinfection and disease exacerbation. The use of sheaths may offer protection.

[1] Csonka GW (1960) *Arth. Rheum.*, 3, 164.
[2] Good AE (1962) *Ann. Int. Med.*, 57, 44.
[3] Sairanen D *et al.* (1969) *Acta Medica Scand.*, 185, 57.
[4] Burns T *et al.* (1983) *Arth. Rheum. Suppl.*, 39.
[5] Farber B *et al.* (1967) *J. Am. Med. Assoc.*, 200, 171.

Psoriatic Arthritis

Psoriatic arthritis is a seronegative polyarthritis seen in 7% patients with psoriasis[1]. The clinical pattern is variable, but radiographic changes tend to be characteristic.

PROGNOSIS

- Overall prognosis is good, with minimal mortality.
- Most patients have predominant distal interphalangeal joint involvement, or a pattern of disease clinically indistinguishable from rheumatoid arthritis, though milder[2].
- 10% develop a severe deforming arthritis.
- Spondylitis develops in 40% and sacroiliitis in 21%[3].
- Extra-articular features are much less common than in rheumatoid arthritis.

TREATMENT

1. Non-steroidal anti-inflammatory agents are usually sufficient to control joint symptoms.
2. Gold and other second line agents may be helpful for resistant cases[4].
3. Immunosuppressive agents, particularly methotrexate, are used as a last resort.
4. Systemic steroids are best avoided but intra-articular injections are frequently helpful.

FOLLOW-UP

Frequency of follow-up is entirely dependent upon the extent and severity of disease.

[1] Leczinsky CG (1948) *Acta Dermatologica-Venereologica*, **28**, 483.
[2] Moll JMH *et al.* (1973) *Ann. Rheum. Dis.*, **32**, 181.
[3] Lambert JR *et al.* (1976) *Ann. Rheum. Dis.*, **35**, 354
[4] Richter MB *et al.* (1980) *Ann. Rheum. Dis.*, **39**, 279

Scleroderma

Scleroderma describes an inflammatory process of the skin causing thickening, tightening, oedema, fibrosis and later, calcinosis. This process may be seen in three major clinical conditions: morphoea, CREST syndrome and systemic sclerosis.

PROGNOSIS

- Morphoea consists of localised patches of scleroderma. It may be widespread and chronic, but the lack of visceral involvement results in a good overall prognosis[1].
- CREST syndrome describes the combination of calcinosis, Raynaud's phenomenon, 'esophageal' dysfunction, sclerodactyly and telangiectasia in association with minimal early visceral involvement, and therefore a relatively good prognosis[2].
- Systemic sclerosis may include the above features as well as bowel and skeletal involvement, cardiomyopathy, pulmonary disease and hypertension secondary to renal damage. Pulmonary fibrosis, reflux pneumonitis, pulmonary hypertension, systemic hypertension with renal disease, truncal scleroderma and age over 40 years are all associated with a poor prognosis. The five-year survival is about 75%.

TREATMENT

1. Morphoea: topical therapy is usually not helpful; physical therapy, and occasionally surgical correction may be indicated for contractures.
2. CREST syndrome and systemic sclerosis do not respond to specific therapy. Treatment is therefore largely palliative. However, systemic steroids may help active cutaneous disease and myositis and possibly early pulmonary fibrosis.
3. Vasodilators (e.g. nifedipine) are occasionally useful for Raynaud's phenomenon. There is no specific therapy for the scleroderma itself. Prompt local treatment of skin ulcers is important.
4. Hypertension should be treated vigorously, and renal failure identified early.
5. Oesophagus: metoclopramide, oesophageal dilatation, or even surgery.
6. Bowel: diet (e.g. bran, stool softeners) for hypodynamic bowel; antibiotics for bacterial overgrowth.
7. Medical therapy (e.g. aluminium hydroxide) for calcinosis is unsuccessful. Occasionally surgery is indicated for large deposits of calcium, e.g. limiting joint movement (notably in CREST syndrome).
8. Physical therapy: muscle exercises for associated muscle weakness; passive exercises to prevent contractures. Gloves for Raynaud's phenomenon and other precautions against the cold.

FOLLOW-UP

Patients should be followed-up 3–6 monthly to provide symptomatic relief. Blood pressure and renal function should be specifically monitored.

---

[1] Curtis AC et al. (1958) Arch. Derm., 78, 749.
[2] Winterbauer RH (1964) Bull. Johns Hopkins Hosp., 114, 361.
[3] Bennett RM et al. (1971) Ann. Rheum. Dis., 30, 581.

Systemic Lupus Erythematosus

Systemic lupus erythematosus (SLE) is a multi-system auto-immune disorder which typically affects women of childbearing age. The aetiology is unknown, but involves genetic, hormonal and environmental factors. With improved diagnostic tests mild cases are now more easily recognised. In the USA the prevalence has been reported as high as 1 in 2000 women aged between 15 and 45 years[1]. In South East Asia it may be more common than rheumatoid arthritis.

PROGNOSIS

- The outlook has changed dramatically in the last few years due to recognition of milder cases.
- Five-year survival may be as high as 98%[2].
- Renal disease is the most important feature affecting prognosis. It usually presents as proteinuria, nephrotic syndrome or microscopic haematuria. The histology on renal biopsy is a helpful predictor of the subsequent course.
- Cerebral disease is the other serious feature. It probably affects more than 70% patients, and may range from psychiatric illness, commonly depression (usually reversible), to epilepsy, cranial neuropathy, strokes and coma.
- Other clinical manifestations are protean. Those directly affecting prognosis include neutropenia (resulting in increased susceptibility to infection), thrombocytopenia, thrombosis and pericardial effusion.
- The arthritis rarely produces serious deformities.
- A distinct syndrome exists with thrombosis, recurrent abortions, thrombocytopenia and neurological disease, associated with high titres of lupus anticoagulant or anticardiolipin antibodies[3,4]. Some of these patients develop pulmonary hypertension[5].
- SLE is characterised by recurrent exacerbations and remissions. For individual patients fresh flares usually resemble earlier ones in their clinical pattern.
- The disease tends to become inactive after the menopause.
- The outlook for males does not in general differ from that for women.

TREATMENT

1. For mild disease, non-steroidal anti-inflammatory agents (e.g. ibuprofen, indomethacin) may be sufficient to control symptoms such as joint aches and pleuritic chest pain. High dose aspirin is best avoided (hepatotoxicity).

2. Antimalarials (e.g. hydroxychloroquine) are often useful for more active disease, especially cutaneous manifestations. Regular eye checks are needed.

3. Corticosteroids are the mainstay of treatment for severe disease. High doses (e.g 60 mg/day) are commonly employed. Dose reduction should be performed gradually with an attempt to achieve as low a dose as possible for maintenance[6]. Initial trials o methylprednisolone given in pulse form i.v are encouraging[7].

4. Azathioprine is useful in active disease particularly as a 'steroid-sparing' agent.

5. Cyclophosphamide (orally or in 'pulse form i.v.) is an important agent for sever lupus, especially glomerulonephritis and cerebral disease.

6. The efficacy of plasmapheresis in SLE is still controversial[8].

7. Hypertension, renal failure, epilepsy an other manifestations of organ dysfunctio should be treated appropriately. The agent normally associated with drug-induced lupus (e.g. methyldopa, phenytoin) are no contraindicated.

8. Certain agents frequently cause flares o SLE and are best avoided. The most common are sulphonamides (including Septrir and penicillin.

9. In patients with drug-induced lupus, withdrawal of the offending drug results in re solution of symptoms.

10. SLE *per se* is not a contraindication to renal transplantation.

FOLLOW-UP

Frequency of follow-up is dependent on severity of disease. Mild disease should be followed-up 6–12 monthly. Patients who have major organ involvement should be monitored closely.

[1] Fessel WJ (1974) *Arch. Int. Med.*, **134**, 1027.
[2] Grigor RR *et al.* (1978) *Ann. Rheum. Dis.*, 37, 121.
[3] Hughes GRV (1983) *Br. Med. J.*, **287**, 1088.
[4] Harris EN *et al.* (1983) *Lancet*, **ii**, 1211.
[5] Asherson RA *et al.* (1983) *Br. Med. J.*, **287**, 1024.
[6] Hughes GRV (1983) *Br. Med. J.*, **287**, 1088.
[7] Kimberley M (1982) *Clin. Rheum. Dis.*, **8**, 261.
[8] Verrier Jones J (1982) *Clin. Rheum. Dis.*, **8**, 243.

Giant Cell Arteritis

Giant cell (or cranial) arteritis (GCA) is a condition affecting those aged over 60 (but occasionally younger) characterised by inflammation in arteries rich in elastic tissue, notably the temporal and other extracranial arteries. This may lead to cranial neuropathies and blindness. There is an overlap between the condition and polymyalgia rheumatica.

PROGNOSIS

- Prognosis depends almost entirely upon the degree of ocular and nervous system damage, which may be largely irreversible. Prompt diagnosis and treatment may prevent the development of such lesions.
- The condition is rarely fatal. Brain stem or cerebral ischaemia occurs very occasionally.
- Involvement of branches of the ophthalmic artery may occur in 40-50%, leading in some cases (10%) to visual loss or blindness[1,2].
- Polymyalgia rheumatica may develop at any time. 40-60% patients with GCA are affected[3].
- Relapses may occur. Occasionally the disease follows a persistent course.

TREATMENT

Corticosteroids are required, initially in high doses (e.g. prednisolone 60 mg daily). These can usually be reduced after a few days, while the clinical state and ESR are carefully monitored. Over several months to two years, the dose may be gradually tailed off to zero, but patients should be followed-up for possible relapse.

FOLLOW-UP

Follow-up should be monthly to monitor the ESR and symptoms until the disease goes into remission. Because of the frequency of relapse, long-term follow-up should be maintained at 6–12 monthly intervals. Patients should be warned to contact the doctor immediately symptoms occur.

[1] Hamilton CR *et al.* (1971) *Medicine (Baltimore)*, **50**, 1.
[2] Hunder GG *et al.* (1969) *Mayo Clin. Proc.*, **44**, 849.
[3] Hunder GG *et al.* (1978) *Bull. Rheum. Dis.*, **29**, 980.

Polyarteritis Nodosa

Polyarteritis nodosa (PAN) is a rare disease characterised by intense inflammation of all three layers of small- and medium-sized arteries, leading to multiple small aneurysm formation, thrombosis and infarction. The wide range of clinical features includes fever, hypertension, renal disease, arthritis, pulmonary infiltration, coronary ischaemia, neuropathy and cerebral involvement.

PROGNOSIS

- In contrast to other systemic vasculitides, patients who recover from an initial life-threatening episode of PAN rarely develop second attacks. Five-year survival is about 60%; however, the majority of deaths occur within the first three months of illness[1].
- The major causes of death in the acute phase are hypertension[1], renal failure (about 25%)[2] and cerebral thrombosis.
- Cardiac involvement (usually coronary arteritis with or without myocardial infarction) occurs in up to 80%, and is the next commonest cause of death[3].
- Nervous system disease may be serious with CNS or cranial nerve involvement in 46%, and peripheral neuropathy in 68%[4]. Cerebral or brainstem lesions may be fatal.

Pulmonary involvement does not necessarily mean a poorer prognosis.

Those patients who survive an acute episode of classical PAN are unlikely to suffer a relapse although residual organ damage may be permanent.

Variants of PAN such as Wegener's granulomatosis and Churg–Strauss syndrome[5], have a more characteristically relapsing course.

Generally patients with visceral organ involvement have a poorer prognosis than those with skin and joint disease[1].

TREATMENT

1. High dose corticosteroids (e.g. prednisolone 60 mg/day) are used in the first instance. 'Pulse' methylprednisolone is now popular.
2. Immunosuppressive therapy in addition to steroids is now the treatment of choice. Cyclophosphamide (2–3 mg/kg/day) is effective in the majority of cases.
3. 'Pulse' intravenous cyclophosphamide (500 mg at increasing intervals) is currently being evaluated. Initial experience is encouraging.
4. Hypertension (a major and often severe problem) should be treated vigorously.
5. Specific organ damage should be managed in the conventional way (e.g. renal failure, myocardial infarction, stroke, bowel infarction) in addition to treatment for the arteritis itself.
6. Steroids and immunosuppressives should be gradually withdrawn if a remission is achieved.

FOLLOW-UP

Regular and frequent follow-up is important to monitor hypertension, renal function and cardiac involvement.

[1] Sack M et al. (1975) J. Rheum., 2, 411.
[2] Rose GA et al. (1957) Q. J. Med., 26, 43.
[3] Holsinger DR et al. (1962) Circulation, 25, 610.
[4] Ford RG et al. (1965) Neurology, 15, 124.
[5] Lanham JG et al. (1984) Medicine, 63, 2.

Ankylosing Spondylitis

Ankylosing spondylitis (AS) is a condition primarily affecting the axial skeleton, with new bone formation, ankylosis, and sacroiliitis. The prevalence for males and females is 4 and 0.5 per 1000, respectively[1]. There is a familial incidence with a polygenic mode of inheritance in 6%. Typical onset is age 15–30.

PROGNOSIS

- Most patients have disease limited to the pelvis and lower spine, and have a good prognosis.
- Severe or total ankylosis occurs in relatively few patients.
- 35% patients develop peripheral joint involvement.
- 25% develop conjunctivitis or iritis[2].
- Heart disease (most commonly aortic regurgitation) occurs in 3% cases following 15 or more years of active AS.
- Upper lobe pulmonary fibrosis is rare and is usually confined to patients with severe thoracic spinal spondylosis[3].
- Possession of HLA-B27 antigen does not affect the severity of the disease[4].

TREATMENT

1. Non-steroidal anti-inflammatory agents (e.g. indomethacin) are the mainstay of drug therapy. They give symptomatic relief and allow mobility to be maintained. Occasionally patients may need phenylbutazone to control pain, but this carries a small but significant risk of bone marrow suppression. All such patients should be monitored with blood counts.
2. Physiotherapy is important to maintain maximum mobility of spine (particularly extension), hips and ribs and to ensure a functional posture should fusion occur. Lying prone for half an hour twice daily is useful to maintain hip extension, an important movement if the spine is involved.
3. Surgery for severe joint disease, e.g. hip replacement.
4. Radiotherapy is now only rarely used owing to the risk of leukaemia.

FOLLOW-UP

Long-term follow-up should be undertaken at 6–12 monthly intervals for management of disease complications. The ESR is an unreliable index of disease activity.

[1] Lawrence JS (1956) Br. J. Clin. Prac., 17, 699.
[2] Blumberg BS et al. (1956) Medicine, 35, 1.
[3] Editorial (1971) Br. Med. J., 3, 492.
[4] Editorial (1978) Br. Med. J., ii, 650.

Polymyositis

Polymyositis is a condition involving chronic inflammation of muscle, with proximal muscle weakness, primarily skeletal. It typically presents in late middle-age. There is an important overlap with dermatomyositis, and many patients have the cutaneous features of that condition.

PROGNOSIS

- The highest proportion of deaths generally occurs in the first two years after diagnosis[1]. These are frequently related to respiratory muscle involvement. One study, however, showed 90% survival at two years and 80% at five years[2].
- Pneumonitis is the worst prognostic feature (usually due to aspiration); its likelihood is increased by oesophageal dysfunction.
- Pulmonary fibrosis is an infrequent complication which may contribute to late mortality. (Associated with the presence of the autoantibody Jo-1.)
- Myocardial involvement is uncommon[3].
- Children have a better prognosis than adults.
- The proportion of cases associated with underlying malignancy is unclear; it may be as low as 9% patients over the age of 40[4].

TREATMENT

1. Corticosteroids: high initial doses (e.g. prednisolone 60 mg/day) for florid cases. This dose may be reduced to the minimum level necessary to maintain a normal serum creatine kinase and symptomatic relief. If this necessitates a prednisolone dose over 10 mg daily, a steroid-sparing agent should be used, e.g. azathioprine.
2. Steroids are usually necessary even if improvement follows the resection of an underlying malignancy.
3. A small proportion of patients do not respond to steroids. Methotrexate, azathioprine or cyclophosphamide may be tried[5,6].
4. Total lymphoid or total body irradiation has been tried in a small number of patients. Initial studies indicate that it may have a place in inducing temporary remission in severely ill patients unresponsive to other therapy.
5. Physiotherapy to help maintain or improve muscle power is important.
6. Therapy may be monitored by myometry[7] and muscle enzymes.
7. It is important to distinguish muscle weakness caused by the disease from that due to steroid side-effects.

FOLLOW-UP

Regular follow-up should continue, even when the disease is in remission, with monitoring of ESR and serum creatine phosphokinase. As the frequency of associated malignancy is small, a routine chest x-ray is worthwhile, but extensive investigations for a primary tumour are not indicated without specific symptoms.

[1] Medsger TA et al. (1971) Arth. Rheum., 14, 249.
[2] DeVere R et al. (1975) Brain, 98, 637.
[3] Adams RD (1975) Diseases of Muscle 3rd edn. London: Harper and Row.
[4] Bohan A et al. (1977) Medicine, 56, 255.
[5] Malaviya AN et al. (1968) Lancet, ii, 485.
[6] Currie S et al. (1971) J. Neurol., Neurosurg. Psych., 34, 447.
[7] Morgan SH et al. (1985) Arth. Rheum., 28, 831.

Polymyalgia Rheumatica

Polymyalgia rheumatica (PMR) is predominantly a disease of the elderly, and is twice as common in women as in men[1]. The aetiology is unknown, although there is some evidence for a viral trigger[2]. It results in muscle stiffness and pain, predominantly in the pectoral girdle. Muscle tenderness is usually mild or absent. There is an important overlap with giant cell arteritis: one report detected the latter in up to 80% cases of PMR.

PROGNOSIS

- The disease tends to remit six months to two years after onset.
- Relapses may sometimes occur; occasionally the disease is persistent.
- Giant cell arteritis may appear at any time during the disease.
- The long-term outlook is good.

TREATMENT

1. In very mild cases non-steroidal drugs such as ibuprofen or indomethacin may be sufficient to control symptoms.
2. Almost all cases require steroids (e.g. prednisolone 20–30 mg per day). The dose should be reduced by 5 mg/month to 10 mg and then by 1 mg/month, if symptomatic relief is maintained and ESR remains below 20–25 mm/hour. The C-reactive protein kinase may also be used to monitor treatment response.
3. Physical therapy in the form of passive exercises to maintain mobility is useful.

FOLLOW-UP

Monthly follow-up to monitor the ESR and disease activity. When the disease is in remission annual follow-up is adequate.

[1] Hunder GG et al. (1978) Bull. Rheum. Dis., **29**, 280
[2] Bell WR et al. (1967) Johns Hopkins Med. J., **121**, 175.

Mixed Connective Tissue Disease

This is a group of disorders[1] with features of two or more of the connective tissue diseases: SLE, polymyositis and scleroderma. High risks to a ribonucleoprotein antigen (RNP) are present and a 'speckled' pattern ANF test. It commonly presents with Raynaud's phenomenon, polyarthritis (especially hands and feet) and abnormal oesophageal mobility[2]. It is commoner in women in the ratio 10:1.

PROGNOSIS

- Prognosis for life is good compared to the other connective tissue diseases[3].
- Renal disease is mild (10%) or absent (90%).
- Five-year survival of 95%[4].
- Morbidity, however, is marked, Raynaud's phenomenon being especially prominent.

TREATMENT

1. It may only require symptomatic treatment, e.g. NSAIDs for polyarthritis, nifedipine for Raynaud's phenomenon.
2. Low dose corticosteroids, e.g. prednisolone 5–10 mg daily.
3. Severe major organ involvement, when it does occur, requires high dose corticosteroids.

FOLLOW-UP

Follow-up should be 3–6 monthly depending on disease activity. Investigations should include blood counts for leucopenia, and renal function tests.

[1] Sharp GC et al. (1972) Am. J. Med., 52, 148.
[2] Bresnihan B et al. (1977) Ann. Rheum. Dis., 36, 557.
[3] Rao KV et al. (1976) Ann. Int. Med., 84, 174.
[4] Wolfe JF et al. (1977) Clin. Res., 25, 488A.

Felty's Syndrome

Felty's syndrome is a complication of rheumatoid arthritis consisting of splenomegaly and neutropenia. Other features may include thrombocytopenia, anaemia, lymphadenopathy, skin pigmentation and chronic leg ulceration. Sjögren's syndrome is frequently present, together with a positive antinuclear factor and high titres of rheumatoid factor. Less than 1% patients with rheumatoid arthritis develop Felty's syndrome. There is a strong association with HLA-DRW4[1].

PROGNOSIS

- The long-term outlook is poor: few patients survive more than 5–10 years.
- Death is usually due to infection (most commonly pulmonary) secondary to neutropenia and impaired neutrophil function.
- The outlook is not usually affected by the activity of the underlying rheumatoid arthritis.

TREATMENT

1. Specific therapy is largely ineffective in the long term.
2. Splenectomy usually reverses haematological abnormalities, but probably does not affect overall prognosis.
3. Prompt antibiotic treatment for bacterial infections is important.
4. D-Penicillamine or gold and immunosuppressives may improve neutropenia[2,3].
5. Lithium stimulates granuloporesis, but lasting benefit has not been demonstrated[4].
6. Corticosteroids are probably ineffective in most cases and predispose to infection.
7. Testosterone stimulates granuloporesis and may be of temporary help in males[5].

FOLLOW-UP

Blood counts should be performed regularly to monitor thrombocytopenia and neutropenia. Patients should be warned to take infections seriously.

[1] Dinant HJ et al. (1980) Arth. Rheum., 23, 1336.
[2] Luthra HS et al. (1981) J. Rheumatol., 8, 902.
[3] Goldberg A et al. (1980) Arth. Rheum., 10, 52.
[4] Gupta RC et al. (1976) Am. J. Med., 61, 29.
[5] Wimer BM et al. (1973) J. Am. Med. Assoc., 223, 671.

Sjogren's Syndrome

Sjögren's syndrome consists of the sicca syndrome (dry eyes and dry mouth) together with a connective tissue disease, usually rheumatoid arthritis[1]. Primary Sjögren's syndrome is generally regarded as a distinct clinical entity, characterised by the sicca syndrome, positive antinuclear factor, high titres of rheumatoid factor and circulating immune complexes, renal tubular acidosis and frequent drug allergies, together with some features of systemic lupus erythematosus (SLE)[2].

PROGNOSIS

- The overall prognosis depends largely upon that of the underlying disease.
- Primary Sjögren's syndrome tends to affect an older age group than SLE, and the outlook is generally good.
- Morbidity from neuropathy, multiple allergies, renal tubular acidosis and other organ involvement may contribute to disability and, occasionally, mortality.
- A small proportion (about 5%) develop lymphoma: this may be intra- or extra-salivary[3].

TREATMENT

1. Symptomatic treatment with methyl cellulose eye drops ('artificial tears'). Acetyl cysteine eye drops should be used if excess mucus is a problem. Surgery (electrocoagulation of the nasolacrimal gland or corneal grafting) is rarely indicated.
2. Increasing oral fluids (e.g. unsweetened lemon juice) helps to alleviate xerostomia. Saliva substitutes are unsatisfactory.
3. The marked tendency to dental caries makes good oral hygiene and regular visits to the dentist essential.

4. Saline soaks help to relieve nasal dryness.
5. Lubricants are required for dysparunia due to vaginal dryness.
6. Infection should be controlled with regular eye swabs; antibiotics for ocular infection, and superinfection of sialectatic parotids; and prompt antibiotic therapy for lung infection secondary to reduced bronchial secretions.
7. Small doses of prednisolone (e.g. 2–5 mg/ day) may relieve many of the symptoms.
8. Higher steroid doses (e.g. prednisolone > 10 mg/day) are required for pulmonary fibrosis or peripheral neuropathy.
9. Immunosuppressives are occasionally used for severe disease.

FOLLOW-UP

Long-term follow-up is unnecessary in isolated Sjögren's syndrome.

---

[1] Bloch KJ et al. (1965) Medicine, 44, 187.
[2] Moutsopoulos HM (1979) Am. J. Med., 66, 733.
[3] Anderson JR et al. (1972) Clin. Exp. Immunol., 10, 199.

Paget's Disease

This is a disorder of unknown aetiology characterised by disorganisation of the normal bony trabecular pattern, bone enlargement and bone deformity. It is usually associated with a raised serum alkaline phosphatase and increased 24 hour hydroxyproline excretion.

PROGNOSIS

- It occurs in 0.5% of the population at age 40, increasing to 10% at 90 years.
- 95% patients with radiological change are asymptomatic.
- 5% complain of chronic symptoms, usually bone pain[1] and deformity; other complications include arthritis of an involved joint, pathological fracture, neural compression from bony enlargement, or high output cardiac failure.
- 1% all patients with Paget's disease develop malignant change, almost always osteogenic sarcoma, but also fibrosarcoma, chondrosarcoma or giant cell tumours. Such cases have a 2% five-year survival.

TREATMENT

1. No treatment is indicated for asymptomatic Paget's disease.
2. Simple analgesics for mild bone pain, or NSAIDs if a joint is involved causing a degenerative arthritis.
3. For troublesome bone pain or nerve compression syndromes: synthetic salmon calcitonin by subcutaneous or i.m. injection 50–100 units, three times a week, and increasing to daily if necessary, usually for 3–6 months. The effect is monitored with symptom response, serum alkaline phosphatase (should fall) and/or urinary hydroxyproline excretion (should fall). The dose may be limited by side-effects—commonly nausea, vomiting, flushing, metallic taste and rash.
4. An alternative to calcitonin is disodium etidronate[2], a diphosphonate. Dosage is 5 mg/kg daily for up to six months. It is given orally as a single daily dose, avoiding food for two hours before and after treatment. Side-effects include nausea and diarrhoea. Response is monitored as in (3).
5. Mithramycin, a cytotoxic agent with considerable risk of toxicity, especially to the liver and to platelets is very rarely used for Paget's disease in view of attendant risks. It is given as an infusion, either daily for 10 days or weekly.
6. Elective surgery. Total hip replacement is the most commonly indicated surgery for Paget's disease. Spinal decompression or neurosurgery for entrapment syndromes, especially to the base of the skull, may occasionally be needed. If possible there should be preoperative treatment with calcitonin or diphosphonates for one month to reduce bone vascularity[3].

FOLLOW-UP

Regular follow-up is unnecessary except in the presence of persistent symptoms.

[1] French WA et al. (1978) Am. J. Med., 56, 592.
[2] Russell RCG et al. (1975) Clin. Orthop. Rel. Res. 108, 241.
[3] Meyers M et al. (1978) J. Bone Jnt. Surg., 60A, 81

Gout

Gout is a condition featuring a raised serum urate (at some stage in the disease), recurrent attacks of a characteristic arthritis, deposits of monosodium urate crystals (tophi), and occasional renal disease and urolithiasis.

PROGNOSIS

- *Acute attack*. Untreated the acute attack of gout will last a few days to a few weeks and resolve completely. Treated with anti-inflammatory drugs the acute attack will resolve usually within 2–5 days.
- Attacks may recur every few weeks or as infrequently as every few years.
- *Chronic tophaceous gout*. This may cause surprisingly few symptoms and require little or no treatment. Allopurinol or uricosuric drugs may slowly reduce the size of the tophi but this can take years.
- There is an increased incidence of coronary and cerebral vascular disease. There is a small risk of associated renal disease. The other associations of obesity and hypertension carry their own prognoses.

TREATMENT

1. *Acute attack*

   a) Non-steroidal anti-inflammatory drugs (NSAIDs) e.g. indomethacin 50 mg tds to be continued until the acute attack has subsided.

   b) Rest (preferably non-weight-bearing) and adequate hydration are required.

   c) Aspiration and intra-articular injection of steroids, if possible should be carried out to accessible joints, e.g. the knee.

   d) Colchicine 500 μg tds if NSAIDs inadequate but gastrointestinal side-effects frequently troublesome.

   e) Allopurinol should never be given alone in the acute attack as this exacerbates it[1].

   f) It is recommended that the patient keeps a supply of NSAIDs to take immediately an attack commences.

2. *Chronic gout*. NSAIDs should be used if the patient is symptomatic, together with allopurinol.

3. Prophylaxis[2] should be considered in the following situations:

   a) More than three or four attacks of gout.

   b) Severe elevation of serum urate e.g. >0.75 mmol/l (normal range 0.1–0.4 mmol/l) which might cause renal lithiasis.

   c) Chronic tophaceous gout. If the tophi are causing symptoms, e.g. risk of skin breakdown, or if patient requiring thiazide diuretic therapy which will worsen the hyperuricaemia.

   d) Prior to or during cytotoxic therapy.

4. Allopurinol 200–300 mg daily as a single dose is used for prophylaxis. NSAIDs should be taken concommitantly for the first month of treatment to avoid precipitating an acute attack. The dose is adjusted according to serum urate.

5. Probenicid is an uricosuric drug which can be used instead of allopurinol or in conjunction with it in cases which are resistant to treatment. It should not be used in patients with renal impairment or urate stones.

6. Restriction of alcohol (of any kind) is recommended as alcohol is associated with increased frequency of attacks and 'bingeing' may directly precipitate an attack. No dietary restrictions are necessary unless there is an excessive protein intake.

7. Surgery occasionally performed for large disfiguring tophi but healing may be a problem leading to chronic sinus formation.

FOLLOW-UP

In patients with significant hyperuricaemia, measure serum uric acid and area levels 6–12 monthly. Patients requiring allopurinol should have the dose tailored according to uric acid levels. Generally patients only need to be seen when they are symptomatic.

---

[1] Boss GR *et al.* (1979) *New Eng. J. Med.*, **300**, 1459.
[2] Liang MH *et al.* (1978) *Ann. Int. Med.*, **88**, 666.

Calcium Pyrophosphate Dihydrate (CPPD) Deposits or Disease (Pseudo-gout)

CPPD crystal deposition causes an acute inflammatory arthritis, similar to gout, or a chronic low-grade inflammatory polyarthritis. Weakly positively birefringent crystals of CPPD are seen in the synovial fluid. There is an equal sex incidence and it usually occurs in the older age group except in the rare familial cases. 10% elderly show x-ray evidence of chondrocalcinosis but only a minority are symptomatic. There is an increased incidence of pyrophosphate arthropathy in hyperparathyroidism, haemochromatosis and Wilson's disease. There is a common association with osteoarthritis, and occasional association with diabetes and gout. Most cases are idiopathic but the following should be measured to exclude the commonest underlying disorders: serum calcium, phosphate, alkaline phosphatase, ferritin, glucose and uric acid[1].

PROGNOSIS

- Prognosis of arthropathy not affected by treatment of any underlying condition.
- *Acute attacks* last weeks and tend to recur at irregular intervals.
- *Chronic type* has similar outcome to osteoarthritis and is usually only slowly progressive.

TREATMENT

1. *Acute attack*

   a) Aspiration of synovial fluid and intra-articular steroid injection (e.g. depot preparation of methylprednisolone)[2].
   b) Non-steroidal anti-inflammatory drugs (NSAIDs) e.g. indomethacin 50 mg tds until the attack subsides.
   c) Rest – non-weight-bearing.

2. *Chronic type*

   a) NSAIDs.
   b) As for osteoarthritis, i.e. joint support, surgery if indicated.

3. No treatment required for asymptomatic patients.

FOLLOW-UP

Regular follow-up is not necessary unless the patient is symptomatic.

---

[1] McCarthy DJ (1976) *Arth. Rheum.*, **19**, 275.
[2] O'Duffy JD (1976) *Arth. Rheum.*, **19**, 349.

Prolapsed Intervertebral Disc

Prolapsed intervertebral disc is usually caused by degenerative disease of the disc, and consists of a herniation of the nucleus pulposus through the ring of the annulus fibrosus. Pain is caused by stretching of the annulus fibrosus and compression of nerve roots, as are motor and sensory disturbance.

PROGNOSIS

- Most lumbar disc herniations respond to conservative management. 90% patients are relieved of pain within six weeks, and eventually return to normal life.
- Despite more aggressive therapy including surgery, permanent neurological impairment may persist in a few patients.
- Central (as opposed to the more common posterolateral) herniation may lead to cord compression: this is particularly serious in cervical lesions.
- There is an increased risk of further disc prolapse.

TREATMENT

1. Bed rest, with monitoring of clinical state, especially neurological.
2. Analgesics, anti-inflammatory agents, muscle relaxants (e.g. diazepam).
3. The usual period of conservative therapy is about two weeks. If symptoms are still severe, or signs are unchanged or worse, more aggressive therapy is probably needed.
4. Traction for root symptoms if symptoms unrelieved by the above. An epidural injection of local anaesthetic and steroid may also be helpful for root symptoms.
5. Manipulation for back pain without root symptoms or signs.
6. Chemonucleolysis (injection of papain into disc space) is indicated for small disc herniations, preferably at one level. About 90% patients improve[1].
7. Laminectomy. Up to 96% patients show improvement, but this is total in only 15%[2].
8. Other manoeuvres such as facet blocks[3], facet denervation[4] and intrathecal steroids[5] may provide symptomatic relief and be suitable for patients who are poor surgical risks.
9. Prompt surgery is important for central disc herniation (especially cervical) and cauda equina compression.

FOLLOW-UP

Follow-up is only necessary in the presence of persistent symptoms. Progressive neurological deficit should be taken seriously.

[1] McCulloch JA et al. (1980) Clin. Orthop., 146, 128.
[2] Hirsch C et al. (1963) Clin. Orthop., 29, 189.
[3] Mooney V et al. (1976) Clin. Orthop., 115, 149.
[4] Shealy CN (1976) Clin. Orthop., 115, 157.
[5] Brown FW (1977) Clin. Orthop., 129, 72.

10

Diseases of the Endocrine System

G. Williams and S. R. Bloom

Hypopituitarism

Clinical hypopituitarism appears after loss of about 75% of the anterior pituitary, due to pituitary and other tumours, surgery, irradiation or infarction (including Sheehan's syndrome). Pituitary failure secondary to hypothalamic disease (e.g. craniopharyngioma, sarcoidosis, histiocytosis X) is usually accompanied by diabetes insipidus. After acute pituitary failure, adrenal failure usually appears within two weeks and hypothyroidism within 4–8 weeks. In progressive hypopituitarism (e.g. expanding tumours), gonadotrophin secretion fails first, followed by growth hormone, TSH and then ACTH. 'Isolated' failure of anterior pituitary hormones (especially gonadotrophins and growth hormone) may occur.

PROGNOSIS

- Highly variable, depending on the underlying pathology.

TREATMENT

1. Hydrocortisone replacement (p. 206) should be started before any thyroxine replacement to avoid adrenal crisis, and may unmask diabetes insipidus; mineralocorticoids are necessary only in a minority of cases.
2. Thyroxine (p. 200).
3. Sex hormone replacement in men

   a) Androgens (e.g. testosterone enanthate 250 mg i.m. every 2–4 weeks) maintain libido, potency, beard growth and well-being and also prevent osteoporosis, but do not restore fertility.
   b) Human chorionic gonadotrophin (HCG; mainly LH activity) combined with menotrophin (FSH) may restore fertility; pulsatile subcutaneous administration of gonadotrophin releasing hormone (LHRH) by a portable infusion pump may be effective in hypothalamic disease with intact gonadotrophs[1].

4. Sex hormone replacement in women

   a) Combined oral contraceptives (30–50 μg ethinyloestradiol) restore libido and menstruation and prevent breast atrophy and osteoporosis.
   b) Ovulation may be induced by FSH followed by HCG or (in hypothalamic disease) by pulsatile LHRH[1].

5. Growth hormone is used by specialist centres to treat children with proven growth hormone deficiency and unfused epiphyses[2]. Human cadaver growth hormone is currently unavailable due to concern over slow virus transmission; synthetic growth hormone (recombinant DNA technology) is now obtainable.

FOLLOW-UP

Review 6–12 monthly for life, more frequently if pituitary damage is progressive. Monitor replacement of sex hormones (libido, potency, secondary sexual characteristics), steroids (p. 206), thyroxine (p. 200) and growth hormone (growth velocity; skeletal x-rays to detect epiphyseal closure).

---

[1] Cutler A et al. (1985) Ann. Int. Med., 102, 643.
[2] Preece MA et al. (1976) J. Clin. Endoc. Metab., 42, 477.

Acromegaly

The prevalence of acromegaly in Britain is about 4 per 100 000. Most cases are due to primary hypersecretion of growth hormone (GH) by anterior pituitary adenomata, mostly eosinophil. A rare cause is GH hypersecretion secondary to production of peptides with GH-releasing factor (GRF) activity by pancreatic and other tumours ('GRF-omas')[1].

PROGNOSIS

- Untreated 40–70% develop hypertension and 15–20% develop diabetes.
- Mortality at all ages is doubled (mainly due to heart disease and stroke).
- The effect of treatment of acromegaly on its prognosis is unknown.

TREATMENT

1. Surgery[2]

   a) Generally first-line treatment; absolutely indicated if vision is threatened.
   b) Trans-sphenoidal adenomectomy for small tumours; mortality and complications (meningitis, CSF leaks) both 1–2%. Transfrontal hypophysectomy for large tumours: mortality up to 20%.
   c) GH normalised in 90% within days.
   d) 80% visual field defects resolve.
   e) Hypopituitarism occurs in 3–15%.

2. Yttrium implantation (50 000–150 000 cGy rods inserted trans-sphenoidally[3])

   a) Suitable for tumours with <10 mm suprasellar extension; contraindicated with partially empty sella turcica (risk of CSF leak).
   b) GH normalised in 50%.
   c) Partial hypopituitarism in 30%.
   d) CSF leaks and meningitis now very rare (<1%).

3. External beam (supervoltage or heavy particle) irradiation; 4000–6000 cGy

   a) For large or invasive tumours, frail patients and previous surgical failures; unsuitable for rapidly-growing tumours or if visual field defects are present.
   b) Slow normalisation of GH levels: e.g. 40% at two years, 70% at five years[4].
   c) Hypopituitarism (10–30%) and temporal lobe damage are commoner with heavy particle treatment.

4. Medical treatments

   a) Current indications: elderly or frail patients; failed surgery or implantation; interim treatment following external beam irradiation.
   b) Bromocriptine (7.5–60 mg/day in 3–4 oral doses) lowers GH levels in 70% acromegalics, often with clinical and metabolic improvement[5]. Long-acting, subcutaneously-injectable somatostatin analogues usefully suppress GH release and relieve sweating and headache[6].

FOLLOW-UP

GH levels after surgery predict outcome. Review after three and six months, and then annually, for recurrence of symptoms, clinical and radiographic signs of tumour re-expansion; reassess need for anterior pituitary hormone replacement (p. 194).

[1] Guillemin R et al. (1982) Science, 218, 585.
[2] Baskin DS et al. (1982) J. Neurosurg., 56, 634.
[3] Cassar J et al. (1981) Acta Endoc., 96, 295.
[4] Eastman RC et al. (1979) J. Clin. Endoc. Metab., 48, 931.
[5] Wass JAH et al. (1977) Br. Med. J., i, 875.
[6] Ch'ng LJC et al. (1985) Br. Med. J., 290, 284.

Prolactinoma

These are the commonest pituitary tumours and mainly affect women, causing galactorrhoea, amenorrhoea and infertility. Microadenomas (<1 cm diameter) are commoner than macroadenomas (>1 cm diameter). A 'partially empty sella' containing CSF, probably following infarction and shrinkage of an adenoma, is found in 20% cases of hyperprolactinaemia.

PROGNOSIS

- Microadenomas: some may regress spontaneously, a minority (5%) enlarge[1].
- Risk of expansion in pregnancy: 5% micro-, 35% macroadenomas[2].
- Worse in men, who tend to present late with larger tumours.

TREATMENT

1. Bromocriptine

    a) Dopamine agonist: lowers prolactin levels, resolves amenorrhoea and galactorrhoea and restores fertility within a year in 80% cases; shrinks some tumours. May be indicated in patients with microadenomas and minimal symptoms, in order to prevent osteoporosis[3].
    b) 1.25 mg nocte, increasing slowly to 2.55 mg tds; taken with food.
    c) Treatment is continued until the tumour has shrunk sufficiently for definitive treatment; or it is continued indefinitely.
    d) Other dopamine agonists: lisuride (short acting), pergolide (long acting).

2. Surgery

    a) Definitive treatment if pregnancy planned, or if bromocriptine ineffective.
    b) Trans-sphenoidal adenomectomy (for microadenoma) or transfrontal hypophysectomy (for macroadenoma).
    c) Menses resume in 60–85% microadenomas, 15–90% macroadenomas.
    d) Hypopituitarism in 10% (microadenoma) to >90% (macroadenomas).
    e) Recurrence in 50% microadenomas, 90% macroadenomas by five years[4].

3. Yttrium implantation[5] (see p. 195)

    a) Definitive treatment for small tumours; prevents tumour expansion in pregnancy.
    b) Spontaneous menses resume in 25%; fertility restored in 15%. With addition of bromocriptine, fertility is restored in 70% patients.
    c) Hypopituitarism in 5%; complications are very rare.

4. External radiotherapy[4]

    a) Definitive treatment for invasive tumours, or following surgery for these.
    b) Normoprolactinaemia in 30% after 1–11 years; interim medical treatment is usually required. Amenorrhoea is rarely cured.
    c) Hypopituitarism is ultimately almost inevitable.

5. Prolactinomas in pregnancy

    a) Macroadenomas must have definitive treatment before pregnancy is advised.
    b) Bromocriptine should be stopped after conception and restarted if the tumour expands; further deterioration requires urgent surgery or implantation.

FOLLOW-UP

Check prolactin levels, anterior pituitary function and visual fields 6–12 monthly (monthly in pregnancy). X-ray pituitary fossa and consider CT scan if there is evidence of tumour expansion or rising prolactin levels.

---

[1] March CM et al. (1981) Am. J. Obstet. Gynec., 9, 835.
[2] Gemzell C et al. (1979) Fertil. Steril., 31, 363.
[3] Klibanski A et al. (1980) New Eng. J. Med., 303, 1511.
[4] Grossman A et al. (1985) Br. Med. J., 290, 182.
[5] Kelly WF et al. (1978) Q. J. Med., 47, 473.

Diabetes Insipidus (DI)

'Cranial' DI (failure of antidiuretic hormone (ADH) secretion) may be idiopathic (30–40% cases), or follow hypothalamic or posterior pituitary damage by surgery or trauma (30%), tumours and histiocytosis X[1]. 'Nephrogenic' DI (insensitivity of renal tubules to ADH) may be primary (mostly familial) or secondary to drugs (demeclocycline, lithium), hypercalcaemia, hypokalaemia, various renal parenchymal diseases and obstructive uropathy. Deficiencies of cortisol and thyroxine (which are permissive to water excretion) may conceal DI and their replacement may precipitate DI.

PROGNOSIS

- Primary cranial or nephrogenic DI are compatible with normal life expectancy if adequately treated.
- Secondary DI: variable prognosis, depending on underlying pathology; post-traumatic DI may last days or weeks but permanent DI may supervene later.

TREATMENT

1. Adequate water intake must be ensured at all times.
2. *Cranial DI*

   a) Mild DI (<3 l/day urine output) requires no specific maintenance treatment.
   b) Desmopressin (DDAVP) 10–20 µg by nasal spray od or bd, or 0.5–2 µg i.m. daily in postoperative or obtunded patients. DDAVP lasts 12 hours and has virtually no vasoconstrictor action. (*Note:* vasopressin tannate, lysine vasopressin and posterior pituitary extract are now obsolete.)
   c) Carbamazepine 200–400 mg od or bd; releases ADH.
   d) Chlorpropamide 100–350 mg/day (adults), 50–200 mg/day (children); releases ADH and sensitises the renal tubules to ADH;

hypoglycaemia (especially dangerous in hypopituitarism) limits its use to occasional cases of mild cranial DI.

3. *Nephrogenic DI*

   a) Thiazides: chlorthalidone (100 mg bd initially, then 50 mg od) or hydrochlorothiazide (50–200 mg/day); their mechanism of action is unknown.
   b) Indomethacin 75–150 mg/day.
   c) DDAVP in high dose (>40 µg/day) may partially overcome tubular ADH resistance in some mild cases.

FOLLOW-UP

Following head injury or cranial surgery, fluid input and DDAVP (if necessary) should be guided by fluid losses and by plasma and urinary electrolytes and osmolality to avoid either dehydration or water overload. Review regularly the need for continuing treatment, which may be withdrawn for a trial period. Patients with 'idiopathic' DI and known hypothalamic or pituitary lesions need careful watching for development of other endocrine deficiencies.

---

[1] Baylis PH (1983) *Clin. Endoc. Metab.*, **12**, 474.

Hyperthyroidism

Thyrotoxicosis affects 2% females and 0.2% males. Most cases are due to Graves' disease (TSH receptors are stimulated by IgG thyroid-stimulating immunoglobulins (TSI) directed against them) or to autonomous thyroid hormone production by an adenoma (toxic nodule) or multinodular goitre. Rare causes include thyroxine administration, thyroiditis and excessive TSH production by the pituitary (TSHoma) or ovarian teratoma.

PROGNOSIS

- Graves' disease

  a) 60–70% have chronic relapsing disease; the rest suffer a single episode.
  b) 50% develop proptosis with or without ophthalmoplegia, often independent of thyroid status or its response to treatment.

- 50% older patients with hyperthyroidism develop atrial fibrillation.

TREATMENT (GRAVES' DISEASE)

1. Antithyroid drugs

   a) Carbimazole inhibits both thyroid hormone and TSI synthesis[1]. 30–45 mg/day (od or tds) is given until euthyroid (4–6 weeks), then 5–20 mg/day (adjusted to maintain euthyroidism) for 12–18 months[2,3]. Skin rashes are quite common (in which case propylthiouracil, 300–450 mg/day should be used); agranulocytosis is very rare (1 per 20 000).
   b) Relapses (50% cases) are treated with one further course of carbimazole or surgery or (if >40 years of age) radioiodine.

2. Beta blockers (sustained-release propranolol or nadolol, both 160 mg/day) partially control symptoms pending surgery or full effect of carbimazole.

3. Subtotal thyroidectomy

   a) Indicated for drug failures, relapses and large goitres.
   b) Préoperatively, carbimazole is given until euthyroid; two weeks preoperatively, there should be a change to aqueous iodine solution (0.1–0.3 ml tds).

   c) Effective in 75% cases; 5% relapse; 20% ultimately become hypothyroid[2,3].
   d) Rare complications (<1%) include acute tracheal compression from haematoma, laryngeal nerve damage, and permanent hypoparathyroidism; 5–10% suffer transient postoperative hypocalcaemia.

4. Radioiodine (180–360 mBq ^{131}I)

   a) Initial treatment or for relapses in patients >40 years of age.
   b) Success rate 75%; failures are treated with further ^{131}I or surgery.
   c) Hypothyroidism occurs in 10–25% at one year, additional 2–4% per year thereafter.

5. Graves' ophthalmopathy

   a) Mild: 1% methylcellulose eye drops, protective spectacles.
   b) Severe (vision threatened): prednisolone 120 mg/day, orbital irradiation, or surgical decompression of the orbit.

6. Treatment in pregnancy and neonate

   a) Carbimazole is not apparently teratogenic but can cause fetal hypothyroidism and goitre. The lowest effective dose is given to maintain normal free T4. Treatment is either for usual 12–18 months with avoidance of breast feeding, or it is stopped four weeks before delivery (when the presence of TSI predicts fetal hyperthyroidism), treating a relapse with further course of carbimazole.
   b) Neonatal hyperthyroidism, due to IgG TSI which cross the placenta, resolves spontaneously when TSI are cleared within a few weeks of birth. Treatment with carbimazole (1 mg/kg/day), pre-

pranolol (2 mg/kg/day) and aqueous iodine solution (0.15 ml/day) may be necessary.

TREATMENT (TOXIC NODULE AND MULTINODULAR GOITRE)

1. Antithyroid drugs are unsatisfactory due to high relapse rate.
2. Partial or hemi-thyroidectomy is indicated for large goitres.
3. Radioiodine treatment (500–1800 mBq ^{131}I) is usually effective and rarely causes hypothyroidism.

TREATMENT (THYROTOXIC CRISIS)

1. Crises are precipitated by surgery or infection in uncontrolled hyperthyroidism.
2. General measures include intravenous fluids, inotropes, intravenous hydrocortisone and antibiotics, and sedation with chlorpromazine 25–50 mg six hourly.
3. Propranolol (1–5 mg i.v. or 80 mg orally, six hourly).
4. Aqueous iodine solution 0.5 ml eight hourly and carbimazole 20 mg eight hourly are given orally or via a nasogastric tube.

FOLLOW-UP

During carbimazole treatment, review every 4–6 weeks until euthyroid and 3–6 monthly thereafter; in pregnancy, every 3–4 weeks. Adjust dose according to clinical state and serum T4 (free T4 if pregnant or taking the oral contraceptive or other medication interfering with thyroxine protein binding). Regular blood counts are unlikely to detect agranulocytosis, but patients should immediately report sore throats or other infections. After a course of carbimazole or surgery or radioiodine treatment, review three monthly for the first year and then annually, for both relapse and development of hypothyroidism.

[1] Weetman AP et al. (1984) Clin. Endoc., 21, 163.
[2] Burr WA et al. (1979) New. Eng. J. Med., 300, 200.
[3] Sugrue D et al. (1980) Q. J. Med., 49, 51.

Hypothyroidism

In Britain the prevalence is about 1%, and the commonest cause is auto-immune disease (atrophic hypothyroidism and Hashimoto's thyroiditis) which has a 6:1 female to male preponderance. Other causes include drugs (lithium, amiodarone), surgical or radioiodine treatment of hyperthyroidism, dyshormonogenesis, pituitary failure and iodine deficiency.

PROGNOSIS

- With correct replacement therapy, life expectancy is normal.
- 12% patients with auto-immune hypothyroidism develop pernicious anaemia.
- Myxoedema coma is rare but has a 50% mortality rate.

TREATMENT

1. Thyroxine, given as a single daily dose; initially, 50 μg/day, increasing by 50 μg/day at 3-4 weekly intervals. In children, old patients and those with ischaemic heart disease the starting dose and increments should be 25 μg.

   a) The dosage is adjusted depending on clinical state and serum T4 concentrations, which should not exceed the normal range[1].
   b) Most patients require 100-200 μg/day although some need 300-400 μg/day. Apparently high or increasing dosages with persistently raised TSH levels suggest poor compliance.

2. Tri-iodothyronine is sometimes used in patients with ischaemic heart disease, since its shorter duration allows more rapid withdrawal if angina develops; 5 μg/day (single daily dose), increasing by 5 μg/day every week; once the patient is clinically euthyroid with normal TSH, there should be a transfer to thyroxine (1 μg tri-iodothyronine = 5 μg thyroxine).

3. Myxoedema coma

   a) Hypothermia is corrected (space blanket); intravenous fluids are administered (with care); antibiotics; and intravenous hydrocortisone hemisuccinate (100 mg six hourly).
   b) Respiratory failure may require ventilation.
   c) Intravenous tri-iodothyronine: 100 μg initially, then 20 μg eight hourly.

FOLLOW-UP

Initially, review clinical state and serum T4 and TSH levels every 3-4 weeks and adjust thyroxine dose as necessary. Once stable, review thyroid status (and cardiovascular function in older patients) once or twice yearly.

---

[1] Jennings PE et al. (1984) Br. Med. J., 289, 1645.

Thyroiditis

The commonest cause is auto-immune damage (Hashimoto's thyroiditis[1]). De Quervain's thyroiditis[2] is due to viral infection (adenoviruses and mumps) and, rarely, bacterial infection may be responsible. Riedel's thyroiditis[3] is dense fibrous infiltration of the thyroid and surrounding tissues, sometimes associated with retroperitoneal and mediastinal fibrosis.

PROGNOSIS

- Hashimoto's: hypothyroidism in 25% at presentation, ultimately over 90%.
- De Quervain's: mild hyperthyroidism for 4–6 weeks (due to leakage of thyroid hormones from the damaged gland), then mild hypothyroidism (repair of gland) before recovery after several months; persistent hypothyroidism in under 10%.
- Riedel's: usually fatal through infiltration of neck structures, e.g. trachea, carotid arteries.

TREATMENT

1. Hypothyroidism: conventional thyroxine replacement (p. 200), which may also shrink the goitre of Hashimoto's thyroiditis.
2. Hyperthyroidism: if necessary, treat symptomatically with beta blockers (p. 198).
3. *De Quervain's:* systemic symptoms and thyroid pain usually respond to non-steroidal anti-inflammatory agents; prednisolone 40–60 mg/day may be needed.
4. *Pyogenic thyroiditis:* systemic antibiotics and surgical drainage.
5. *Riedel's thyroiditis:* excision and wedge resection for tracheal obstruction.

FOLLOW-UP

Hashimoto's: 6–12 monthly review of thyroid status and size of goitre. De Quervain's: every 2–4 weeks until thyroid function is normal. Riedel's: 6–12 monthly review of thyroid status; regular surgical follow-up for tracheal obstruction.

---

[1] Moens H *et al.* (1978) *New Eng. J. Med.*, **299**, 133.
[2] Stancek D *et al.* (1975) *Med. Microbiol. Immunol.*, **161**, 133.
[3] Lee JG (1935) *Arch. Surg.*, **31**, 982.

Hyperparathyroidism

Primary hyperparathyroidism has a prevalence of 1 per 1000 and is a common cause of hypercalcaemia, accounting for 50% cases detected by routine screening. There is a two to threefold female preponderance. Most cases are asymptomatic. Excessive PTH secretion is due to a single adenoma in over 80% cases, to generalised hyperplasia of all four glands in 15% (especially in the multiple endocrine neoplasia (MEN) syndromes) and to parathyroid carcinoma in about 1%. Secondary hyperparathyroidism is compensatory PTH hypersecretion following hypocalcaemia due to renal failure or vitamin D deficiency.

PROGNOSIS (UNTREATED PRIMARY HYPERPARATHYROIDISM)

- 40%–50% develop renal stones, nephrocalcinosis and finally renal failure.
- 10–25% develop bone disease, mostly mild and asymptomatic.
- 5–10% develop peptic ulceration (due to hypercalcaemia *per se*; also Zollinger–Ellison syndrome in MEN 1).
- 5% develop clinically-significant depression and/or muscle weakness.
- Asymptomatic patients (detected by routine screening): after five years 60% show no deterioration; 20% require surgery for progressive disease[1].
- Parathyroid carcinoma usually secretes PTH and is fatal in 1–15 years due to renal failure; rare non-secreting tumours cause rapidly-fatal carcinomatosis.

TREATMENT (PRIMARY HYPERPARATHYROIDISM)

1. Medical maintenance treatment

    a) Indicated in asymptomatic patients with serum Ca concentration <2.8 mmol/l and normal renal function and bone density; and in patients unfit for surgery.
    b) Low calcium diet – no dairy products or white bread; softened water should be drunk.
    c) Frusemide 40–80 mg/day with potassium supplements; adequate hydration.
    d) Sodium cellulose phosphate 5 g eight hourly with meals; causes diarrhoea.

2. Emergency treatment of hypercalcaemia

    a) Rehydration and promotion of diuresis: 4–10 l of saline daily with frusemide (up to 100 mg two hourly by slow intravenous infusion to reduce ototoxicity); monitor cardiovascular status (including central venous pressure); serum electrolyte and magnesium concentrations should also be monitored.
    b) Mithramycin: single intravenous dose of 25 μg/kg; repeated after a few days if necessary. The development of nephrotoxicity, hepatotoxicity (prolonged prothrombin time) and thrombocytopaenia should be considered[2].
    c) Calcitonin (1–2 MRC units/kg subcutaneously or i.m. six hourly) may help some patients for a short time[3].
    d) Aminodipropylidene diphosphonate (ADP) 15 mg/day i.v.
    e) Haemo- or peritoneal dialysis: with phosphate replacement.
    f) Other drugs (used less commonly): intravenous phosphate (e.g. 500 ml of 0.1 M phosphate buffer given over 10 hours causes severe metastatic calcification; EDTA is highly nephrotoxic. Steroids are ineffective.

3. Surgery

    a) Indicated if serum Ca > 2.8 mmol/l or if there is significant renal, bone or neuropsychiatric disease.
    b) Parathyroid glands may sometimes be localised preoperatively with ultrasound

CT scanning, thallium-technetium subtraction scanning, angiography or selective venous sampling for PTH; 10% adenomas are ectopic.

c) A single adenoma or carcinoma is removed; if hyperplasia is found, 3½ glands are removed.

d) The success rate is 90%. Permanent hypoparathyroidism occurs in 1%. Transient hypocalcaemia with hypophosphataemia and hypomagnesaemia occurs in patients with extensive bone disease ('hungry bone syndrome'), due to accelerated remineralisation of the depleted skeleton; it is treated with calcium and magnesium supplements and alfacalcidol 1–10 μg/day.

FOLLOW-UP

During medical treatment, six monthly review for symptoms, serum calcium concentration, renal function (urea, creatinine; evidence of calculi); loss of bone mass (skeletal radiography). Postoperatively, measure serum calcium daily initially; patients with the 'hungry bone syndrome' will need calcium, magnesium and vitamin D treatment until blood biochemistry (including alkaline phosphatase) is normal and there is radiographic evidence of bone healing. Serum calcium and renal function should be reviewed annually in postoperative patients; delayed recurrence of disease is common with parathyroid carcinoma. Patients and their first-order relatives should be screened for MEN.

[1] Purnell DC et al. (1974) Am. J. Med., 56, 800.
[2] Elias E et al. (1972) Ann. Surg., 175, 431.
[3] West TET et al. (1971) Lancet, i, 675.

Hypoparathyroidism

Permanent hypoparathyroidism complicates 1% neck explorations for hyperparathyroidism and 1% total thyroidectomies. Idiopathic hypoparathyroidism is probably auto-immune and is associated with other auto-immune endocrine diseases (mainly Addison's disease) alopecia, vitiligo and chronic mucocutaneous candidiasis[1]. Di George's syndrome (very rare) is agenesis of the parathyroids and thymus. Pseudohypoparathyroidism is not due to PTH deficiency, but to insensitivity of the target tissues (bone and kidney) to PTH.

PROGNOSIS

- 20% develop calcification of the basal ganglia but parkinsonism is uncommon.
- Over 50% have cataracts due to lens calcification.
- 20% children have subnormal intelligence which may improve with treatment.
- Intractable convulsions or laryngeal spasm may be fatal.

TREATMENT

1. Calcium supplements to provide total daily intake of 25–50 mmol.
2. Vitamin D

   a) Calciferol (1–3 mg/day) takes 4–12 weeks to be fully effective.
   b) 1-α-hydroxycholecalciferol (alfacalcidol: 0.5–2 μg/day) acts more quickly but is more likely to cause hypercalcaemia.

3. Emergency treatment of severe tetany: 10–20 ml of 10% calcium chloride solution injected i.v. over five minutes or 0.5 mmol/kg infused i.v. over four hours. The ECG is monitored in digitalised patients.
4. Pseudohypoparathyroidism is treated similarly, using alfacalcidol.

FOLLOW-UP

Measure serum calcium concentration frequently while adjusting vitamin D dosage, and 3–6 monthly once stable. Aim to maintain serum calcium in the lower half of the normal range while avoiding hypercalciuria (>12.5 mmol/day), which predisposes to nephrolithiasis. In idiopathic hypoparathyroidism watch for possible development of adrenal failure and other auto-immune diseases.

---

[1] Schneider AB et al. (1975) Metabolism, 24, 871.

Phaeochromocytoma

Phaeochromocytomas account for 0.5% cases of hypertension. Males and females are equally affected, mostly in early to middle adult life. 10% (more in children) occur outside the adrenals and 3% lie outside the abdomen. 10% are malignant and 25% are multiple; those associated with medullary carcinoma of the thyroid in the multiple endocrine neoplasia (MEN) 2 syndrome are often bilateral, multifocal and malignant.

PROGNOSIS

- Death may occur from hypertension, cardiac arrhythmia and myocarditis (50% autopsy cases). Hypertension is sustained in 50% cases.

TREATMENT

1. Preoperative preparation and medical treatment

   a) Medical treatment is indicated in frail patients or those with metastases.
   b) Phenoxybenzamine 10 mg bd initially, increasing by 10 mg daily to up to 80 mg bd until hypertension is controlled.
   c) Propranolol 10–40 mg/day is then added if needed to control hypertension or cardiac arrhythmias. Previous α-blockade is essential to prevent hypertensive crisis due to unopposed α-stimulation.
   d) α-methyltyrosine 1–2 g/day blocks catecholamine synthesis and is used to treat benign and malignant tumours unresponsive to alpha and beta blockade[1].

   e) Streptozotocin is occasionally useful in malignant phaeochromocytoma[2].

2. Surgery

   a) Phenoxybenzamine with or without propranolol for at least two weeks before surgery; intravascular volume is restored with blood and plasma.
   b) Sodium nitroprusside (up to 1 μg/kg/minute) by intravenous infusion will control peroperative hypertension; circulatory support (fluids, pressors) may be needed after removal of the tumour.
   c) Surgery is usually curative but recurrences are common in MEN.

FOLLOW-UP

Lifelong, regular review for recurrence of symptoms, hypertension and elevated urinary VMA excretion. Screen relatives for MEN 2.

---

[1] Sjoerdsma S et al. (1965) Lancet, ii, 1092.
[2] Hamilton BPM et al. (1977) Arch. Int. Med., 137, 762.

Hypoadrenalism

Hypoadrenalism is either primary (destruction of the adrenal cortex by auto-immune disease, tuberculosis, malignant infiltration, etc.) or secondary to pituitary failure (p. 194). The prevalence in Britain is about 4 per 100 000; women predominate because of the auto-immune variety (60% cases).

PROGNOSIS

- Untreated total adrenal failure is fatal.
- Even with full replacement therapy, avoidable deaths still occur through failure to increase steroid dosage during intercurrent illness.

TREATMENT

1. Maintenance

    a) Hydrocortisone (10–40 mg/day, usually in two doses, the larger in the morning) and fludrocortisone (0.05–0.2 mg mane) are adjusted individually.
    b) Hydrocortisone overdosage causes insomnia, weight gain and cushingoid features; underdosage causes loss of energy, weight loss, anorexia and postural hypotension. An extra midday dose counters cortisol deficiency in the late afternoon. Alternative glucocorticoids are cortisone, prednisolone and dexamethasone.
    c) Fludrocortisone overdosage causes oedema, hypertension and hypokalaemia; underdosage produces postural hypotension, raised urea and hyperkalaemia. Plasma renin activity measurements may help dose adjustments[1]. Fludrocortisone is not usually needed when hypoadrenalism is due to pituitary failure.
    d) A steroid card and emergency supply of steroid tablets should be issued.

2. Emergency treatment

    a) Significant intercurrent illness (fever and systemic symptoms): the hydrocortisone dosage should be doubled; vomiting demands urgent parenteral treatment, intravenous fluids and medical advice.
    b) Trauma and surgery: hydrocortisone hemisuccinate 100 mg i.m. six hourly and intravenous fluids until eating and drinking normally; the dose is tapered to usual maintenance dose over 3–4 days[2]. Fludrocortisone is not needed when hydrocortisone dosage exceeds 100 mg/day.
    c) Acute adrenal insufficiency: hydrocortisone 100 mg i.v. initially, then six hourly as above; urgent intravenous rehydration with saline; hypoglycaemia and infection are treated as necessary.

FOLLOW-UP

Every 6–12 months and at short notice if necessary. Check for evidence of under- or overdosage and (with auto-immune adrenal failure), the development of hypothyroidism, diabetes and pernicious anaemia. Check steroid card and emergency steroid supply.

---

[1] Smith SJ et al. (1984) Lancet, i, 11.
[2] Plumpton FS et al. (1969) Anaesthesia, 24, 12.

Cushing's Syndrome

Cushing's disease is due to excessive ACTH production by the pituitary (usually a basophil or chromophobe adenoma) and accounts for 80% Cushing's syndrome in adults; there is a 4:1 female to male preponderance. Other causes of cortisol excess include 'ectopic' ACTH production by neuroendocrine tumours (small cell carcinoma of the lung and carcinoid) and cortisol production by adrenal adenoma or (rarely) carcinoma. A common cause is overtreatment with glucocorticoids.

PROGNOSIS (UNTREATED CUSHING'S SYNDROME)

- *Cushing's disease* increases mortality several-fold through hypertension, diabetes and infection (up to 50% mortality at five years).
- In the *ectopic ACTH syndrome*, survival varies from weeks (small cell carcinoma) to years (carcinoid).
- *Adrenal carcinoma* has a median survival time of 1–2 years.

TREATMENT

1. *Cushing's disease*

a) The logical treatment – ablation of the pituitary tumour – is usually practicable, although a pituitary cause may be difficult to prove.

b) Trans-sphenoidal surgery (adenomectomy or hypophysectomy): cure rate 60–90%, recurrence rate 10%, hypopituitarism rate 5–10%[1].

c) Yttrium implantation (p. 195; 20 000–150 000 cGy): cure rate 80–100% in selected patients; recurrence rate zero; hypopituitarism rate 40%[2].

d) External beam irradiation (4000–5000 cGy): cure rate 25–60% (after several months; interim medical treatment may be necessary); hypopituitarism rate 10–40%[3].

e) Bilateral adrenalectomy followed by life-long adrenal replacement (p. 206): recurrences rarely occur due to residual or ectopic adrenal tissue. Nelson's syndrome (unrestrained expansion of the pituitary adenoma with massively elevated ACTH levels) occurs in 10% cases; pituitary irradiation may prevent its development; ACTH secretion may be blocked with cyproheptadine but invasive tumours require surgery or radiotherapy[4].

f) Cortisol synthesis blockade (metyrapone, 0.75–4 g/day; aminoglutethimide and trilostane may also be used) is used as interim treatment or long term in patients unsuitable for definitive treatment; adrenal replacement may be necessary. Metyrapone may cause nausea, vomiting and hirsutism.

g) Suppression of ACTH release by drugs (cyproheptadine 12–24 mg/day; bromocriptine 10 mg/day; sodium valproate 200–300 mg/day) is under investigation.

2. *Ectopic ACTH syndrome*

a) Tumours may be treated with surgery (may be curative, e.g. with carcinoids), radiotherapy or chemotherapy (small cell carcinoma).

b) Cortisol synthesis blockade (metyrapone).

3. *Adrenal tumours (adenomas and carcinomas)*

a) Surgical resection (with radiotherapy for carcinoma).

b) Cortisol synthesis blockade (above).

c) Cytotoxic agents for carcinoma: *op'* - DDD (2–8 g/day) causes adrenal atrophy and reduces cortisol levels after some weeks, and prolongs survival in 30% cases; methotrexate, doxorubicin and streptozotocin are being evaluated.

d) External beam irradiation is used to treat adrenal carcinoma.

Contd.

FOLLOW-UP

Regular and lifelong, for recurrence, development of adrenal insufficiency, appearance of Nelson's syndrome (pigmentation and expansion of the fossa) after adrenalectomy, and pituitary failure after pituitary surgery or irradiation.

[1] Bigos ST *et al.* (1980) *J. Clin. Endoc. Metab.*, **2**, 348.
[2] White MC *et al.* (1982) *Br. Med. J.*, **285**, 280.
[3] Aristizabel S *et al.* (1977) *Int. J. Radn. Oncol. Biol. Phys.*, **2**, 47.
[4] Moore TJ *et al.* (1976) *Ann. Int. Med.*, **85**, 731.

Primary Aldosteronism

Primary aldosteronism (excessive secretion of aldosterone) accounts for about 1% all cases of hypertension, but for 50% those with spontaneous hypokalaemia. Hypertension is occasionally accelerated; 80% cases have hypokalaemia[1]. Most cases are due to a solitary adrenal adenoma (=Conn's syndrome; 60%) or to bilateral hyperplasia of the zona glomerulosa (30%); the latter may rarely be ACTH-dependent ('glucocorticoid-suppressible aldosteronism'[2]). Rare causes are multiple adenomata and adrenal carcinoma.

PROGNOSIS

- Surgical resection of an adenoma cures hypertension for over one year in 70% patients and permanently in 50–60%.
- Bilateral hyperplasia: surgery cures hypertension in only 30% cases.

TREATMENT

1. *Solitary adenoma (Conn's syndrome)*. Spironolactone 300–400 mg/day is given for 3–4 weeks preoperatively to control hypertension and replenish potassium, and long term in patients unsuitable for surgery. Patients whose hypertension responds to spironolactone are more likely to respond to surgery.

2. *Bilateral hyperplasia*

   a) Spironolactone 300–400 mg/day initially; maintenance dose may be lower due to long-term inhibition of aldosterone secretion.

   b) Amiloride 10–40 mg/day may be added to reduce spironolactone dosage if side-effects (gynaecomastia, impotence) are troublesome.

FOLLOW-UP

Regular, lifelong review of blood pressure and plasma potassium concentrations.

---

[1] Sutherland DJA *et al.* (1966) *Can. Med. Assoc. J.*, 95, 1109.
[2] Conn JW *et al.* (1966) *J. Am. Med. Assoc.*, 195, 21.

Congenital Adrenal Hyperplasia

This group of rare disorders is due to enzyme defects in steroid synthetic pathways. Cortisol deficiency causes a compensatory increase in ACTH secretion, leading to the characteristic adrenal hyperplasia and accumulation of steroid precursors 'upstream' of the enzyme block. Effects of the precursors include virilisation, increased urinary sodium losses (by blocking the action of aldosterone) and hypertension[1]. Clinical manifestations depend on the site of the block and hence the precursors which accumulate. The commonest variety, partial 21-hydroxylase deficiency, causes virilisation; complete 21-hydroxylase deficiency also causes excessive urinary salt loss. 11-α-hydroxylase deficiency produces virilisation and hypertension without salt loss.

PROGNOSIS

- Life expectancy is normal in mild forms.
- Salt-losing forms cause potentially fatal adrenal crises soon after birth.
- Life-threatening hypoglycaemia may occur during febrile illness, especially in salt-losing forms[2].
- Adequate treatment normalises life expectancy and restores fertility.

TREATMENT

1. Glucocorticoids correct cortisol deficiency and suppress excessive ACTH production and hence precursor accumulation. Hydrocortisone (25 mg/m^2 of body surface area) or dexamethasone (0.5–1.5 mg/day) in two or three daily doses; a larger evening dose may maximise the suppressive effect. Dosages are adjusted to normalise plasma or urinary steroid precursor concentrations.
2. Mineralocorticoids (e.g. fludrocortisone, 50–200 μg/day) are indicated in salt-losing forms.
3. Hypertension (in 11-α-hydroxylase deficiency) responds to glucocorticoids.

FOLLOW-UP

Lifelong, regular review of replacement treatment (see p. 206). Patients should carry a steroid card, have an emergency supply of steroids and be aware of the risk of hypoglycaemia.

[1] Bongiovanni AM *et al.* (1967) *Rec. Prog. Horm Res.*, **23**, 375.
[2] Hinde FRJ *et al.* (1984) *Br. Med. J.*, **289**, 1603.

Carcinoid and Other Gastrointestinal Endocrine Tumours

These rare tumours, characterised by cytoplasmic hormone secretory granules and neurone-specific enolase activity[1], mostly arise from the gut and pancreas and frequently metastasise to the liver. They secrete peptides and amines which produce characteristic syndromes. Midgut carcinoids produce serotonin and other mediators which cause the classical carcinoid syndrome; VIPomas secrete vasoactive intestinal polypeptide, causing watery diarrhoea; gastrinomas cause recurrent peptic ulceration and diarrhoea; insulinomas cause hypoglycaemia; glucagonomas cause diabetes and a migratory necrolytic rash.

PROGNOSIS

- Very variable; survival may be prolonged even with disseminated metastases.
- Carcinoid: most metastasise; five-year survival 33% (hindgut), 99% (midgut).
- Insulinoma: 85% are benign; removal of a lone primary is usually curative.
- VIPoma, gastrinoma and glucagonoma: 60–90% are malignant.

TREATMENT

1. In the absence of metastases, the primary tumour (e.g. insulinoma) should be removed.
2. Hepatic and other metastases

   a) Arterial embolisation with microspheres or a suspension of dura mater[2].
   b) Chemotherapy: streptozotocin and 5-fluorouracil are being evaluated[3].
   c) Surgical debulking is palliative but may improve symptoms.

3. Specific medical treatments

   a) Carcinoid: serotonin antagonists, e.g. cyproheptadine (up to 32 mg/day in divided doses); short courses (<6 months) of methysergide (2–6 mg/day); p-chlorophenylalanine is still experimental.
   b) Insulinoma: frequent meals and diazoxide (5 mg/kg/day in divided doses).
   c) VIPoma, gastrinoma, glucagonoma: long-acting subcutaneously-injectable somatostatin analogues suppress peptide hormone release[4].
   d) VIPoma: prednisolone 40–60 mg/day.
   e) Gastrinoma: H_2-blockers (e.g. cimetidine 800–1600 mg/day) and omeprazole (a proton pump inhibitor; 20–60 mg/day) both inhibit acid secretion.
   f) Glucagonoma: zinc sulphate 200 mg eight hourly may improve the rash.

FOLLOW-UP

Regular monitoring of tumour markers (peptide hormones, urinary 5HIAA) and of tumour bulk (serial CT or ultrasound scanning). Patients and their first-order relatives should be screened for MEN 1.

[1] Polak JM, Bloom SR (1985) *Endocrine Tumours*. London: Churchill Livingstone.
[2] Allison D J *et al*. (1977) *Lancet*, **ii**, 1323.
[3] Moertel CG *et al*. (1980) *New Eng. J. Med.*, **303**, 1189.
[4] Wood SM *et al*. (1985) *Gut*, **26**, 438.

11

Metabolic Diseases

H. Keen and D. L. Cohen

Diabetes Mellitus

Insulin dependent diabetes, lethal in the absence of treatment, differs in many respects from the non-insulin dependent type. Insulin dependent diabetes mellitus (IDDM, Type 1) affects about 1 per 1000 children under age 16. Peaks of onset occur in autumn and winter months. Susceptibility is inherited with HLA DR3 and DR4 antigens. An auto-immune attack upon insulin producing cells, perhaps triggered by viral infection(s) may be responsible for the insulin deficiency. This is relevant to attempts to slow or reverse the process in recently diagnosed IDDM with immunomodulatory drugs. Non-insulin dependent diabetes mellitus (NIDDM, Type 2) prevalence rises with age, peaking in the 60s in Europeans and 10–20 years earlier in Asians. Symptoms vary from moderate to trivial. It is often associated with obesity and is commonly familial.

PROGNOSIS (IDDM)

- Insulin treatment usually prevents early metabolic fatalities but life expectancy is reduced by the complications of diabetes. Loss of expected years of life, approximately 20–30 in those with youthful onset, lessens with increasing age at diagnosis.
- Most diabetologists believe that good metabolic control lowers the incidence of some complications. This is based largely on clinical observations that 'better controlled' patients are less likely to develop severe complications, and experiments suggesting that renal and retinal lesions are less likely to affect better treated diabetic animals. However some poorly-controlled diabetics escape complications and some well-controlled patients fall victim. Individual genetic or environmental factors are probably important. The main arguments are summarised by West[1].
- About 40% youthful onset IDDM will develop renal failure due to diabetic nephropathy. About half of these will reach end-stage renal failure and either die of it or receive renal support.
- Coronary heart disease, occurring twice as often in diabetics as in matched non-diabetics, is a major cause of premature mortality and affects both sexes equally. Peripheral arterial disease contributes to chronic foot ulceration, intermittent claudication and gangrene in 5–10% long-term IDDM patients.
- Diabetic neuropathy also contributes to chronic foot ulceration and occasionally causes Charcot arthropathy. Visceral neuropathy causes episodic diarrhoea, postural hypotension and is implicated in male impotence although this may be psychogenic[2].
- Diabetic retinopathy is the cause of most blindness registrations in middle-aged people, and affects about 10% diabetic surviving 20 years or more of the disease. Timely photocoagulation should reduce this risk. Regular screening for high-risk features of retinopathy (early new vessels or large superficial haemorrhages) is essential.
- Diabetic ketoacidosis may complicate the course of IDDM and cause death particularly in older patients. Severe hypoglycaemia may also be lethal or leave serious neurological defects such as hemiparesis or mental impairment.
- Enhanced susceptibility to chronic and sometimes unusual infections may cause severe disability. Pulmonary tuberculosis, chronic urinary tract infections and destructive sepsis in the feet should be anticipated.

TREATMENT (IDDM)

1. Treatment for the acutely ill

a) In the newly diagnosed severely ketoacidotic patient, hospital admission, rehydration, insulin administration, electrolyte and cardiovascular monitoring and treatment of coexistent infection is life saving. The comatose patient will require up to 5 or 6 l of intravenous saline in the first 24 hours and intravenous insulin delivered continuously at a rate of 3–6 units per hour with supplements of potassium chloride (20–30 mmol with each litre

214

saline) during the first few hours of treatment and when plasma potassium falls. Intravenous sodium bicarbonate is rarely indicated. Emptying the stomach by nasogastric suction will prevent aspiration of vomit, and catheterisation may be needed for urinary retention. When glucose falls to 10 or 11 mmol/l insulin administration should be slowed and 5% glucose added to the i.v. regime.

b) Accurate fluid replacement requires a central venous line and intensive care.

c) A precipitating cause for ketoacidosis in new or known diabetics must always be sought. Common viral or bacterial infections often affecting the urinary or respiratory tracts, may be responsible. Sputum, urine and blood should be cultured routinely, but 'best guess' antibiotics started only if bacterial infection is likely or the patient very ill. In the older patient ketoacidosis may be associated with painless myocardial infarction only revealed by an ECG.

d) In hyperosmolar states with dramatically high blood glucose levels, hypernatraemia and raised urea, subcutaneous heparin to prevent thromboses should be given as well as insulin and normal or half-normal saline i.v. fluids.

2. Maintenance treatment

a) Maintenance insulin should ideally be given at least twice daily. Regimens should provide insulin peaks from soluble insulin to coincide with main meals, and basal levels between meals and overnight from slower acting preparations. Commonly a mixture of soluble and either isophane or lente insulin in the proportion 40:60 is given 20 minutes before breakfast and before the evening meal. Alternatively a daily dose of ultralente insulin provides the basal levels upon which peaks of soluble, taken before main meals, are superimposed. The insulin regimen must take the life style and preferences of the patient into account.

b) Diet should be as near to normal for the patient as possible. Carbohydrate, largely unrefined, should provide 50–55% calories; fats, some polyunsaturated, 30–35% calories, and protein the remainder[3].

c) Porcine insulins are less immunogenic than bovine, and human insulins even less so. Many physicians use human insulin for patients receiving injections temporarily and for new diabetics. Established patients may be confused by the quicker onset of action of the human preparations and should not be changed without good reason.

d) Self-management should be encouraged by teaching the patient to measure blood glucose with strips, how to improve control and the need to continue insulin even when ill, balanced if necessary by glucose drinks. Hypoglycaemia from delayed meals or extra exertion should be explained and emergency action suggested. Systematic education is vital for good control.

e) Pregnancy and contraception should routinely be discussed with young female diabetics. The combined oral contraceptive is not contraindicated but blood pressure and lipids should be monitored. Diabetic women should aim for normal blood sugars before planning a pregnancy and should maintain tight control throughout. This is thought to reduce the risk of fetal abnormality, abnormally large babies and obstetric problems[4].

PROGNOSIS (NIDDM)

- The risk of arterial disease (coronary heart disease, peripheral vascular disease and stroke), the main hazard in NIDDM, is approximately doubled compared with non-diabetics. Fatality rates from myocardial infarction are doubled. The risk of gangrene in toes and feet is 20 times increased.

- Visual disability from retinopathy, especially maculopathy, from cataract or from both is common.

- Though initially controlled with diet or oral agents 25% NIDDM patients will later require insulin. Stress such as trauma or infection may lead to a period of ketoacidosis during which insulin is necessary.

Contd.

TREATMENT (NIDDM)

1. A diet similar to that in IDDM, restricted in calories in the obese, may initially control blood glucose.

2. Sulphonylureas such as tolbutamide up to 1 g bd for older milder cases, or glibenclamide up to 15 mg bd will be required if diet fails. They may cause weight gain in which case metformin, a biguanide, in doses up to 1 g bd may control glycaemia, either by itself or with sulphonylureas. Hypoglycaemia, though uncommon, may be a problem especially in the elderly.

3. Failure to respond to diet and drugs or loss of initial response is an indication for insulin. The thin middle-aged NIDDM patient may require insulin from the beginning.

4. Associated hypertension and hypercholesterolaemia should be sought and corrected.

5. Retinopathy, which often affects the macular region threatening central vision, is treatable by photocoagulation. Patients should have their fundi examined through dilated pupils regularly.

6. Urinary tract infection should be suspected and eradicated in poorly controlled NIDDM patients.

7. Those with neuropathy should be taught correct foot care and have regular chiropody[5].

FOLLOW-UP

A system of regular annual review is an essential minimum for all diabetics. This should include fundoscopy through dilated pupils and visual acuity testing, measurement of blood pressure and examination of the feet for neuropathy. Other visits to improve control and dietary adherence may be needed. Most NIDDs are best followed by interested GPs sharing care with the hospital[6].

[1] West KM (1982) In *Complications of Diabetes* 2nd edn. (Keen H, Jarrett RJ eds.). London: Edward Arnold.
[2] Hosking DJ et al. (1979) *Br. Med. J.*, 2, 1394.
[3] Mann JI (1984) *Diabetic Medicine*, 1, 191.
[4] Kalkhoff RK (1985) *Diabetes*, 34 Suppl. 2, 97.
[5] Ward JD (1982) *Diabetologia*, 22, 141.
[6] Home P (1984) *Br. Med. J.*, 289, 713.

The Hyperlipidaemias

Hyperlipidaemia includes raised plasma cholesterol, raised fasting triglycerides or both and indicates abnormality of the lipid-carrying proteins. The condition may be primary due either to a single gene abnormality or more commonly polygenic when diet and obesity are important factors. If hyperlipidaemia occurs secondary to another disease such as hypothyroidism, alcohol abuse or chronic renal disease, recognition and treatment of this underlying cause is important.

PROGNOSIS

- Raised cholesterol, in low or intermediate density lipoproteins, probably leads to arterial disease by direct deposition in the arterial intima. The risk of atherosclerosis increases with rising cholesterol values, that of coronary heart disease being 2–4 times higher above 6.7 mmol/l than below this level. The rates of stroke and gangrene are also correlated with total serum cholesterol in people under 65.
- Skin and tendon xanthomas are more often found in the rarer single gene disorders. In the commoner polygenic cases of hypercholesterolaemia the risk of arterial disease is lower, family history less striking, and skin lesions less common.
- In severe hypertriglyceridaemia an eruptive xanthomatous skin rash and lipaemia retinalis may occur and uncommonly, attacks of abdominal pain (Zieve syndrome) and acute pancreatitis.
- Close relatives of index cases should be screened and treated if affected.

TREATMENT[1,2]

1. Diet

    a) Reduction of total fat intake to 30–35% calories.
    b) Increase of the ratio of polyunsaturated to saturated fatty acids to 0.7–1.0 : 1.0.
    c) Replacement of fat calories with unrefined carbohydrate especially legumes,

e.g. beans. Greatly raised triglycerides require restriction of dietary fats and their partial replacement by medium-chain triglyceride supplements.

2. If diet is ineffective a drug should be used. Cholestyramine is the first choice for severe hypercholesterolaemia, probucol an alternative. Clofibrate or nicotinic acid are used for raised triglycerides.
3. Patients with severe hypercholesterolaemia who are resistant to drug treatment may be suitable for plasmapheresis or surgical diversion of portal blood to the systemic circulation. Xanthomata may require surgical removal.
4. Prevention of CHD in large populations may depend on reduction of fat intake by the population at large and this advice has been adopted by many national health agencies[3,4].

FOLLOW-UP

Patients on a diet require frequent brief consultations for accurate weighing, correction of dietary errors and moral support. Drug treatment should be stopped if ineffective because of doubt about long-term unwanted effects.

[1] *Drugs Ther. Bull.* (1982) **20**, 41.
[2] Buckley BM *et al.* (1982) *Br. Med. J.*, **285**, 1293.
[3] Prevention of coronary heart disease (1983) *J. Roy. Coll. Phys.*, **17**, 66.
[4] Prevention of coronary heart disease. Report of a World Health Organisation expert committee (1982) Technical report series 678. Geneva: WHO.

Osteoporosis

Osteoporosis[1] refers to loss of bone mass and may be secondary to other disorders such as thyrotoxicosis, or to steroid therapy. In women bone mass decreases rapidly in the first three years after the menopause and more slowly thereafter. Initial bone mass is greater in Africans so depletion takes longer. Clinically it contributes to the occurrence of femoral neck, wrist and vertebral crush fractures.

PROGNOSIS

- The prevalence of femoral neck, spine, and wrist fractures is 0.6%, and 2.5%, and 5% in 60-year-old white women and 6%, 7.5%, and 15% at age 80. Fracture healing is normal.
- The overall mortality from femoral neck fractures is 30%.

TREATMENT[1]

1. Underlying causes should be treated.
2. Vertebral crush fractures require 2–3 weeks bed rest with a pillow to hyperextend the site of fracture for one hour twice daily. The patient should be taught improved postural use of the back.
3. There is no proven way to restore bone mass or strength after a fracture.
4. Prevention of further bone loss, either prophylactically around the menopause or after a fracture, can be achieved with oestrogen replacement and calcium supplements.
5. Cyclical oestrogen replacement, with added progestogen to reduce the possible risk of endometrial cancer, is effective but carries all the unwanted effects of oestrogen therapy, including monthly withdrawal bleeds, and the need for supervision by a gynaecologist. It should be offered to all women who have a premature menopause.
6. The optimum duration of oestrogen replacement has never been properly eval-

uated. The benefit of treatment is probably maintained when treatment is stopped.
7. Recent evidence suggests that other 'fast bone losers' may be detectable by a urinary hydroxyproline >0.1 mmol/24 hours or a serum alkaline phosphatase >130 i.u./l.
8. Most Western women have daily calcium intakes less than 1.5–2 g daily. Calcium supplements should be given to raise the daily intake to this value. Three tablets of Sandocal provide 1 g and should be taken between meals. This reduces bone loss and vertebral fracture rate[2].
9. Reducing protein intake to <60 g/day reduces the obligatory urinary calcium loss and therefore conserves body calcium.
10. Fluoride may be effective but has a high incidence of minor side-effects.
11. Vitamin D is indicated only in patients with calcium malabsorption.

FOLLOW-UP

The number of women at risk is enormous and treatment unproven once bone loss has occurred. Simple advice on maintaining a high calcium intake and making the environment safer for the elderly may be as valuable as routine hormone replacement therapy.

---

[1] Nordin BEC (1985) *Metabolic Bone and Stone Disease* 2nd edn. London: Churchill Livingstone.
[2] Matkovic V et al. (1979) *Am. J. Clin. Nutr.*, **32**, 540.

Osteomalacia

Osteomalacia in adults and rickets in children is due to lack of vitamin D. In the UK osteomalacia most often occurs in Asian immigrants and the elderly[1], mainly due to lack of exposure to sunlight. It presents with bone pain or proximal myopathy or is detected after biochemical screening. It may be secondary to malabsorption or renal disease.

PROGNOSIS

- If treatment is given before deformities have occurred recovery is complete.
- In rachitic children treated before the age of four deformity may also resolve.

TREATMENT

1. In the absence of malabsorption, treatment is with oral vitamin D as calcium and vitamin D tablets 1 bd, which provides 1000 u vitamin D daily. Myopathy and pain improve within a month. Bone healing takes about 10 months. Therapy should continue for at least a year, and in the two major groups at risk a long-term supplement is worthwhile. Recently a single intramuscular injection of 600 000 u vitamin D has been shown to restore and maintain normal biochemistry for at least six months and avoid the need to take tablets[2].

2. Causes of malabsorption should be corrected if possible. Therapy is with higher doses of potent vitamin D preparations, e.g. calciferol, high strength 40 000–100 000 u daily or i.m. vitamin D. Calcium should also be given.

3. Osteomalacia due to renal tubular disorders or vitamin D resistance requires 1,25 OH vitamin D 1 μg/day with phosphate supplements in the former. These disorders need specialist supervision.

4. The treatment of renal osteodystrophy is complicated and should be managed by a specialist. A high calcium intake is maintained, with aluminium hydroxide as a binder to reduce phosphate absorption. When plasma phosphate falls to less than 2 mmol/l, vitamin D, most conveniently as 1,25 OH D, is indicated.

FOLLOW-UP

In those at risk serum vitamin D should be measured annually and supplements given as necessary. Patients with malabsorption or renal disease should be followed in out-patients.

---

[1] Sharland D (1982) *J. Roy. Coll. Phys.*, **16**, 502.
[2] Burns J *et al.* (1985) *Br. Med. J.*, **290**, 281.

Hyperuricaemia and Gout

Hyperuricaemia can give rise to several clinical problems: acute gouty arthritis, chronic gouty arthritis or uric acid stones. It may be asymptomatic. Symptoms result from crystallisation of sodium urate in synovial fluid or urine. Rare enzyme deficiencies, haematological malignancy and its treatment, and drugs, commonly thiazides, may cause hyperuricaemia. Most patients have a genetic tendency influenced by environmental factors such as alcohol or obesity[1].

PROGNOSIS

- With current treatment gout carries no excess mortality.
- Untreated chronic gouty arthritis may lead to deformity and loss of function.
- On balance there is no good evidence that the treatment of asymptomatic hyperuricaemia has any effect on the incidence of ischaemic heart disease, renal failure or gouty arthritis.

TREATMENT[2]

1. Acute arthritis: Indomethacin 50 mg tds or colchicine 1 mg stat plus 0.5 mg two hourly until attack subsides or diarrhoea occurs. Allopurinol is contraindicated. Other non-steroidal anti-inflammatory drugs may also be effective.
2. Chronic arthritis: Allopurinol in a dose sufficient to return the serum urate to normal. Indomethacin or colchicine may be prescribed concurrently for the first two months to prevent acute attacks.
3. Sulphinpyrazone and probenecid are uricosuric and therefore contraindicated in stone disease and ineffective in renal failure. They are now used less often.

4. Renal stones are managed by increasing fluid intake and lowering urate excretion with allopurinol as above. While the urate concentration is still high, stone formation can be reduced by raising urine pH to >6.2 using oral alkalis.
5. Long-term lowering of serum urate is only indicated in:

   a) Frequent acute attacks of arthritis.
   b) Gout with chronic joint changes or tophi.
   c) Gout with evidence of renal damage.
   d) Gout with a serum urate consistently $>480\,\mu mol/l$.

6. In completely asymptomatic hyperuricaemia long-term treatment is indicated only if urate $>540\,\mu mol/l$ (see *Prognosis*).

FOLLOW-UP

When long-term treatment is indicated, follow-up should be frequent until urate levels are normal and then twice yearly.

[1] Scott JT (1983) *Gout Ann. Rheum. Dis.*, **42** Suppl 16.
[2] Scott JT (1980) *Br. Med. J.*, **281**, 1164.

Porphyrias

This group of disorders is due to deficient enzymes in the pathway of haem biosynthesis leading to the accumulation of intermediates – porphyrins. Inheritance is autosomal dominant. Acute porphyrias – acute intermittent, variegate and coproporphyria – present with abdominal pain, predominantly motor neuropathy and acute psychiatric disturbances. Porphyria cutanea tarda (PCT) and erythropoietic protoporphyria present with skin photosensitivity. PCT is almost always associated with liver disease, usually alcoholic.

PROGNOSIS

- Women have more attacks than men, often related to menstruation or oral contraceptives.
- Most deaths are due to the adult respiratory distress syndrome but they are now rare in major centres.
- There may be residual wrist or foot drop.

TREATMENT[1]

1. Acute attacks can be prevented by avoidance of all drugs (except those known to be safe), and of dieting or starvation. Sulphonamides, barbiturates, phenytoin and oestrogens are common culprits[2].
2. Relatives should be screened and taught about the disease if affected.
3. Acute attacks often present with abdominal pain and vomiting or neuropathy. Most resolve with supportive treatment and a high carbohydrate intake (400 g/day) with supplements of Hycal or 20% fructose 2 l/day into a central vein if nausea prevents normal feeding. Alcohol and drugs known to precipitate acute attacks must be avoided.
4. Pain is treated safely with aspirin or morphine, anxiety with chlorpromazine, hypertension and tachycardia with propranolol. Acid-base and electrolyte abnormalities are monitored and corrected. Respiration is monitored – mechanical ventilation may be needed for respiratory paralysis.
5. Paralysed limbs need splinting and passive physiotherapy. Active physiotherapy should start with recovery.
6. If the attack is worsening after 1–2 days, haematin, prepared from red cells and infused intravenously, leads to clinical or biochemical improvement in 50–80% patients. It is not usually helpful once assisted ventilation has been required.
7. Sunlight should be avoided in patients with photosensitive rashes. Sunscreens have to be highly coloured to be effective as the photosensitivity lies in the visible spectrum.
8. In porphyria cutanea tarda venesection until haemoglobin falls below 12 g/dl or until no new skin lesions appear will induce remission which may last three years. Chloroquine can be used where venesection is contraindicated. 250 mg twice weekly induces an acute hepatitic reaction and resolution of symptoms.

FOLLOW-UP

Patients should be warned always to alert all doctors as to their condition. They should be followed in hospital out-patients where the current state of their illness can be updated and passed on to relatives and GPs.

---

[1] Goldberg A et al. (1980) Clin. Haemat., 9, 2.
[2] Magnus IA (1984) Br. Med. J., 288, 1474.

12

Viral Diseases

J. E. Banatvala and J. M. Welch

Measles

Meales is an acute infectious disease caused by a paramyxo-like virus classified as a morbillivirus and is characterised by fever, coryza, cough, conjunctivitis, enanthem and rash. Complications are common, particularly in malnourished or immunosuppressed patients. Before the advent of vaccination in the UK there were about 500 000 notifications of measles in each epidemic year. Although a safe and effective vaccine is now available, only about 60% children in the UK receive it, and this poor uptake is insufficient to control the disease; there are still up to 100 000 cases of measles each year and 20 deaths. In the USA vaccination is a condition of school entry and so 97% children entering kindergarten have been vaccinated; in 1982 only 2000 cases of measles were notified.

PROGNOSIS

- In developing countries the mortality is up to 12%. In the UK 7% have a serious complication, and 1 in 5000 die.
- Croup is a complication of the prodromal period which rarely causes respiratory obstruction.
- Viral involvement of the respiratory tract occurs in almost all cases and resolves within a few days. Respiratory complications such as secondary bacterial pneumonia, bronchiolitis and severe bronchitis occur in 4%, and are the most common reasons for patients with measles being admitted to hospital in the UK[1].
- Febrile convulsions are the commonest neurological complication. Postinfectious encephalomyelitis occurs in 0.1% and causes demyelination; 60% recover completely, 25% have brain damage and 15% die. Coma or convulsions indicate a poor prognosis.
- Measles infection in immunocompromised patients may be atypical with a prolonged incubation period and no rash. Giant cell pneumonia and measles encephalopathy are relatively common and usually fatal.
- The incidence of sub-acute sclerosing panencephalitis is 0.2 per million, but the disease is becoming even rarer since the advent of measles vaccination. This disease is progressive and fatal.
- Measles virus is not teratogenic.

TREATMENT AND PREVENTION

1. Uncomplicated measles is treated with bed rest and analgesia if necessary. Fluids are encouraged. Humidification is helpful in infants.
2. Antibiotics given prophylactically do not prevent superinfection, and so should be reserved for bacterial complications such as pneumonia, otitis and conjunctivitis.
3. Live attenuated vaccine evokes a persistent antibody response in 95% and complications are rare. It should be given to all healthy children at one year, but is contraindicated in immunosuppressed patients.
4. Measles vaccine or human normal immunoglobulin, given within 72 hours of exposure, will prevent or attenuate the disease. Measles vaccine should be given to healthy contacts and immunoglobulin to immunocompromised patients.

FOLLOW-UP

Follow-up is unnecessary once the patient is better.

---

[1] Carter H et al. (1985) Br. Med. J., i, 1717.

Rubella

Rubella is classified as a non-arthropod-borne togavirus (rubivirus). Infection with rubella may cause a mild febrile illness with rash, lymphadenopathy and conjunctivitis; it is asymptomatic in up to 25% cases. Other viruses can produce a similar picture, e.g. parvoviruses. Rubella is rarely complicated, except if acquired *in utero* when it may induce a persistent and generalised infection and result in a wide spectrum of anomalies which include nerve deafness, cataract, cardiac abnormalities and mental retardation.

PROGNOSIS

- Arthralgia/arthritis occurs in up to 60% women but is less common in men and children; it seldom persists beyond 10 days, and there is no evidence of permanent sequelae.
- Encephalitis is very rare, but the mortality is said to approach 20%.
- The incidence and type of congenital defect depend on the stage of pregnancy in which infection is contracted. Following rubella in the first trimester 90% fetuses are infected and almost all of these are affected[1]; spontaneous abortion occurs in up to 20%. Cardiac and eye abnormalities occur in over 50% of those infected in the first two months. The risk declines thereafter, but deafness may occur following infection up to the twentieth week.

TREATMENT AND PREVENTION

1. Live attenuated vaccines produce persisting immunity in over 90%. Congenital rubella can be prevented by ensuring that all women are immune before becoming pregnant.
2. Therapeutic abortion should be offered to women who have serologically-proven rubella during the first 3–4 months of pregnancy.
3. Human normal immunoglobulin reduces, but does not eliminate, risk to the fetus[2]. High titre rubella immunoglobulin is available from the Scottish Blood Transfusion Service, and may be more effective. Immunoglobulin should be given to susceptible pregnant women who have been exposed to rubella but would refuse abortion.
4. Joint involvement is treated with analgesics or non-steroidal anti-inflammatory drugs.

FOLLOW-UP

Infants with intrauterine infection, even though apparently healthy at birth, should be reviewed regularly to detect late sequelae, particularly deafness. Review of acquired rubella in a non-pregnant patient is only necessary if joint involvement is severe and prolonged.

---

[1] Miller E *et al.* (1982) *Lancet*, ii, 781.
[2] Peckham CS (1974) *Br. Med. J.*, i, 259.

Mumps

Mumps is an acute febrile illness caused by a paramyxovirus. Characteristically the salivary glands are affected but involvement of other glandular tissue and the CNS is not uncommon. The disease is usually mild in children; adults are more prone to complications.

PROGNOSIS

- Parotitis resolves within 10 days.
- Epididymo-orchitis occurs in 20% postpubertal males, and is unilateral in over 90%. Sterility rarely results.
- Oophoritis is not uncommon; sterility has not been described.
- Pancreatitis is common but usually mild, resolving within seven days.
- Aseptic meningitis occurs in 10% and may precede parotitis. It is often asymptomatic. Complete resolution within seven days is usual.
- Postinfectious encephalomyelitis is rare, severe and potentially fatal.
- Deafness is very rare, usually unilateral, and irreversible. It is generally preceded by vertigo, tinnitus and vomiting.

TREATMENT AND PREVENTION

1. Uncomplicated mumps requires only symptomatic treatment.
2. The pain of orchitis responds to hydrocortisone (100 mg 1m tds); a scrotal support also helps.
3. Live attenuated mumps vaccine is given routinely to all children in the USA, is safe and produces prolonged immunity in up to 99%. In the UK consideration of vaccination may be given to adults at risk such as non-immune male medical staff.
4. Neither vaccine nor mumps-specific immunoglobulin protects susceptible contacts following exposure.

FOLLOW-UP

Follow-up is unnecessary once the patient is better.

Herpes Viruses

Herpes virus infections generally occur in childhood and, with the exception of varicella, are usually asymptomatic. After primary infection, these DNA viruses become latent, but may reactivate later, especially if immunity is impaired.

Herpes simplex virus (HSV)

HSV infections are characterised by vesicles but can be protean, particularly in the immunosuppressed. HSV-II causes the majority of genital herpes, whereas HSV-I is isolated from most lesions elsewhere; HSV-II genital lesions recur more frequently than those caused by HSV-I. Viraemia occurs in primary disease and causes systemic symptoms, which are rare during reactivation.

PROGNOSIS

- Primary infection is usually oral, but may occur elsewhere on the face or body. It is usually asymptomatic but may also result in a variety of clinical manifestations. The commonest is a gingivostomatitis which in infants can cause feeding problems and occasionally dehydration. Spontaneous resolution occurs within 10–14 days. The frequency of recurrence is widely variable, but the site affected tends to be constant.
- A primary herpetic whitlow often increases in size and severity for 7–10 days before subsiding over the next month; recurrences may occur.
- Primary ophthalmic HSV may cause an acute follicular conjunctivitis or keratoconjunctivitis, often with surrounding vesicles. This usually settles within one month, but up to 15% develop a chronic blepharoconjunctivitis which lasts for months[1]. Reactivation produces dendritic or stromal keratitis which can progress to scarring and blindness.
- Patients with eczema or burns may develop a generalised infection with HSV (eczema herpeticum). In severe cases the lesions become atypical and confluent, and the mortality approaches 10% without treatment.
- Herpes encephalitis is rare but serious; treatment with acyclovir reduces the mortality from 50% to 19%, but 30% of the survivors are disabled[2]. Poor prognostic features are coma and age over 30.
- Primary genital herpes is often asymptomatic but may cause severe pain and retention of urine; resolution is complete in 2–6 weeks. Recurrences occur in 50%; the average frequency is 3–4 times/year.
- Neonatal HSV is more severe when acquired from a primary maternal genital infection since virus concentrations are high and the baby is unprotected by maternal antibody; dissemination occurs in 80% and the mortality is then 70%.
- Immunosuppressed patients may develop large ulcers which often take weeks to heal. Disseminated disease may occur and is frequently fatal without treatment.

TREATMENT

1. Mild herpetic lesions in immunocompetent patients warrant only symptomatic treatment. The use of expensive specific therapy may often be obviated by skilled counselling relating to risks of transmission and factors inducing reactivation.
2. Topical acyclovir (ACV) (5% ACV cream five times/day) has a limited role in treating genital and non-genital infections. Patient-initiated treatment during the prodrome is most likely to be successful, and once ulcers or vesicles are visible treatment is useless.
Contd.

ACV is the treatment of choice in ocular herpes (3% ACV ointment five times/day), being more effective than vidarabine or idoxuridine. Trifluorothymidine is available on a named patient basis for patients who develop sensitivity to ACV.

3. Oral ACV (200 mg five times/day for five days) may accelerate healing in disabling infections such as gingivo-stomatitis, herpetic whitlow, primary genital herpes, and ulceration in immunosuppressed patients. Prophylactic oral administration suppresses reactivation, and is useful to cover severe immunosuppressive events such as bone marrow transplantation (BMT). Long-term (e.g. 3-4 months) oral therapy is effective in suppressing recurrent genital lesions but this should be reserved for patients who have frequent severe episodes.

4. Intravenous ACV (5 mg/kg tds for 5-7 days) is indicated in eczema herpeticum, severe primary genital herpes complicated by urinary retention, and disseminated disease. Adenosine arabinoside improves survival in neonatal herpes, but preliminary studies of ACV are encouraging. A higher dose of ACV (10 mg/kg tds) is needed for herpes encephalitis, and this should be continued for 10 days.

5. Idoxuridine and adenosine arabinoside have now been superseded by acyclovir. Topical idoxuridine (5% in dimethyl sulphoxide) is of limited value in treating cutaneous HSV. Adenosine arabinoside is relatively insoluble and therefore cumbersome to administer, and is much less potent than ACV.

6. A DNA-free HSV-II subunit vaccine has been shown to boost cell-mediated immunity and antibody titres in patients with recurrent HSV-I or HSV-II, and to reduce significantly the frequency and duration of their recurrences[3].

FOLLOW-UP

Most HSV infections are self-limiting and follow-up is necessary only if recurrences are likely to lead to permanent damage, e.g. ocular herpes, morbidity or severe genital herpes. Consultations are often patient-initiated.

[1] Darougar S et al. (1985) Br. J. Ophthalmology, 69, 2.
[2] Skoldenberg B et al. (1984) Lancet, ii, 707.
[3] Cappel R et al. (1985) J. Med. Virol., 16, 137.

Varicella/zoster (VZ)

Primary infection causes varicella (chickenpox), and reactivation produces zoster (shingles). Varicella is a febrile illness with a vesicular rash; in children it is characteristically mild but in adults may be more severe. Asymptomatic infection is rare, but as a sparse rash is often missed or forgotten, 20-40% individuals with no history of varicella actually have antibodies to VZ.

The incidence and severity of shingles increases with age. Patients with markedly impaired cell-mediated immunity are particularly prone to serious and often life-threatening complications of both varicella and zoster.

PROGNOSIS (VARICELLA/CHICKENPOX)

- Resolution without complications within 14 days is usual in almost all children and most adults.
- Fetal damage complicating varicella in early pregnancy has been reported in about 20 cases. Ultrasound and fetoscopy may be of value in determining whether fetal damage has occurred.
- Neonatal varicella is likely to be severe if the disease is acquired from a maternal infection occurring in the five days before or month following delivery.
- Abnormal chest x-rays are common in adults with varicella and pulmonary calcification may be permanent; overt pneumonia is rare but causes death, often suddenly, in up to 30%.
- Post-infectious encephalomyelitis affects children more frequently than adults and characteristically results in cerebellar ataxia. The mortality is up to 5%; over 80% recover completely although the remainder may have psychological and neurological sequelae. Coma indicates a poor prognosis.
- Thrombocytopenia or coagulation defects may cause bleeding into the rash and elsewhere, and may be fatal.

- Untreated varicella in leukaemic children has a mortality of up to 30%; pneumonia occurs commonly. Patients immunosuppressed for other reasons fare better.

TREATMENT AND PREVENTION (VARICELLA/CHICKENPOX)

1. Recent trials with live attenuated varicella vaccines have shown that they are well tolerated and protective if given to seronegative medical staff or leukaemic children in remission or between courses of chemotherapy. One dose is adequate in healthy patients but leukaemics may need boosters. Currently the vaccine is available for named patients.
2. Uncomplicated varicella merits symptomatic treatment only.
3. Anti-varicella-zoster immunoglobulin (ZIG) may prevent or attenuate infection if given within five days of exposure. It is indicated for neonates exposed to maternal varicella (see above), and is also available for non-immune immunosuppressed patients and pregnant women exposed to varicella or zoster. There is no evidence that ZIG is valuable in established infection.
4. As acyclovir (ACV) is less potent against VZ than against herpes simplex, higher dose intravenous therapy (10 mg/kg tds, adjusted in renal failure) is needed to reach therapeutic levels for serious infections. As in-patient treatment is required, and ACV is expensive, it should be reserved for life-threatening disease such as varicella pneumonia or varicella in an immunocompromised patient. It should be started within three days of the onset of the illness if possible.
5. Adenosine arabinoside is effective against varicella in immunosuppressed patients, but has now been superseded by the easier to administer and more potent ACV.
6. Experimentally, interferon (α) has been shown to limit local spread and dissemination of infection in immunocompromised patients.

PROGNOSIS (ZOSTER/SHINGLES)

- Uncomplicated zoster resolves within two weeks.

- Dissemination occurs in up to 10%, producing a varicelliform rash of varying severity which generally resolves within 7–10 days. It is most common in patients who are elderly or have impaired cell-mediated immunity for other reasons. Widespread visceral involvement is rare but life threatening.
- As zoster is not a marker of occult malignancy, an intensive search for a tumour is not justified[1].
- Ocular involvement complicates 50% cases of ophthalmic zoster: most tissues of the globe can be affected causing a variety of lesions many of which, such as episcleritis, scleritis and keratitis, often become chronic or relapse up to six years later. Iritis occurs in 52%; 12% of these develop permanent sphincter damage. External ocular muscle palsies occur in 31%; symptomatic resolution is usual within three months. Optic neuritis occurs in 1%; the prognosis for vision is poor.
- Facial nerve involvement causes paralysis, which is usually complete. Improvement may continue for over a year; recovery is full in 50% and good in a further 39%[2].
- Bladder or rectal dysfunction complicating sacral zoster usually resolves completely within four months.
- Post-herpetic neuralgia is more common over the age of 65, and especially complicates ophthalmic involvement. It usually settles in weeks or months, but may persist indefinitely. Severe and disabling pain may result in suicide.

TREATMENT AND PREVENTION (ZOSTER/SHINGLES)

1. Vaccination may prove useful in older people to prevent shingles by boosting cell-mediated immunity.
2. Mild zoster requires only simple analgesia.
3. Topical idoxuridine, if given within the first three days, may reduce the duration of pain in the acute illness and accelerate healing but its use is limited by inconvenience, cost and side-effects.
4. High doses of oral ACV (e.g. 800 mg five times/day) if given early may arrest progress

Contd.

of the disease and reduce pain, but it is absorbed poorly and erratically and the optimum dose is not yet established. Amino (hydroxyethoxymethyl) purine is a prodrug of ACV under trial which may prove useful as its oral absorption is excellent[3]. There is no evidence that ACV reduces the incidence of post-herpetic neuralgia.

5. Steroids (e.g. prednisolone 40 mg daily for 10 days, reducing to none over the next three weeks) have been shown to diminish the incidence of post-herpetic neuralgia in elderly patients if given early[4]. In the absence of contraindications this is a safe and effective treatment.

6. Intravenous ACV (10 mg/kg tds, reduced in renal failure) should be reserved for patients who have severe complications or are immunocompromised.

7. Eye involvement should be treated with topical ACV (3% eye ointment, five times/day), and with systemic ACV if it is severe and new skin lesions are still forming; the patient should also be seen by an ophthalmologist.

8. Analgesics, combinations of an antidepressant with a major tranquilliser, transcutaneous nerve stimulation, and acupuncture may all be useful in individual patients. In otherwise intractable cases injection or surgical ablation of the nerve may be necessary.

FOLLOW-UP

Follow-up is unnecessary for uncomplicated varicella or zoster, but patients with severe post-herpetic neuralgia will benefit from support and perhaps referral to a pain clinic, and those with chronic ocular lesions may need regular ophthalmic review.

[1] Ragozzino MW et al. (1982) New Eng. J. Med., 7, 393.
[2] Heathfield KWG et al. (1978) Br. Med. J., i, 343.
[3] Selby P et al. (1984) Lancet, ii, 1428.
[4] Keczkes K et al. (1980) Br. J. Derm., 102, 551.

Cytomegalovirus (CMV)

Acquisition of antibody to CMV is related to age and social class; in general about 60% young adults have evidence of previous infection with CMV. Infection is usually subclinical but occasionally heterophile antibody-negative infectious mononucleosis-like illness or hepatitis may result. In transplant recipients and other immunocompromised patients CMV may produce fever, pneumonitis, leucopenia, hepatitis and retinitis, and sometimes prove fatal. Intrauterine infection by CMV is the commonest microbial cause of psychomotor retardation. Iatrogenic transmission of CMV can occur via transfusions of blood and blood products, and allografts.

PROGNOSIS

- Congenital CMV infection occurs in 0.3–0.4% infants; 5–15% of these have detectable CNS sequelae at five years, usually the result of primary maternal infection. Infection at any stage of pregnancy can cause damage.

- 60–90% renal transplant recipients have evidence of active CMV infection. 80% primary infections and 10–30% secondary infections are clinically overt. Primary infection is the more likely to cause serious illness and death, but the risks have been reduced by changes in immunosuppressive regimens[1].

- Up to 50% bone marrow transplant (BMT) recipients who survive more than three weeks develop symptomatic CMV infection, which has a mortality of 40–70%. Death usually results from interstitial pneumonia.

TREATMENT AND PREVENTION

1. Interferon may prove useful for prophylaxis of CMV infections in transplant recipients
2. A report that oral acyclovir (ACV) was effective in prophylaxis has not been confirmed
3. Dihydroxypropoxy methylguanine (DHPG)* is a derivative of ACV which has greater potency against CMV.
4. Foscarnet (trisodium phosphonoformate hexahydrate)* appears promising in transplant recipients with life-threating CMV infections[2]. It is virostatic and so early and prolonged administration is required.
5. Intravenous high titre anti-CMV immunoglobulin* prevents[3] or attenuates CMV infec

* Under trial in immunosuppressed patients.

tion when given prophylactically to BMT recipients. It has also been used with success in immunosuppressed patients with severe disease[4].

6. Live attenuated vaccine reduces the severity of CMV infection in renal transplant recipients[5], but it seems unlikely that such a vaccine will become generally available.
7. Iatrogenic CMV infection can be prevented by giving only blood, blood products, and organs from seronegative donors to seronegative transplant recipients and neonates.
8. Congenital disease is not preventable at present, as although primary infections can be diagnosed serologically, no markers of fetal damage are available.

FOLLOW-UP

Babies with congenital CMV may require repeated developmental assessment. Once postnatally-acquired CMV infection has resolved, follow-up is not necessary unless the patient is immunocompromised and symptoms recur.

[1] Kurtz JB et al. (1984) Q. J. Med., **211**, 341.
[2] Ringden O et al. (1985) Lancet, **i**, 1503.
[3] Condie RM et al. (1984) Am. J. Med., **76**, 134.
[4] Blacklock HA et al. (1985) Lancet, **ii**, 153.
[5] Plotkin SA et al. (1984) Lancet, **i**, 528.

Epstein–Barr virus (EBV) (including infectious mononucleosis)

Infection with EBV is usually subclinical but in adolescents and young adults commonly results in infectious mononucleosis (IM), a febrile illness with lymphadenopathy, pharyngitis, and often splenomegaly. In healthy individuals the illness is self-limiting and complications are rare. Immunocompromised patients may, however, develop a severe primary or recrudescent infection. EBV may also be involved in the pathogenesis of lymphomas in some of these patients. EBV infection is fatal in patients with X-linked lymphoproliferative syndrome (Duncan disease) in whom specific T-cell responses are impaired.

PROGNOSIS

- IM usually resolves completely within six weeks.
- Nasopharyngeal oedema is usual but rarely causes respiratory obstruction.
- Splenomegaly occurs in 50%; ruptured spleen is rare but potentially fatal.
- Although abnormal liver function tests occur in 95% patients, jaundice occurs in only 5% and is usually mild.
- Rash results in 90% patients given ampicillin and does not necessarily denote penicillin allergy.
- Neurological complications (e.g. meningitis, facial nerve palsy) are uncommon, but occur more frequently in adults than children; complete resolution is usual but occasional fatalities have been reported.
- Myocarditis and pericarditis are very rare, but transient asymptomatic ECG abnormalities are common.
- Although mild thrombocytopenia occurs in 25–40%, purpura is rare. Haemolytic anaemia is uncommon and usually self-limiting.
- Although prolonged malaise is unusual, vague debilitating symptoms are often too readily attributed to a previous episode of IM.

TREATMENT AND PREVENTION

1. Uncomplicated IM is treated with rest and aspirin.
2. Prednisolone (40 mg daily, reducing over 12 days) speeds resolution and improves wellbeing[1]; it is probably better reserved for such circumstances as students approaching final examinations.
3. Parenteral hydrocortisone (100 mg bd for three days) usually reduces severe nasopharyngeal oedema, and may obviate the need for tracheostomy.
4. Steroids are also indicated for neurological and cardiac complications, thrombocytopenia and haemolytic anaemia.
5. Ruptured spleen is life threatening, and treatment of shock, including blood transfusions, and surgery are required.
6. Immunocompromised patients with acute

Contd.

EBV infection may benefit from acyclovir (i.v. 10 mg/kg tds for 7–10 days).

7. Prolonged symptoms may be relieved by a 2–3 month course of antidepressants (e.g. amitryptiline, starting with 10 mg nocte, and increasing until the patient feels slightly sleepy in the mornings).

8. A subunit vaccine is currently in preparation and trials may be carried out involving students without EBV antibodies.

FOLLOW-UP

Follow-up is unnecessary once the patient has recovered.

---

[1] Bolden KJ (1972) *J. Roy. Coll. Gen. Prac.*, **22**, 87.

Human Papillomaviruses (HPV) (Warts)

These are potentially oncogenic DNA viruses; about 30 genotypes have been identified and each appears to be associated with a certain type of wart. Over the last 10 years the prevalence of genital warts and of cervical cancer and precancer has increased dramatically; there is mounting evidence that cervical dysplasia and cancer *in situ* are linked with genotypes 16 and 18.

PROGNOSIS

- Most warts eventually disappear spontaneously, but may recur.
- Laryngeal papillomas often recur and cause progressive damage to the vocal cords.
- Skin papillomas do not become malignant: laryngeal papillomas may rarely do so.
- 30% women with vulval genital warts have associated cervical intraepithelial neoplasia (CIN)[1] as do 32% sexual partners of men with penile HPV[2].
- Epidermodysplasia verruciformis is a rare autosomal recessive disorder in which multiple warts are induced by papillomaviruses (particularly 5 and 8). Squamous cell carcinomas develop in nearly a third of patients, especially in areas exposed to the sun.

TREATMENT

1. Salicylic acid in collodion is a useful initial treatment for skin and plantar warts.
2. Formaldehyde or glutaraldehyde solution may be used as an alternative for plantar warts.
3. The initial treatment of genital warts is with trichloracetic acid or podophyllin. The latter is an antimitotic agent and is contraindicated in pregnancy. Several treatments are required, and these are painful.
4. Cryotherapy with liquid nitrogen or dry ice is an effective treatment for all types of wart, and is the method of choice when facilities permit. It is time-consuming if multiple lesions are present, and the more rapid liquid nitrogen cryospray is under trial. Cryoprobes are available for cervical application.
5. Laser treatment appears promising but is still under assessment.
6. Parenteral interferon has been shown to be effective in the treatment of laryngeal papillomas, but cessation of therapy may be followed by recurrences.

FOLLOW-UP

Patients with laryngeal papillomatosis may need regular ENT review. All women with genital warts should have cervical smears taken each year, and may also require colposcopy.

---

[1] Walker PG *et al.* (1983) *Br. J. Vener. Dis.*, **59**, 327.
[2] Campion MJ *et al.* (1985) *Lancet*, **i**, 943.

Respiratory Syncytial Virus (RSV)

RSV is classified as a pneumovirus and is the commonest cause of severe respiratory infection in infancy. Outbreaks occur in winter, and are the commonest cause of acute bronchiolitis and pneumonia among infants admitted to hospital. Infection in older children and adults usually only results in coryzal symptoms, but may cause exacerbations of chronic bronchitis, and pneumonia in elderly patients. Nosocomial infection can be a serious problem in paediatric wards.

PROGNOSIS

- The mortality of bronchiolitis and pneumonia in infants is up to 5%. Sudden death is not uncommon.
- Serious illness is less common in breast-fed babies.
- Children with certain pre-existing conditions fare badly; these include severe combined immunodeficiency, cystic fibrosis, and congenital heart disease, particularly if pulmonary hypertension is present.
- Bronchiolitis usually resolves within a few days, but up to 50% affected infants may develop recurrent wheezing during childhood.

TREATMENT

1. Skilled supportive treatment is essential, and should include oxygen and humidity.
2. Early trials of ribavirin given by aerosol to infants with pneumonia and bronchiolitis have been encouraging[1,2].
3. There is no evidence that steroids are of benefit.
4. No vaccine is available; the incidence of bronchiolitis and pneumonia in infants given an inactivated vaccine was higher than in controls.

FOLLOW-UP

Follow-up is unnecessary once the patient has recovered.

---

[1] Hall CB et al. (1983) New Eng. J. Med., 308, 1443.
[2] Taber LH et al. (1983) Paediatrics, 72, 613.

Rotavirus

Rotaviruses are ubiquitous and are the commonest cause of acute diarrhoeal disease in infants. In temperate climates rotaviruses occur most commonly in winter, and affect children aged 6–24 months. Nosocomial infection is common, but infection is usually mild or asymptomatic in neonates in whom breast feeding is protective.

PROGNOSIS

- Symptoms usually subside within five days and, although some individuals excrete virus for 10-14 days, prolonged diarrhoea is uncommon.
- Desalination occurs in about 15% infected children admitted to hospital in the UK: it is usually mild and deaths are rare. In tropical countries profound dehydration may occur and be fatal.
- Immunocompromised infants (e.g. with severe combined immunodeficiency) exhibit persistent rotavirus excretion with diarrhoea and may be viraemic.

TREATMENT AND PREVENTION

1. Most cases respond to rehydration with oral glucose-electrolyte solution (e.g. dioralyte) for 1-2 days, followed by resumption of normal diet.
2. If desalination is severe, or fluids cannot be tolerated orally, treatment should be given intravenously.
3. Prophylactic oral human immunoglobulin reduces the severity of rotavirus infection in low birthweight babies[1].
4. An oral live attentuated vaccine is under trial; preliminary results are promising.

FOLLOW-UP

Follow-up is unnecessary once symptoms have resolved.

---

[1] Barnes GL *et al.* (1982) *Lancet*, i, 1372.

Lassa Fever

This arenavirus is endemic in West Africa, and occasional cases enter the UK during the incubation period. Infection is usually subclinical or mild, especially in children, but may be severe with high fever, headache, vomiting, pharyngitis, myocarditis, encephalopathy and haemorrhage.

PROGNOSIS

- Patients admitted to hospital in Africa with Lassa fever have a mortality of 15–30%.
- A high level of viraemia ($>10^4$ TCID$^{50/ml}$) and a high aspartate transaminase (>150 i.u./l) are indications of a poor prognosis.
- Deafness is the only long-term complication.

TREATMENT

1. Good nursing care and supportive therapy are essential.
2. High dose intravenous ribavirin (under trial) reduces the mortality of severe Lassa fever from 50% to 14%[1]. If possible it should be given within the first six days of illness.
3. Convalescent plasma appears to reduce mortality, but the plasma used should contain therapeutic concentrations of neutralising antibodies and must therefore be collected late in convalescence.

FOLLOW-UP

Follow-up is unnecessary once resolution has occurred.

---

[1] McCormick JB et al. (1985) New Eng. J. Med. **314**(1), 20.

13
Infectious Diseases

D. Reid and I. W. Pinkerton

Amoebiasis

Amoebiasis is caused by the protozoan *Entamoeba histolytica*. After an incubation period which ranges from a few days to several months (commonly 2–4 weeks) the patient may develop intestinal or extraintestinal disease although many remain asymptomatic[1]. Common clinical features are fever, bloody or mucoid diarrhoea and abdominal pain. In the UK 100–200 imported cases are reported each year. Distribution is worldwide but especially in areas containing poor sanitation, mental institutions and sexually promiscuous male homosexuals.

PROGNOSIS

- Amoebic granulomata (amoeboma) may occur on the wall of the large intestine in patients with long-standing disease.
- Perianal ulceration may rarely result from direct extension from the intestinal lesion[2].
- Abscesses of the liver or less commonly of the lung or brain can be caused by intravenous dissemination.
- Relapse and the carrier state can occur.
- Mortality in the UK is 1–2%.

TREATMENT

1. Metronidazole 800 mg tds for 5–10 days or emetine 1 mg/kg daily i.m. up to a maximum of 65 mg.
2. In severe infections combine one of the above with diloxanide 500 mg tds orally for 10 days.
3. Carriers may be treated with metronidazole 400–800 mg tds for five days.
4. Liver abscesses should be aspirated if large and metronidazole given.

FOLLOW-UP

Known carriers should be told about the importance of personal hygiene. Close contacts should be screened. 'High risk' excreters should be excluded from occupations involving handling food until shown to be clear.

---

[1] Hoare CA (1958) *Roy. Soc. Health J.*, **78**, 681.
[2] Wilcocks C (1967) *Abs. World Med.*, **41**, 241.

Anthrax

Anthrax is an acute bacterial infection predominantly affecting the skin in the form of a lesion which progresses over a few days from a papule to an ulcer with a characteristic black eschar surrounded by oedema. It occurs worldwide[1] and affects virtually all mammals including man. The disease is caused by *Bacillus anthracis* and has been known by a variety of names through the ages, e.g. malignant pustule, malignant oedema, woolsorters' disease and ragpickers' disease, the latter two terms giving some indication of the environmental hazards associated with this infection. The incubation period is usually 2–5 days. Human anthrax has become much less frequent in the UK and other industrialised countries (in the 20 years between 1961 and 1980 only 145 cases have occurred in the UK). It is still prevalent in many parts of Africa, Iran, Iraq and Turkey.

PROGNOSIS

- The prognosis depends on the form of infection – cutaneous, pulmonary, intestinal or meningeal. Although many cutaneous cases are self-limiting and heal spontaneously, about 20% have dissemination of infection.
- Penicillin therapy usually results in the cutaneous lesion being sterile in 48 hours but scabs may take many weeks to separate.
- Most cases of pulmonary, intestinal and meningeal anthrax have a fatal outcome.

TREATMENT

1. Penicillin is the drug of choice – usually 1 mega unit given six hourly i.m. In severe cases this should be given i.v. during the first 24 hours.
2. Treatment should be started as soon as possible and continued for seven days.
3. If allergy to penicillin is suspected alternative drugs are tetracycline or erythromycin, 2 g daily in divided doses for each drug.
4. Chloramphenicol and streptomycin are alternative treatments.
5. Supportive therapy may be required in severe cases. This includes intravenous fluids, blood transfusion and tracheostomy if the patient has respiratory obstruction.

FOLLOW-UP

In the UK the disease should be notified to the Local Health Authority. If appropriate, the veterinary authorities and Factory Inspectorate should be informed. An alum-precipated vaccine is available and is recommended for workers exposed to anthrax-infected material, e.g. bone meal production and hide preparation[2].

---

[1] Glassman HN (1968) *Pub. Health Reps., US Dept. Health Educ. Welf.,* 73, 22.
[2] Turner W (1966) *Med. Officer,* 116, 81.

Botulism

A serious intoxication of the nervous system involving cranial nerve paralysis due to toxins produced by *Clostridium botulinum*. The organism is widely distributed in soil, water and the intestinal tracts of animals and fish. Toxin is produced when foods are improperly processed under anaerobic conditions[1]. Symptoms appear from 12–48 hours after eating contaminated food. The condition is uncommon in the UK but is encountered in the USA in association with home canning of fish, fruit and vegetables[2].

PROGNOSIS

- 60% cases die within a week, from respiratory or cardiac failure, in the absence of intensive care facilities.
- The shorter the incubation period the worse the prognosis.

TREATMENT

1. Trivalent antitoxin (types A, B and C) should be injected as soon as available.
2. Intensive therapy facilities are required for general support and mechanical ventilation.

FOLLOW-UP

Cases should be notified to the Local Health Authority. Contacts who may have eaten contaminated food should be located and kept under observation. Early administration of antitoxin may be helpful and gastric lavage and/or purgation should be considered. Contaminated food should be sterilised by boiling before being discarded.

[1] Ball AP *et al.* (1979) *Q. J. Med.*, **48**, 473.
[2] Horwitz MA (1977) *J. Infect. Dis.*, **136**, 153.

Brucellosis

Acute brucellosis may affect most systems of the body and initially the patient complains of fever, headache, night sweats, extreme fatigue, muscle and joint pains, anorexia and loss of weight. Relapses can occur and some patients develop the chronic form of the disease. Four members of the *Brucella* species are pathogenic to man (*B. melitensis*, *B. suis*, *B. abortus* and *B. canis*). The incubation period is variable, usually 5–30 days but can be several months. In the UK the number of new cases of *B. abortus* infection has decreased dramatically following the eradication of brucellosis from cattle. Cases nowadays are mostly attributed to chronic brucellosis or infection among returning travellers, usually caused by *B. melitensis* – 26 such cases were reported in the UK in the five years 1979–83. Imported dairy products have also been known to cause outbreaks.

PROGNOSIS

- Acute brucellosis may last several weeks but occasionally a relapsing and prolonged illness may occur.
- Chronic brucellosis may develop in a patient who has had the acute form of the disease but some patients present for the first time with a history of symptoms which started insidiously.
- Persons who have been repeatedly exposed to infected secretions (e.g. veterinarians) may develop allergic skin conditions[1].
- Mortality is 2–3%.

TREATMENT

1. Tetracyclines have been used most often and have been effective in doses of 2 g daily for a minimum of three weeks.
2. Because relapse rates of 5–10% have been reported with tetracyclines the addition of streptomycin 1 g daily i.m. for three weeks has also been recommended[2].
3. Co-trimoxazole has also been used extensively but reported relapse rates have been higher than with tetracyclines.
4. Doxycycline and minocycline are also effective and promising results have been obtained with rifampicin.
5. The response of chronic brucellosis to antibiotic treatment is often disappointing.
6. Brucella endocarditis usually requires the replacement of the affected valve.

FOLLOW-UP

The disease should be reported to the Local Health Authority so that the source may be identified and control measures taken.

---

[1] Loue WC *et al.* (1983) *Update*, **27**, 2153.
[2] Elberg SS (1981) *Vet. Pub. Health*, **81**, 31.

Cholera

Cholera is an enteric disease of sudden onset characterised by profuse watery stools, occasional vomiting, rapid dehydration, acidosis and circulatory collapse. Asymptomatic or mild cases are very common. There are several biotypes of *Vibrio cholerae* (the causative organism). The El Tor strain is now epidemic and has superseded the classical biotype. The incubation period ranges from a few hours to five days, usually 2–3 days. Very occasionally cases are imported into Europe but further spread occurs only rarely.

PROGNOSIS

- In severe, untreated cases death may occur within a few hours and the mortality rate may be over 50%.
- With appropriate treatment the mortality rate is under 1%.

TREATMENT

1. Rapid electrolyte and fluid replacement is vital to counteract dehydration[1].
2. Tetracycline 500 mg six hourly should be given for 48 hours.
3. If resistant strains are present chloramphenicol 500 mg six hourly may be substituted.

FOLLOW-UP

A notifiable disease in the UK. Household contacts should be placed under observation for five days, screened bacteriologically and possibly given tetracycline prophylaxis[2]. Cases and contacts should be excluded from handling food until three negative specimens taken at 48 hourly intervals have been collected.

---

[1] Damluji SF *et al.* (1964) *J. Trop. Med. Hyg.*, **67**, 220.
[2] Communicable Diseases Surveillance Centre and Communicable Diseases (Scotland) Unit (1985) *Community Med.*, **i**, 305.

Diphtheria

Diphtheria is a bacterial disease caused by *Corynaebacterium diphtheriae* which usually affects the pharynx, tonsils or larynx. In the UK 63 cases (with five deaths) occurred between 1970–79 – nearly all were in unimmunised or inadequately immunised children and imported infections were evident. The incubation period is usually 2–5 days but can be longer.

PROGNOSIS

- The prognosis depends on the immune state of the patient and the ability of the bacterium to produce toxin. If the membrane is limited to the nostrils, toxicity is negligible. Severe complications occur in those with more extensive involvement.
- If there is haemorrhage into the lesion the outlook is grave.
- Myocarditis can occur and death from cardiac arrest or circulatory failure may follow. For those who recover, cardiac function usually becomes normal.
- Diphtheritic paralysis may occur after 14 days but if the patient survives the paralytic stage ultimate recovery is usual.
- Mortality for non-cutaneous diphtheria is 5–10%[1].

TREATMENT

1. Antitoxin should be given immediately; patients with nasal lesions should receive 8000 units i.m.; with tonsillar and/or laryngeal lesions, 30 000–40 000 units i.m. (if the tonsillar lesions are severe 60 000 units should be given; half i.m. and half i.v.); the dose may be doubled if nasopharyngeal lesions are present.
2. Penicillin 250 000 units six hourly for 5 days i.m. or erythromycin 250 mg six hourly for 5 days by mouth is given to eradicate the organism.
3. The patient should be isolated.
4. During the first three weeks of severe diphtheria strict bed rest is advisable to avoid cardiac complications.
5. Humidification of the atmosphere may help to ease laryngeal obstruction, otherwise a tracheostomy may be required.
6. If pharyngeal paralysis is present the patient may not be able to swallow and a per-nasal intragastric tube is required for feeding purposes.

FOLLOW-UP

Patients should be segregated until they have had at least three consecutively negative throat and nose swabs taken at intervals of 2–3 days[2]. Nose and throat swabs should be taken from close contacts and carriers. Unimmunised close contacts should be given erythromycin 250 mg six hourly by mouth for 5 days as well as the first dose of a primary course of three doses of toxoid. Previously immunised contacts under 10 years of age should be given a booster dose of toxoid. Adult type toxoid is given to those aged 10 years or over.

---

[1] Galbraith NS *et al.* (1980) *Br. Med. J.*, **281**, 489.
[2] Emoud RTD (1975) *Medicine*, **2**, 88.

Hookworm

Hookworm is a chronic debilitating disease with anaemia and hypoproteinaemia due to nematode infestations of the small bowel. The cause is most commonly *Necator americanus* or *Ancylostoma duodenale*.

PROGNOSIS

- Infection, if of moderate severity, may be asymptomatic in otherwise adequately nourished individuals.
- Chronic infection may retard mental and physical development of children.
- Pulmonary reactions may occur on exposure to infective larvae.
- Hookworm infection is not a direct cause of mortality.

TREATMENT

1. Tetrachloroethylene is still widely used for this condition but has been superseded by less toxic drugs.
2. Bephenium in a single dose of 2.5 g, repeated after two days, is not absorbed and has few side-effects[1].
3. Mebendazole 100 mg bd for three days or as a single dose of 1 g has proved effective.
4. Anaemia should be treated with oral iron[2].

FOLLOW-UP

Examine stools to confirm effectiveness of treatment. Improve sanitation to avoid soil contamination with infected human faeces.

---

[1] Nagaty H *et al.* (1959) *J. Trop. Med. Hyg.*, **12**, 284.
[2] Woodruff AW (1964) *Practitioner*, **193**, 138.

Hydatid Disease

Hydatid disease is caused by the development in humans of larval cysts of the tapeworm Echinococcus whose adult forms occur in dogs and other carnivores. Found most commonly where dogs are used to herd grazing animals which act as intermediate hosts[1]. Incubation period varies from months to years.

PROGNOSIS

- Symptoms depend on the site of cysts, most frequently in the lungs or liver, and on their rate of growth.
- General health may be little disturbed and calcified cysts may be found by routine x-ray or at autopsy.
- Dangerous effects include pulmonary collapse, rupture into the peritoneum, fracture of bone and cerebral compression.

TREATMENT

Surgical removal of a cyst if accessible, with care not to disperse infective contents[2].

FOLLOW-UP

In the UK the disease should be reported to the Local Health Authority. Slaughtering practice should be improved and the feeding of infected offal to dogs avoided. The dog population should be reduced to the essential level and the remaining dogs treated with anthelmintics.

---

[1] Chisholm IL *et al.* (1983) *J. Hyg.*, **90**, 19.
[2] Morris DL (1981) *Br. J. Hosp. Med.*, **25**, 586.

Legionnaire's Disease

Legionnaire's disease derives its name from the outbreak of predominantly respiratory illness which occurred in Philadelphia in 1976 among veterans of the American Legion[1]. The disease is caused by members of the legionellaceae, of which there are an increasing number of designated serogroups and species, the commonest pathogen being *Legionella pneumophila*. These organisms may be found in a wide variety of environmental sources – mud and natural water courses, cooling towers, air-conditioning units and piped water supplies especially in fittings such as shower heads and taps. The incubation period is 2–10 days. About 250 cases occur each year in the UK. Males are more likely to be affected than females in the ratio 2.5:1.

PROGNOSIS

- The illness is characteristically associated with a severe pneumonia which in favourable cases resolves in 2–3 weeks.
- Prognostically unfavourable complications include disseminated intravascular coagulation, gastrointestinal bleeding, rhabdomyolysis, respiratory failure, encephalopathy, shock and renal failure.
- Increasing age, smoking and possibly alcohol consumption are factors in the more seriously ill.
- Immunosuppressed patients are at increased risk of a fatal outcome.
- Mortality is 10–25% during outbreaks.

TREATMENT

1. Since formal diagnosis may depend on serological evidence treatment must be commenced on clinical suspicion.
2. Erythromycin is the drug of choice. The dosage varies from 2–4 g daily given orally or i.v. depending on the severity of the illness[2].
3. Rifampicin may be given in addition to erythromycin in a seriously ill patient with pneumonia.
4. Some patients will develop gastrointestinal bleeding, respiratory and renal failure and these complications will require appropriate supportive therapy.
5. Because case-to-case spread of Legionnaire's disease appears to be rare, there is usually no need to treat the patient in isolation facilities.

FOLLOW-UP

Although not a notifiable disease in the UK, it may be useful to the Local Health Authority for details of the case to be reported in order to identify and render safe possible environmental sources. Enquiries should be made about additional cases as outbreaks are relatively common (about a third of cases are associated with outbreaks). Careful follow-up of the patient should be undertaken.

---

[1] Fraser DW *et al.* (1977) *New Eng. J. Med.*, 2? 1189.

[2] Sanford JR (1979) *New Eng. J. Med.*, 300, 654.

Leishmaniasis

A protozoal infection of rodents, foxes and domestic dogs spread to man by the bite of sandflies. Cutaneous leishmaniasis occurs mainly in Africa, the Middle East and in Central and S. America. Incubation period is a few days to several weeks. Visceral leishmaniasis (Kala-azar) is found in the Mediterranean area, India and the Far East in addition to those areas where the cutaneous variety occurs. It has an incubation period of 3–6 months but may occasionally be shorter. A febrile illness becomes established and as systemic effects of the infection extend, debility worsens.

PROGNOSIS

- Variable, depending on the strain of leishmania, the geographical area involved and the resistance of the patient.
- Single lesions may heal spontaneously in 3–12 months but subsequent scarring develops.
- Multiple nodules are common and may persist for years. Ulceration and secondary infection occurs.
- Cutaneous leishmaniasis is disfiguring rather than dangerous.
- In the absence of treatment for visceral leishmaniasis, death from exhaustion or intercurrent infection occurs after a period of many months.

TREATMENT

1. Pentavalent antimony compounds are the mainstay of treatment for all forms of the disease[1]. Sodium antimony gluconate 2 g (containing 600 mg antimony) is given by i.v. or i.m. injection. Six daily injections are usually adequate for Indian kala-azar but for all other forms 30 daily injections are recommended.
2. Antimony-resistant cases are given diamidine compounds such as hydroxystilbamidine isethionate 250 mg daily i.v. for 10 days followed by a rest period of a week and the course repeated twice.
3. Amphoteracin B has been used with success in cases resistant to other forms of treatment.
4. Splenectomy is occasionally necessary.

FOLLOW-UP

Notify to Local Health Authority in the UK. Control sandfly population[2]. Permanent antimalarial cover is required for splenectomised individuals depending upon geographical location.

---

[1] Bray RS (1972) *Br. Med. Bull.*, **28**, 39.
[2] Chance ML (1981) *Br. Med. J.*, **283**, 1245.

Leprosy

Leprosy is a chronic disease affecting the skin, nasal mucosa and peripheral nerves caused by *Mycobacterium leprae*. In lepromatous leprosy, nodules, papules, macules and diffuse infiltrations are extensive and involvement of the nasal mucosa may lead to obstructed breathing. In tuberculoid leprosy, skin lesions are few but peripheral nerve involvement tends to be relatively severe. The incubation period is about four years for tuberculoid leprosy and eight years for lepromatous leprosy. The world prevalence is estimated to be about 12 million and the main endemic areas are south-east Asia, Tropical Africa, some Pacific Islands and some areas of Latin America.

PROGNOSIS

- Modern treatment has radically changed the outlook for the leprosy patient.
- Hospital admission is usually now only required for treatment of ulcers and surgical correction of deformities in unaesthetic limbs.
- Patients with lepromatous leprosy have a continuing risk of eye lesions, particularly iridocyclitis. Regular ophthalmic examination is advisable.
- Collapse of the nasal bridge and deformity or loss of digits may occur.
- There is an increased risk of other infections including tuberculosis, hepatitis B and amyloid disease.
- Although leprosy is generally not considered to be a fatal disease, mortality rates are elevated in lepromatous patients. Death usually results from intercurrent infection or amyloidosis.

TREATMENT

1. Patients with *lepromatous leprosy* require treatment for life with annual bacteriological review, even after clinical quiescence has been achieved.
2. Patients with *tuberculoid leprosy* can usually cease taking anti-leprotic drugs after regular treatment for 2–3 years.
3. Most patients can be treated as out-patients with no danger to themselves or others[1].
4. Dapsone in daily doses of 50–100 mg should be used in combination with rifampicin 600 mg per day (because of the increasing incidence of dapsone resistance) during the first 6–18 months of treatment. Immunological reactions occurring during the course of treatment, e.g. erythema nodosum leprosum may require corticosteroid therapy.
5. Reconstructive surgical measures and the prevention of trauma to unaesthetic limbs may be required.

FOLLOW-UP

Prophylactic dapsone and annual examination for five years should take place for household contacts of lepromatous patients[2]. If the contact is a child or adult sharing sleeping accommodation with the patient, examination should take place every three months. BCG vaccine should be offered to any child or young adult (not strongly tuberculin-positive) who has been in close contact with a leprosy patient.

[1] Jopling WH (1974) *Br. J. Hosp. Med.*, **11**, 43.
[2] Filice GA *et al.* (1978) *Ann. Int. Med.*, **88**, 538.

Leptospirosis (Weil's Disease, Canicola Fever)

A group of zoonotic infections caused by various leptospirae, e.g. *Leptospira icterohaemorrhagica* (causing Weil's disease) and *L. canicola* (causing canicola fever). After an incubation period of 4–19 days (usually about 10 days) the patient may develop fever, headache, vomiting, myalgia, conjunctival suffusion, meningitis, rash or uveitis. More severe cases may progress to jaundice, renal insufficiency, haemolytic anaemia and haemorrhage into the skin and mucous membranes. About 40 cases per year occur in the UK.

PROGNOSIS

- Relapses occur in about a third of cases of Weil's disease.
- Older patients have a poorer prognosis and males may do less well than females.
- Mortality in Weil's disease may be as high as 20% but is much lower in canicola fever.

TREATMENT

1. To be effective in clearing the blood of leptospirae, penicillin, the drug of choice, must be given within the first few days of illness. Antibiotics given after the first week are unlikely to influence the course of the illness[1].

2. If renal failure develops, dialysis may be required.
3. Blood transfusion may be necessary if haemorrhagic features are severe.

FOLLOW-UP

A notifiable disease in the UK. Rodent control may be necessary[2]. In canicola fever enquiries about ill dogs should be made and veterinary examination requested. Immunisation of those at risk of Weil's disease (e.g. sewage workers) should be considered.

---

[1] Lawson JH (1978) *Medicine*, 5, 252.
[2] Robertson MH *et al.* (1981) *Lancet*, ii, 626.

Malaria

A disease caused by one of four types of the protozoa of the genus *Plasmodium*; these are *P. falciparum, P. vivax, P. malariae* and *P. ovale*. The most serious of these is falciparum malaria (malignant tertian) which may present with fever, chills, sweats and headache. The other human malarias – vivax (benign tertian), malariae (quartan) and ovale do not carry the same risk. Falciparum malaria predominates in Africa, parts of South America and Indonesia while vivax malaria is particularly common in the Indian subcontinent and ovale malaria in West Africa. The female anopheline mosquito is the definitive host for plasmodia and the incubation period is about 12 days for *P. falciparum*, 14 days for *P. vivax* and *P. ovale* and 30 days for *P. malariae*. With some strains of *P. vivax* there may be a much longer incubation period (8–10 months) and even longer with *P. ovale*. Occasionally infection can be spread by blood transfusion[1], contaminated syringes or from mother to fetus (congenital malaria). In the UK up to 2000 cases may occur each year[2].

PROGNOSIS

- Relapses occur commonly with vivax and ovale infections at irregular intervals for up to two and five years, respectively.
- Malarial infections may persist for many years with recurrent recrudescences.
- Falciparum malaria may produce haemolysis causing haemoglobinaemia, haemoglobinuria (black water fever), cerebral symptoms (cerebral malaria), renal damage, disseminated intravascular coagulation or pulmonary oedema.
- Mortality in falciparum malaria in children and untreated adults may be greater than 10%.

TREATMENT AND PREVENTION

1. Local measures. Mosquito bites should be avoided by keeping arms and legs covered when outdoors after sundown. Sleeping accommodation should be suitably screened, otherwise a mosquito net can be used.
2. Chemoprophylaxis. The choice of anti-malaria prophylaxis will vary according to the country to be visited as strains of plasmodia resistant to chloroquine and even to the newer combination drugs containing pyrimethamine and dapsone or sulfadoxine have emerged. If travelling to a country where there are resistant strains consideration should be given to prescribing two drugs, e.g. proguanil (daily) plus chloroquine (weekly). Prophylaxis should be started before (about one week) the visit, and continued until one month afterwards. Because of the rapidly changing resistance patterns up-to-date advice should be sought from a designated centre.
3. Prompt and effective treatment is especially vital in *falciparum malaria*.

   a) If the organism is sensitive to chloroquine then 600 mg should be given orally followed by 300 mg after six hours followed by 300 mg daily for two days.
   b) If the organism is resistant to chloroquine, quinine dihydrochloride or bisulphate 600 mg orally should be prescribed every eight hours for at least four doses followed by a single oral dose of Fansidar (pyrimethamine and sulphadoxine).

4. If *cerebral malaria* is present then quinine should be used by i.v. infusion over four hours in a dose of 5–10 mg/kg base. Chloroquine base, 200 mg i.v. every 12 hours may be used as an alternative. Hydrocortisone or dexamethasone may also be required in cerebral malaria; and if renal failure is present, peritoneal dialysis or haemodialysis.
5. In *vivax, malariae or ovale malaria* chloroquine base is indicated 600 mg orally followed by 300 mg after six hours then 300 mg daily for two days.
6. The exoerythrocytic phase should be eradicated with primaquine 7.5 mg bd orally for two weeks.

FOLLOW-UP

A notifiable disease in the UK. Patients should be warned about the hazards to others of donating blood or sharing syringes. If a history of recent blood transfusion or sharing syringes is obtained from the patient then appropriate investigation should be arranged.

[1] Bruce-Chwatt LJ (1982) *Trop. Dis. Bull.*, 79, 827.
[2] Public Health Laboratory Service Communicable Diseases Surveillance Centre and the Communicable Diseases (Scotland) Unit (1983) *Community Med.*, 5, 148.

Meningitis (Pyogenic)

The main causes of pyogenic bacterial meningitis are *Neisseria meningitidis, Haemophilus influenzae, Streptococcus pneumonia* and in neonatal life *Escherichia coli*. Other less frequently encountered organisms are *Staphylococcus aureus, Klebsiella aerogenes, Leptospira spp.* and *Listeria monocytogenes*.

PROGNOSIS

- Meningococcal infection may be confined to the nasopharynx and remain asymptomatic.
- Meningococcal meningitis, usually a disease of young children, also occurs in adolescents and other adults.
- In the absence of treatment mortality is high.
- Fulminant cases occur with septicaemia and haemorrhagic rash, which may be fatal despite treatment.
- Haemophilus meningitis, mainly confined to children under five years, may be slower in onset with consequent delay in recognition and treatment.
- Recovery is usual if treatment is started without delay.
- Pneumococcal meningitis occurs at all ages and may be secondary to focal infection in the sinuses or middle ear.
- Mortality is higher in pneumococcal than in meningococcal or haemophilus infection[1], especially at the extremes of life.
- All forms of bacterial meningitis may be followed by persisting neurological damage[2]. Deafness is the most commonly encountered effect.

TREATMENT

1. *Meningococcal meningitis* is treated with penicillin 120 mg/kg daily in divided doses four hourly, i.v. or i.m. Treatment is continued for 10 days.
2. *Haemophilus meningitis* is most effectively treated with chloramphenicol in a dose of 50–100 mg/kg daily in divided dosage for 10 days. (Ampicillin resistance is encountered sufficiently often to make this an unacceptable choice.)
3. *Pneumococcal cases* are given large doses of parenteral penicillin. For an adult 24 g of penicillin may be given daily in divided doses four hourly for the first few days, reducing according to response.
4. Coliform and other Gram-negative organisms may be treated with a combination of amoxycillin (100 mg/kg/day) and an aminoglycoside such as gentamicin (5 mg/kg/day in divided doses, eight hourly).

FOLLOW-UP

Notify to Local Health Authority in the UK Treat family contacts of meningococcal cases with rifampicin 5–10 mg/kg daily for two days

[1] Goldacre MJ (1976) *Lancet*, **i**, 28.
[2] Davey PG *et al.* (1982) *J. Hygiene*, **88**, 383.

Paratyphoid

Paratyphoid (which with typhoid is termed enteric fever) is caused by one of three salmonellae – *Salmonella paratyphi A*, *S. paratyphi B* and *S. paratyphi C*. Paratyphoid B is commonest, A is less frequent and C extremely rare. After an incubation period of 1–10 days the patient may have fever, headache, splenic enlargement, rose spots on trunk, vomiting and diarrhoea. In the UK about 60 cases of paratyphoid B and 50 of paratyphoid A are diagnosed each year – most having been infected overseas[1].

PROGNOSIS

- Paratyphoid is usually milder and shorter than typhoid with fewer complications.
- Relapses occur in about 3% cases.
- Under good conditions and appropriate therapy, mortality is usually negligible.

TREATMENT

1. The patient should be treated in an infectious diseases unit with isolation facilities.
2. Chloramphenicol is usually the antibiotic of first choice and is given in a daily dose of 2 g for an adult or 50 mg/kg body weight for a child[2].
3. Amoxycillin in a dose of 2 g six hourly provides a less toxic alternative and is particularly appropriate when organisms resistant to chloramphenicol are encountered. Co-trimoxazole can also be used.
4. Antibiotics should be continued for two weeks to reduce the chance of relapse.
5. Blood transfusion and surgery may be necessitated by the complications of intestinal haemorrhage or perforation.
6. Persistently positive stool cultures over several months warrant consideration of an extended course of amoxycillin for 2–3 months.
7. Chronic carriers may require cholecystectomy after investigation of the biliary tract.

FOLLOW-UP

A notifiable disease in the UK. The case must be reported promptly to the Local Health Authority. To ensure that the patient is free from infection at least three consecutive negative faecal and urine samples must be obtained at least 48 hours apart and not earlier than 2–3 weeks after the last possible exposure to infection. If any of these are positive, the samples should be repeated at intervals of one month until at least three negative specimens are obtained. Exclusion from work of food handlers is important until they are shown not to be chronic carriers. At least 12 faecal samples (six after magnesium sulphate purges) should be obtained before return to food handling duties. Typhoid vaccine may be given to family, household and nursing contacts. Two negative faecal and urinary cultures (with a 24-hour interval) should be obtained from contacts who are food handlers in the household. The source and vehicle of infection should be sought. Routine administration of typhoid vaccine to the community is not recommended.

[1] Public Health Laboratory Service Communicable Disease Surveillance Centre (1983) *Br. Med. J.*, **287**, 1366.
[2] Department of Health and Social Security (1972) *Memorandum on Typhoid and Paratyphoid Fevers*. Norwich: HMSO.

Plague

Plague is a zoonosis in which man is infected by *Yersinia pestis*, a bacillus transmitted between rodents and to man by fleas. After an incubation period of 2–6 days there is lymphadenitis, lymphadenopathy (buboes) and fever (bubonic plague) followed by pneumonia, mediastinitis or pleural effusion (pneumonic plague). Person-to-person spread can result in outbreaks. Urban plague has been controlled in most countries[1].

PROGNOSIS

- Untreated septicaemic plague or pneumonic plague is invariably fatal.
- Untreated bubonic plague has a mortality rate of about 50%.
- Mortality is low with appropriate and prompt treatment.

TREATMENT

1. Patients with pneumonic plague should be strictly isolated with precautions against airborne spread of disease until three days have elapsed after starting appropriate antibiotic therapy.
2. Tetracycline or streptomycin or chloramphenicol therapy is very effective if given early enough[2]. Tetracycline is the drug of choice. Initially 1.5 g should be given six hourly i.v. to adults for the first 48 hours followed by 2.0 g daily in divided doses for seven days. Streptomycin is given i.m. in a dose of 500 mg every 4–6 hours, according to clinical improvement.

FOLLOW-UP

A notifiable disease in the UK. Close contacts should be disinfested and, if in contact with pneumonic plague, should be given appropriate chemoprophylaxis, e.g. tetracycline (15–30 mg/kg body weight, daily) for seven days while being kept under observation. Anti-rodent measures should be instituted.

---

[1] Centers for Disease Control (1982) *Morb. Mort. Weekly Rep.*, **31**, 301.
[2] World Health Organisation Expert Committee on Plague (1970) *Tech. Rep. Ser.*, **447**.

Psittacosis

An acute generalised infection due to *Chlamydia psittaci*, with fever, headache and pneumonitis as the usual presenting features. Infection usually comes from pet birds[1]. There is a wide spectrum of severity from trivial symptoms to life-threatening illness with myocarditis[2] and renal failure. The incubation period is about 10 days.

PROGNOSIS

- Most cases recover without treatment.
- Older patients are at greater risk of dangerous complications such as myocarditis and renal failure.

TREATMENT

1. Tetracycline 2 g daily in divided dosage for 10 days is effective.
2. Chloramphenicol is also effective in similar dose.

FOLLOW-UP

In the UK the disease should be reported to Local Health Authority. The possible source, including origin of affected birds, should be investigated.

[1] Erooga MA (1968) In *Some Diseases of Animals Communicable to Man in Britain* (Graham-Jones O ed.) p. 143. Oxford: Pergamon Press.
[2] Thomas DJB *et al.* (1977) *Practitioner*, **218**, 394.

Salmonellosis

The numerous members of the animal-associated group of salmonellae are important causes of food-borne infection worldwide. Cases occur singly or in outbreaks, the latter often associated with residential institutions. The incubation period is 1–2 days.

PROGNOSIS

- Infection is followed by a wide spectrum of effects, varying from asymptomatic faecal excretion through a few days of diarrhoea to life-threatening septicaemia.
- Achlorhydria, associated with pernicious anaemia, gastric surgery or alcoholism, predisposes to more severe illness[1].
- States of impaired immunity either due to drugs or disease worsen the prognosis.
- Pre-existing inflammatory bowel disease may be exacerbated.
- Septicaemia occurs in about 5% adult infections and may be associated with shock.
- Focal abscesses occur in bone, soft tissues and viscera.
- Asymptomatic excretion continues for several weeks during convalescence.

TREATMENT

1. Anti-diarrhoeal agents to reduce motility such as codeine, morphine, diphenoxylate or loperimide give some symptomatic relief.
2. Antibiotics are not indicated for uncomplicated cases as the period of convalescent excretion is prolonged[2].
3. For septicaemic illness or those in poor prognostic categories, an appropriate antibiotic should be given, chosen if possible in the light of known sensitivity. Amoxycillin, chloramphenicol and co-trimoxazole are most commonly employed. Treatment should be continued for 10 days.

FOLLOW-UP

Report to Local Health Authority in the UK. In convalescence, usually three negative stool cultures, taken on alternate days, are required to confirm clearance for food handlers.

---

[1] Sharp JCM et al. (1982) Update, 25, 213.
[2] Dixon JMS (1965) Br. Med. J., ii, 1343.

Schistosomiasis

Schistosomiasis is a group of diseases caused by trematodes of the genus *Schistosoma*, widely distributed in the rural tropics and infecting many millions throughout the world. Man is the definitive host with freshwater snails acting as passive intermediate hosts. Incubation period is about 4–6 weeks after infection.

PROGNOSIS

- In severely infected individuals, 25% die as a direct result of the disease and in 50% it is a contributory cause.
- While many infected individuals remain asymptomatic, cystitis, haematuria, calcification of the bladder and obstruction leading to hydronephrosis, hypertension and renal failure may occur.
- *S. haematobium*, most prevalent in Africa, Egypt and the Middle East, predominantly involve the veins of the urinary system.
- *S. mansoni*, most prevalent in Tropical Africa and S. America and *S. japonicum* in the Far East locate mainly in the mesenteric veins.
- Fever and blood-stained diarrhoea occur in the early stages.
- Polyposis and anaemia are common manifestations. Hepatic cirrhosis and portal hypertension may develop as late features.
- In all forms of disease prior to fibrosis and calcification, considerable benefit can be expected from treatment.

TREATMENT

1. Praziquantel is the most effective treatment for all forms of infection in a single oral dose of 40 mg/kg.
2. For *S. mansoni* an alternative treatment is oxamniquine 15 mg/kg on two consecutive evenings.
3. For *S. haematobium*, metriphonate in a single dose of 7.5 mg/kg given on three occasions at intervals of 2–3 weeks. A once-only dose together with a single dose of niridazole may be as effective and more practical for mass treatment.

FOLLOW-UP

The disease should be reported to the Local Health Authority and stools or urine examined for continued egg excretion four weeks after treatment. Eosinophilia should fall after successful treatment, and should be monitored. Sanitation must be improved to protect water courses[1], and snail-breeding areas treated with molluscicides. Safe water supplies for drinking and bathing are vital[2]. Mass treatment of population in highly endemic areas may be considered.

---

[1] Macdonald G (1965) *Trans. Roy. Soc. Trop. Med. Hyg.*, **59**, 489.
[2] Pitchford R J (1970) *South Afr. Med. J.*, **44**, 475.

Shigellosis (Bacillary Dysentery)

Shigellosis is a bacterial disease involving the large and small intestine and causing diarrhoea, fever, vomiting, abdominal pain and tenesmus. The incubation period is 1–7 days, usually 1–3 days. There are four species of shigellae – *Shigella sonnei, S. flexneri, S. boydii* and *S. dysenteriae. S. sonnei* is common in the West whereas the other species account for most isolates in the Third World. In the UK between 3000 and 4000 cases of dysentery are notified annually, mostly involving children.

PROGNOSIS

- In sonnei dysentery the outlook is nearly always good except in debilitated babies or elderly patients already suffering from another disease.
- Dysentery due to *S. flexneri* or *S. dysenteriae* has a poorer prognosis, especially the latter where mortality rates of 20% have been reported.

TREATMENT

1. Antibiotics are not indicated in mild infections[1].
2. Clear fluids and a light, low residue diet should be given.
3. In severe attacks intravenous fluids should be administered and antibiotics may become indicated at this stage – the type depending on bacteriological sensitivity.

FOLLOW-UP

A notifiable disease in the UK. Hygiene and health education measures should be undertaken at schools and nurseries to prevent spread of infection[2]. In convalescence, usually three negative stool cultures, taken on alternate days, are required to confirm clearance for food handlers.

[1] Weissman JB *et al.* (1973) *J. Infect. Dis.*, **127**, 611.
[2] Weissman JB *et al.* (1975) *Lancet*, **i**, 88.

Streptococcal Infection

This is an extremely common infection most usually recognised as exudative follicular tonsillitis but may also infect the skin and genital tract. Incubation period 1–3 days. Asymptomatic human carriers are the reservoir of infection.

PROGNOSIS

- Nasopharyngeal infection may be asymptomatic and remain infective for 10-21 days.
- Untreated tonsillitis usually settles in about a week.
- Susceptible individuals may develop scarlet fever due to toxin from some strains of organism. An erythematous rash accompanied by characteristic tongue coating is followed by desquamation in about 1-2 weeks.
- Skin lesions are accompanied by lymphangitis and regional adenitis.
- Erysipelas is the most characteristic form of dermal infection.
- Septic complications include peritonsillar abscess, otitis media, orbital cellulitis and ethmoiditis.
- Non-septic sequelae such as acute rheumatism[1], glomerulonephritis[2] and erythema nodosum may follow infection at any site although the throat is the most common. Skin infection is rarely followed by acute rheumatism.

TREATMENT

1. Streptococcal throat infection should be treated with penicillin, initially by injection in a dose of 0.3-1.2 g, followed by oral penicillin V 250-500 mg, six hourly for 10 days. (Children 25 mg/kg/day.)
2. Erythromycin should be substituted for penicillin in allergic subjects.

FOLLOW-UP

The Local Health Authority should be notified in the UK. For young patients with known heart lesions or following acute rheumatism, prophylactic oral penicillin should be prescribed until the age of 20 years.

[1] Colling A et al. (1980) J. Hyg., 85, 331.
[2] Weinstein L et al. (1971) J. Infect. Dis., 124, 229.

Tetanus

Tetanus (lockjaw) is characterised by painful muscular contractions often first appearing in the masseter and neck muscles before spreading to the trunk. Severe spasms may produce opisthotonos and in the face, risus sardonicus. Infection is caused by *Clostridium tetani* usually gaining entry following an injury but a history of trauma may be lacking. Infection of the umbilical stump is a common occurrence in primitive communities resulting in tetanus neonatorum. The incubation period is normally 4–21 days depending on the type of wound. Most cases have symptoms within 14 days (average 10 days). About 100 cases a year occur in the UK. Worldwide the annual mortality has been estimated at 50 000.

PROGNOSIS

- Shorter incubation periods (<7 days) are in general associated with a poorer prognosis as they tend to occur in patients with more heavily contaminated wounds and severe disease.
- The interval between the onset of symptoms and the development of generalised convulsions (the period of onset) is a useful prognostic indicator. The outlook is more favourable if this is over two weeks but less so if under one week.
- Satisfactory control of convulsions is essential for recovery and early resort to tracheostomy and relaxant drugs in severe cases improves prognosis.
- A poorer prognosis is usual in the very young (especially neonates) and the old. Young adults have the best outlook.
- Mortality rates range from 10 to 60% depending on the immune state of the population and the availability of skilled medical and nursing care.

TREATMENT

1. Wound excision to remove damaged tissue and foreign material[1].
2. Benzyl penicillin 1 mega unit i.m. six hourly for one week is the antibiotic of first choice[2].
3. Antitoxin in the form of human tetanus immune globulin 30–300 i.u./kg body weight or equine antitoxin 10 000–20 000 units i.m. should be given.
4. Sedation with diazepam and/or chlorpromazine should be given.
5. Pethidine 50 mg every 4–6 hours i.m. may be required.
6. Tracheostomy may be needed to ensure a safe airway and facilitate mechanical ventilation if muscle relaxants are required.

FOLLOW-UP

All cases require active immunisation with tetanus toxoid during convalescence as the disease itself does not confer immunity. Where appropriate in communities where umbilical sepsis is common, health education should take place.

---

[1] Laurence DR *et al.* (1966) *Br. Med. J.*, **i**, 33.
[2] Edmondson RS (1980) *Br. J. Hosp. Med.*, **23/6**, 596.

Toxoplasmosis

Toxoplasmosis is caused by the protozoan *Toxoplasma gondii* which occurs worldwide in mammals, birds and humans. Primary infection is frequently asymptomatic but acute disease results in fever, lymphadenopathy and lymphocytosis. Rarely cerebral signs, pneumonia, myocarditis or a rash may develop. If infection occurs during pregnancy fetal damage – chorioretinitis, intracerebral calcification, hydrocephaly, microcephaly, fever, jaundice and hepatosplenomegaly – can result. The incubation period is 10–23 days.

PROGNOSIS

- Most acquired infections in adults are mild.
- Mortality in infancy is about 12%.
- Uveitis may occur in 20% cases but chorioretinitis is a rare manifestation.
- Occasionally acquired toxoplasmosis can result in a long debilitating illness but death rarely occurs.
- In congenital infection 60% develop chorioretinitis, hydrocephalus and intracranial calcification[1].

TREATMENT

1. Treatment is usually unnecessary.
2. Pyrimethamine 25–50 mg and sulphadimidine 4–8 g daily for 2–4 weeks if symptoms are other than mild.
3. Spiramycin 2–4 g daily for 2–6 weeks should be preferred in pregnancy.
4. Where the eye is affected, prednisolone may be used in combination with pyrimethamine and sulphadimidine as there is often failure to respond to these latter drugs possibly due to hypersensitivity to toxoplasma[2].

FOLLOW-UP

If infection occurs during pregnancy therapeutic abortion should be considered. In congenital cases, determine antibodies in the mother.

[1] Eichenwald HF (1957) *Am. J. Dis. Child.*, **94**, 411.
[2] Beverley JKA (1975) *Medicine*, **3**, 132.

Trypanosomiasis

A protozoal infection of man and both wild and domestic animals, transmitted in Tropical Africa by the tsetse fly and in S. America by the faeces of blood-sucking bugs. Highly endemic in infected areas[1].

PROGNOSIS

- In Africa two geographically defined organisms occur:

  a) *T. rhodesiense*, with incubation period of 2–3 weeks, may cause rapidly progressive disease with early CNS involvement ('sleeping sickness') and death in a few months.

  b) *T. gambiense* has incubation period of many months with a protracted course of several years.

- Prognosis is good in African trypanosomiasis if treatment is begun before CNS involvement. If not, more toxic drugs are required and mortality is at least 10%.

- American trypanosomiasis (Chagas' disease) is caused by *T. cruzi*. Incubation period 14 days. Prognosis is variable. Acute febrile symptoms commonly settle but there is a risk of continuing subacute disease with development of cardiomyopathy which may be fatal, mega-colon and mega-oesophagus are late complications.

TREATMENT (AFRICAN TRYPANOSOMIASIS)

1. Suramin 1 g i.v. in 10% solution freshly prepared. Dose repeated every few days to a total of 6 g.
2. Pentamidine may be preferred for *T. gambiense* infections. 400 mg in 10% solution i.m. daily for 10 days.
3. Melarsoprol is used in advanced cases. Courses of daily i.v. injections of 3.6 mg/kg are given for four consecutive days, with a rest period of one week between courses. Three courses of treatment are given. When toxic encephalopathy is observed smaller doses are indicated in the initial stages of treatment.
4. Nitrofurazone is used in relapses. It is given orally in a dose of 500 mg three times daily for 7 days. Courses may be repeated after a rest period of a week.

TREATMENT (AMERICAN TRYPANOSOMIASIS)

1. No wholly satisfactory treatment is available[2].
2. Nifurtimox is used in acute disease in a dose of 10 mg/kg daily for three months.
3. Alternatively benznidazole may be given 5 mg/kg daily for 30 days.

FOLLOW-UP

The disease should be notified to the Local Health Authority in the UK. Serological follow-up of cases to detect persisting infection. Insecticide attack on insect vectors in affected localities.

---

[1] World Health Organisation and Food and Agriculture Organisation (1979) *Tech. Rep. Ser.*, **635**.
[2] Lumsden WHR (1972) *Br. Med. Bull.*, **28**, 34.

Tuberculosis (Extrapulmonary)

Extrapulmonary tuberculosis may involve the lymphatic, skeletal, genito-urinary, alimentary or central nervous systems[1]. Extrapulmonary tuberculosis has not matched the decline in respiratory tuberculosis. About 30% cases of tuberculosis in the UK are non-respiratory. The main human pathogens are *Mycobacterium tuberculosis* and rarely the bovine type *Mycobacterium bovis*. The incubation period of tuberculosis (from infection to primary lesion) is about 4–12 weeks; progressive disease is greatest within a year or two after infection. Extrapulmonary tuberculosis is generally not communicable.

Note: for *Pulmonary tuberculosis* see p. 18.

PROGNOSIS

- The most hazardous period for the development of overt disease is the first 6–12 months after infection. The risk is highest in those under three months old, lowest in later childhood, and high again in adolescents and young adults.
- Tuberculosis of the spine can result in paraplegia and deformity.
- If the kidneys are infected there may be impairment of renal function.
- Tuberculosis of the female genital tract is an important cause of infertility (45%) associated with tubal obstruction.
- Alimentary tuberculosis is insidious and progressive and may require surgical intervention.
- Tuberculous meningitis carries the risk of neurological sequelae and mortality[2].
- Mortality increases with age and is higher in males especially among the poor in urban areas.

TREATMENT

1. The aim is to treat the patient promptly and to maintain an acceptable therapeutic regime of sufficient duration to make relapses unlikely. A further objective is to minimise the possibility of the development of drug resistance. This is achieved by administering drugs in combination.
2. There is usually an initial eight-week course using isoniazid and rifampicin supplemented by ethambutol or possibly streptomycin.
3. Treatment is continued for 6–18 months with two drugs, one of which should be isoniazid (which should always be accompanied by pyridoxine to reduce the risk of peripheral neuropathy). The second may be rifampicin or ethambutol.
4. In tuberculous meningitis corticosteroids are helpful in inhibiting fibrosis at the base of the brain.
5. Surgical advice should be sought for renal, bone or joint disease.

FOLLOW-UP

Tuberculosis is a notifiable disease in the UK. Contacts should be examined, x-rayed and tuberculin tested. BCG is given to those shown to be tuberculin negative. Young contacts may be given prophylactic isoniazid. Newborn infant contacts do not need to be tuberculin tested but should be given BCG without delay.

---

[1] Kennedy DH (1983) *Update*, **27**, 671.
[2] Medical Research Council (1980) *Br. Med. J.*, **281**, 895.

Typhoid

Typhoid is a systemic disease with a wide variety of clinical features (e.g. fever, headache, splenomegaly, rose spots etc.) which, with paratyphoid, is termed 'enteric fever'. Infection is caused by *Salmonella typhi* which gains access to the patient by mouth and is usually transmitted by contaminated food and water, occasionally resulting in large outbreaks. Approximately 200 cases occur in the UK each year and about 80% of these patients derive their infection from abroad, especially the Indian subcontinent[1]. The incubation period is usually 10–14 days.

PROGNOSIS

- The illness may take many weeks to settle. In most patients the febrile period lasts about one month.
- 5–15% cases relapse, usually during the second week after the temperature returns to normal.
- Intestinal haemorrhage occurs in 2–8% cases (usually in the third week).
- Perforation in 3–4% cases (usually towards the end of the third week) causes approximately a quarter of all deaths.
- Osteomyelitis, cholecystitis and myocarditis can occur but are relatively rare.
- Approximately 1–2% cases continue to excrete organisms as chronic carriers.
- Antibiotic therapy has reduced mortality from 10% to <1%.

TREATMENT

1. The patient should be treated in an infectious diseases unit with isolation facilities.
2. Chloramphenicol is usually the antibiotic of first choice and is given in a daily dose of 2 g for an adult or 50 mg/kg body weight for a child[2].
3. Amoxycillin in a dose of 2 g six hourly provides a less toxic alternative and is particularly appropriate when organisms resistant to chloramphenicol are encountered. Co-trimoxazole can also be used.
4. Antibiotics should be continued for two weeks to reduce the chance of relapse.
5. Blood transfusion and surgery may be necessitated by the complications of intestinal haemorrhage or perforation.
6. Persistently positive stool cultures over several months warrant consideration of an extended course of amoxycillin for 2–3 months.
7. Chronic carriers may require cholecystectomy after investigation of the biliary tract.

FOLLOW-UP

A notifiable disease in the UK. The case must be reported promptly to the Local Health Authority. To ensure that the patient is free from infection at least three consecutive negative faecal and urine samples must be obtained at least 48 hours apart and not earlier than 2–3 weeks after the last possible exposure to infection. If any of these are positive, the samples should be repeated at intervals of one month until at least three negative specimens are obtained. Exclusion from work of food handlers is important until they are shown not to be chronic carriers. At least 12 faecal samples (six after magnesium sulphate purges) should be obtained before return to food handling duties. Typhoid vaccine may be given to family, household and nursing contacts. Two negative faecal and urinary cultures (with a 24-hour interval) should be obtained from contacts who are food handlers in the household. The source and vehicle of infection should be sought. Routine administration of typhoid vaccine to the community is not recommended.

[1] Public Health Laboratory Service, Communicable Diseases Surveillance Centre (1983) *Br. Med. J.*, 287 1205.
[2] Sharp JCM *et al.* (1981) *Update*, 7, 737.

Typhus

Typhus is a febrile illness with an associated rash (which may become haemorrhagic) due to a number of rickettsiae in different parts of the world; variously transmitted by lice, fleas, ticks and mites. Classical louse-borne epidemic typhus has a human reservoir, the others are rodent-associated zoonoses. The incubation period is usually within the range 5–15 days.

PROGNOSIS

- Epidemic louse-borne typhus has a mortality of 10–40% increasing with age. Outbreaks are rare but occur in disaster areas with breakdown in hygiene.
- Illness is often mild in children.
- Mite borne (scrub typhus) of south-east Asia: untreated cases remain febrile for three weeks. Mortality varies from 10 to 40%. Myocarditis is a feature.
- Tick typhus occurs in Asia, Africa[1] and as Rocky Mountain Spotted Fever in the USA[2]. Renal, hepatic and pulmonary involvement occur. Mortality about 20% if untreated.
- Flea-borne typhus occurs worldwide. It is a much milder disease with mortality about 2%.

TREATMENT

Tetracycline or chloramphenicol is curative if given early. A loading dose of 3 g is followed by 500 mg four hourly until temperature is normal for 72 hours. Course usually lasts about six days.

FOLLOW-UP

Report to Local Health Authority in the UK. Insecticide treatment of contacts and their belongings. Contacts are kept under observation for 15 days. Rodent control should be instituted.

[1] Maegraith B (1965) *Exotic Diseases in Practice*. London: William Heinemann Medical Books.
[2] Grundy JH (1979) *Medical Zoology for Travellers*. Hampshire: Noble Books.

14
Genito-urinary Diseases
J. R. W. Harris and G. E. Forster

Syphilis

Syphilis, caused by the spirochaete *Treponema pallidum*, is usually sexually transmitted. In 1982, there were 3929 new cases in Great Britain. Numbers have declined since 1978 due, in part, to a fall in homosexually acquired disease.

PROGNOSIS

- In pre-antiobotic era: 30-40% cases developed late symptomatic disease within 3–40 years (15% gummata; 10% cardiovascular syphilis; 10% neurosyphilis).
- With antibiotic treatment: 95% early and late infection 'cured'; progression of late disease halted – underlying pathology unchanged.
- Immunosuppression may reactivate avirulent/low virulent treponemes present in lymph nodes, aqueous humour and cerebrospinal fluid (CSF).
- Prior yaws or pinta confers some immunity[1].

TREATMENT

1. Early and latent infection: Treatment of choice is intramuscular aqueous procaine penicillin G for 10 days in early infection (total dose 6 megaunits), 15–20 days in later stages (total dose 9–12 megaunits), achieving a minimum serum concentration of 0.03 μg/ml. Benzathine penicillin may be given in early (total dose 2.4 megaunits) and latent infection (total dose 7.2 megaunits). Tetracycline or erythromycin is substituted, in patients allergic to penicillin, in early disease (total dose 30 g) and latent disease (total dose 60 g).
2. Late infection: Aqueous procaine penicillin G (total dose 12 megaunits) for cardiovascular syphilis, neurosyphilis (CSF examination essential to confirm diagnosis). New regimes include high dose intravenous penicillin, with oral probenecid, for 14 days. Tetracycline may be used if patient allergic to penicillin (total dose 60 g).
3. Syphilis in pregnancy: Penicillin is given in dosage appropriate to the stage of the disease. Erythromycin (not estolate) is used if the patient is penicillin allergic, but it has poor placental penetration, therefore the infant should be treated at birth with penicillin.
4. Congenital syphilis: CSF examination, then aqueous procaine penicillin G (50 000 units/kg for 10 days).
5. Jarisch–Herxheimer reaction: 'All or none phenomena' 3-12 hours after first dose of any treponemicidal drug. Rare in late syphilis, may cause morbidity. Steroid cover in cardiovascular disease and neurosyphilis of doubtful value.

FOLLOW-UP

Serological testing: All sexual contacts within preceding 3–6 months in early infection; regular partner in late disease; children of infected mother. Serological surveillance of patient: Monthly for three months, then three monthly for two years following early infection; 6–12 monthly for two years, then annually after late infection. CSF examination: 6–12 months after treatment of neurosyphilis. Retreatment considered if: Symptoms/signs persist or recur; titre of non-treponemal test demonstrates either (1) fourfold increase, or (2) fails to show fourfold decrease within one year[2].

[1] Adler MW (1984) *Br. Med. J.*, **288**, 551.
[2] CDC (1982) *Morb. Mort. Week. Rep.*, 31 Suppl. 2 50S.

Gonorrhoea

Gonorrhoea is caused by the Gram-negative intracellular diplococcus, *Neisseria gonorrhoeae* and is usually sexually transmitted, affecting the mucosal surfaces of the genital tract, rectum and oropharynx. In 1982, there were 58 778 reported cases in Britain, post-pubertal gonorrhoea having declined since the mid-1970s.

PROGNOSIS

- In industrialised countries, 80–90% gonococcal infection is uncomplicated, with good prognosis.
- Asymptomatic infection occurs in 5–10% cases in men and 50% cases in women attending Sexually Transmitted Disease clinics (the true prevalence is unknown).
- 35–50% men with gonorrhoea develop postgonococcal urethritis (PGU), caused in the majority by coinfection with *Chlamydia trachomatis*.
- Rectal infection frequently occurs in homosexual men, with varying symptoms and signs. 40% women with gonorrhoea have rectal infection, being the only site involved in 5% cases.
- Oropharyngeal infection is found in about 25% homosexual males and 5% heterosexual patients with genital gonorrhoea.
- Local complications (e.g. epididymitis, Bartholinitis) are uncommon.
- 10–15% female patients develop pelvic inflammatory disease (PID)[1]. Late complications include infertility, ectopic pregnancy and chronic salpingitis. Tubal occlusion develops in 75% cases after three or more episodes of PID. Risk of ectopic pregnancy increases seven times after one or more episodes of salpingitis[2].
- 1% untreated cases develop disseminated gonococcal infection (DGI), the commonest cause of bacterial arthritis in young adults[3].
- No long-term immunity develops after infection.

TREATMENT

1. Choice of effective therapy depends upon the prevalence of penicillinase producing *Neisseria gonorrhoeae* (PPNG) and the development of chromosomally mediated antibiotic resistance within the community[2]. Single-dose treatment is preferred, being cheap, with good patient compliance and reduced side-effects.

2. Uncomplicated adult infection: Penicillin is the treatment of choice with cure rates of 93–98.3%, e.g. ampicillin 3.5 g, probenecid 1.0 g stat by mouth. Alternative therapy includes spectinomycin 2.0 g intramuscularly stat (cure rate 96.3%).

3. Rectal infection: Co-trimoxazole (trimethoprim 80 mg, sulphamethoxazole 400 mg) 4 tablets bd for two days or amoxycillin 500 mg orally tds for five days.

4. Oropharyngeal infection: Co-trimoxazole 2 tablets bd for five days or amoxycillin (as for rectal infection).

5. Complicated infection

   a) Pelvic inflammatory disease – Spectinomycin stat followed by oral doxycycline (100 mg) and metronidazole (400 mg) bd for 10–14 days (treats possible chlamydial infection).

   b) DGI – Benzyl penicillin 1 megaunit intramuscularly/intravenously followed by oral ampicillin 500 mg qds with oral probenecid for 10 days. Co-trimoxazole, 2 tabs. bd substituted in patients allergic to penicillin.

6. Other gonococcal infections

   a) Ophthalmia – Systemic penicillin for 7–10 days.

   b) In children – reduced adult dosage (exclude infection in parent(s) and sexual assault).

   c) In pregnancy – penicillin in conventional dosage or oral erythromycin 500 mg qds for 7–10 days[4].

Contd.

7. New developments

   a) Third-generation cephalosporins, e.g. cefotaxime. Isolated resistance reported in Far East.
   b) Quinolone derivatives, e.g. ciprofloxacin. Effective against PPNG and infection in extragenital sites.
   c) Monobactams, e.g. aztreonam. Effective against PPNG.
   d) Possible vaccine[2].

FOLLOW-UP

Examine all recent sexual contacts, treat as appropriate. Exclude other sexually transmitted diseases, e.g. *Chlamydia trachomatis*. Repeat cultures from all sites at 7 and 14 days, whilst patient abstaining from coitus.

[1] Rees E *et al.* (1969) *Br. J. Ven. Dis.*, **45**, 205.
[2] Hook EW *et al.* (1985) *Ann. Int. Med.*, **102**, 229.
[3] Anon (1984) *Lancet*, **i**, 832.
[4] CDC (1982) *Morb. Mort. Week. Rep.*, **31** Suppl. 2, 37S.

AIDS

The acquired immune deficiency syndrome (AIDS), caused by the human T-cell lymphocytotropic virus 3 (HTLV-3), is characterised by opportunistic infections (OI) and malignant neoplasms (e.g. Kaposi's sarcoma (KS)) in patients without known cause for immunodeficiency[1]. AIDS is part of a wide spectrum of clinical states associated with HTLV-3 infection. These include symptom-free carriers, patients with persistent generalised lymphadenopathy and seronegative virus-positive persons. The epidemiology of the disease is changing. At first, AIDS was recognised in certain 'at-risk groups', but it is now behaving like any other sexually transmitted infection. It is generally transmitted sexually but occasionally by transfusion or inoculation with blood products[2].

PROGNOSIS

- Overall fatality rate: 40–50% in cases reported between 1979–84.
- Incubation period: Prolonged, ranging from 15–57 months (median 27.5 months).
- Kaposi's sarcoma: 25% AIDS cases have KS at presentation, 6–8% develop it. 20% with limited KS survive two years (median 18 months).
- Opportunistic infections: commonest presentation, unusual and multiple. 1–2% survive two years (median 7–8 months). *Pneumocystis carinii* found in 80% cases, 60% at presentation.
- Pregnancy: Accelerates progression of disease. Risk of affecting subsequent pregnancy is 65% if mother is HTLV-3 positive.
- Health personnel: Minimal risk in the absence of other risk factors (if recommended safety guidelines followed).

TREATMENT

1. Empirical: Pathogenesis of disease not fully delineated.
2. *Kaposi's sarcoma:* Widespread skin, visceral and lymph node disease. Excision, radiotherapy or alpha-interferons.
3. *Opportunistic infections:* Affecting lungs, central nervous system, gut and skin

   a) Protozoan
      i) *Pneumocystis carinii* pneumonia: high dose co-trimoxazole for 21 days. 46–70% develop allergic rash. Chest radiograph resolution within 3–6 weeks. Pentamidine may be used[3].
      ii) *Toxoplasma gondii*: Pyrimethamine and sulfadoxine (Fansidar).
      iii) Cryptosporidium: Often resistant to therapy, e.g. spiramycin.

   b) Viral
      i) Herpes simplex: Acyclovir. Low dose maintenance therapy once remission is obtained.
      ii) Cytomegalovirus: Foscarnet (trisodium phosphonoformate); acyclovir analogue, DHPG.

   c) Fungal
      i) *Candida albicans*: Oral nystatin, amphotericin or ketoconazole. Intravenous amphotericin B for systemic fungal infections.

   d) Bacteria
      i) Atypical mycobacteria: Often resistant to conventional antituberculous therapy.

4. Non-specific manifestations, e.g. recrudescence of atopy presenting as seborrhoeic eczema: Conventional therapy.

5. Future prospects in treating HTLV-3 viraemia:

   a) Agents that block HTLV-3 replication, including leucocyte interferons and certain rifamycins, e.g. suranim.
   b) Placebo controlled studies of isoprinosine in AIDS-related diseases.
   c) Development of safe, protective vaccine[4].

FOLLOW-UP[5]

Regular out-patient review; early treatment of any opportunistic infection. Counselling and
Contd.

education of AIDS patients, their families and friends.

[1] CDC (1982) *Morb. Mort. Week. Rep.*, **31**, 507.
[2] *Acquired Immune Deficiency Syndrome – Aids* (1985) DHSS: London.
[3] Anon (1985) *Lancet*, **i**, 676.
[4] Seligmann M *et al.* (1984) *New Eng. J. Med.*, **311**, 1286.
[5] Miller D, Weber J, Green J (eds.) (1986) *The Management of AIDS Patients*. London: Macmillan.

Nongonococcal Urethritis

Nongonococcal urethritis (NGU) refers to any urethritis not caused by gonorrhoea. It has a complex aetiology, being sexually acquired, secondary to other genito-urinary conditions or associated with non-infectious causes.

PROGNOSIS

- NGU is often a self-limiting condition when untreated.
- Infective causes of NGU include *Chlamydia trachomatis* (30–50%) and *Ureaplasma urealyticum* (10–40%). No causative agent is found in 20–25% cases[1].
- Local complications (e.g. epididymitis, Bartholinitis) are uncommon.
- The incidence of prostatitis developing after NGU is unknown, but is thought to be low.
- Sexually acquired reactive arthritis (SARA) rarely follows an attack of NGU (1% cases). Urethritis may be a component of enteric Reiter's syndrome.
- At least 20% men require more than seven days treatment although this is sufficient to cure chlamydial infection. Tetracycline-resistant ureaplasmas may be responsible in a few cases.
- At least 10% men relapse without necessarily being reinfected. Exclude anxious self-examiners and underlying structural disease (e.g. urethral stricture) if symptoms persist for longer than four weeks[2].

- No long-term immunity develops after infection.

TREATMENT

1. Similar therapy is effective in postgonococcal urethritis, chlamydia-positive and chlamydia-negative NGU.
2. Treatment of choice is oral tetracycline (e.g. oxytetracycline 500 mg six hourly or triple tetracycline 300 mg 12 hourly for seven days), may be repeated for a second week if symptoms persist.
3. Erythromycin stearate 500 mg 12 hourly used for 7–14 days if tetracycline fails.

FOLLOW-UP

Examine all recent sexual contacts, epidemiological treatment preferred. Exclude other sexually transmitted diseases. Tests of cure should be performed on completion of therapy, patient having abstained from coitus.

[1] McCutchan JA (1984) *Rev. Infect. Dis.*, 6, 669.
[2] Anon (1985) *Lancet*, i, 145.

Trichomoniasis

Trichomoniasis, caused by the protozoon *Trichomonas vaginalis*, is a sexually transmitted infection of the lower genital tract, commonly affecting women.

PROGNOSIS

- Treatment failure in 5% patients, attributable to reinfection, poor compliance, inactivation of nitroimidazole by other vaginal microorganisms and development of antibiotic resistance[1].
- No long-term immunity develops after infection.

TREATMENT

1. Systemic: Nitroimidazole derivatives, e.g. metronidazole or nimorazole 2.0 g by mouth in a single dose. Longer courses may be given.
   NB. Nitroimidazoles not recommended during first trimester of pregnancy[1].

2. Local

a) Vaginal preparations, e.g. clotrimazole pessaries and cream.
b) Rectal suppositories, e.g. metronidazole 2.0 g in a single dose[2].

FOLLOW-UP

Epidemiological treatment recommended for male contacts[3]. Exclude other sexually transmitted diseases, e.g. gonorrhoea. Tests of cure, whenever possible, at seven days.

---

[1] Robbie MO *et al.* (1983) *Am. J. Obstet. Gynaec.*, **145**, 865.
[2] Panja SK (1982) *Br. J. Ven. Dis.*, **58**, 257.
[3] Mindel A *et al.* (1985) *Eur. J. Sex. Trans. Dis.*, **2**, 91.

Candidosis

Candidosis affects the lower genital tract, being more common in women and usually caused by *Candida albicans*. Sexual contact plays a minor role in transmission.

PROGNOSIS

- Treatment is effective in 75–80% cases.
- Traditional risk factors predisposing to recurrent infection (e.g. oral contraceptives) have been queried.
- Short courses of antifungal therapy may be helpful in recurrent infection[1].

TREATMENT

1. Imidazole derivatives: Topical, e.g. clotrimazole pessaries and cream (500 mg as single dose or 200 mg daily for three days)[2]. Other formulations include tampons. Systemic therapy, e.g. oral ketoconazole has no benefit over topical therapy except in immunocompromised host. Side-effect of hepatotoxicity (1 in 15 000 cases[3]).

2. Polyene derivatives: Topical, e.g. nystatin. Less patient acceptability although similar cure rates. Some strains of candida have developed resistance. Systemic therapy includes oral nystatin. No additional therapeutic benefit has been shown.

3. New developments: Clinical trials with third generation imidazoles.

FOLLOW-UP

Exclude other sexually transmitted diseases. Follow-up is unnecessary unless patient remains symptomatic.

[1] Davidson F *et al.* (1978) *Br. J. Ven. Dis.*, **54**, 176.
[2] Mendling W *et al.* (1982) *Chemotherapy*, **28** Suppl. 1, 43.
[3] Hay RJ (1985) *Br. Med. J.*, **290**, 260.

Chlamydial Infection

The obligate intracellular bacterium *Chlamydia trachomatis* is the commonest sexually transmitted microorganism worldwide. Serovars A–C are the cause of trachoma, whilst serovars D–K cause urogenital infections and conjunctivitis. Clinical manifestations are similar to gonorrhoea[1].

PROGNOSIS

- Untreated infection may persist for years.
- Infection is asymptomatic in 30–50% cases in women, 20% cases in men.
- Commonest cause of nongonococcal urethritis and postgonococcal urethritis.
- Local complications (e.g. epididymitis, Bartholinitis) are uncommon.
- 10–15% infected women develop pelvic inflammatory disease, management similar to gonococcal salpingitis.
- Perihepatitis is a rare but recognised systemic complication.
- 1% untreated cases develop sexually acquired reactive urethritis[2], 50% have acute chlamydial infection at onset of Reiter's disease.
- Adult ophthalmia results from autoinoculation. Blindness does not occur in contrast to hyperendemic trachoma.
- 30–50% infants of chlamydia-positive mothers are colonised; 30% develop conjunctivitis and/or nasopharyngeal infection.
- Commonest cause of pneumonia in newborns in the USA (3–4 per 1000).
- No long-term immunity develops after infection[3].

TREATMENT (See also gonorrhoea, nongonococcal urethritis)

1. *Uncomplicated adult infection:* Tetracycline is the treatment of choice. Erythromycin should be used in pregnancy.
2. *Neonatal infection:* Ophthalmia neonatorum – erythromycin syrup (50 mg/kg/day) in divided doses for 14 days. Chlamydial pneumonia – as above, for 21 days.
3. *Lymphogranuloma venereum:* Prolonged course of tetracycline recommended (e.g. doxycycline 100 mg bd for 21 days).

FOLLOW-UP

Examine all recent sexual contacts; epidemiological treatment preferred. Exclude other sexually transmitted diseases. Reassess uncomplicated cases at seven days for compliance, side-effects and clinical progress. Repeat cultures 3–6 weeks later if poor compliance suspected. Complicated cases require more frequent follow-up.

[1] Jones BR (1983) *Br. Med. Bull.*, **39**, 107.
[2] Taylor-Robinson D *et al.* (1980) *J. Clin. Path.*, **33**, 205.
[3] Thomas BJ *et al.* (1984) *J. Clin. Path.*, **37**, 812.

Condyloma Acuminata

Condyloma acuminata (genital warts) are usually sexually transmitted and associated with human papillomavirus (HPV) types 6, 11 and (less frequently) 16.

PROGNOSIS

- Vulval warts: Cervical condylomata co-exist in 5% cases. Cytological/colposcopic evidence of flat warts (HPV 6) in 50% cases. Therapy advised.
- Cervical intraepithelial neoplasia: HPV 6 and/or 16 demonstrated in 60% biopsies.
- Juvenile laryngeal papillomas: Genital warts (HPV 6) in 70–80% mothers.
- There is an association with carcinoma: HPV 16 and 18 found in invasive cervical, penile and vulval carcinomas[1].

TREATMENT

1. External genital/perianal: Topical application of 10–25% podophyllin.
2. Urethral/meatal: Podophyllin if accessible. Urethroscopy when upper limit not seen. Intraurethral 5% 5-fluorouracil considered.
3. Cervical: Cytology/colposcopy before therapy. Use cryotherapy, electrodiathermy or laser.
4. Alternative therapies: Cryotherapy, electrosurgery, surgical excision.
5. Podophyllin *contraindicated* on cervix and during pregnancy[2].

FOLLOW-UP

Exclude other sexually transmitted diseases. Examine sexual partners. Annual cervical smear recommended in women.

[1] Singer A *et al.* (1984) *Br. Med. J.*, **288**, 735.
[2] CDC (1982) *Morb. Mort. Week. Rep.*, **31** Suppl. 2, 48S.

15

Psychiatric Diseases

M. A. Reveley

Depressive Illness

Depressive illness is a disorder characterised by a dysphoric mood such as feeling depressed, sad, blue, despondent or discouraged, associated with poor appetite, weight loss, difficulty with sleeping (such as interval or terminal insomnia), loss of energy, agitation or psychomotor retardation, loss of interest in usual activities, feelings of self-reproach or guilt, loss of concentration, recurrent thoughts of death or suicide[1]. Symptoms lasting 2–4 weeks are necessary for the diagnosis. When depressive illness is accompanied by prominent biological symptoms it is called 'endogenous'; when accompanied by delusions or hallucinations it is 'psychotic'; when associated with mania it is 'bipolar' and when there is no history of mania it is 'unipolar'. When there is no previous history of psychiatric disorder it is called 'primary', and when it occurs during another psychiatric disorder it is 'secondary' depression. About 5% men and 9% women have major depression at some time in their lives. About 10% of these are bipolar and 90% unipolar.

PROGNOSIS

- The mean age of onset is about 40. For bipolar patients the mean age is in the early thirties.
- About two-thirds of depressives have only a single attack; in 5–10% the illness is chronic[2].
- Between episodes of illness most patients function well although there are occasional residual symptoms.
- The length of individual episodes is extremely variable ranging from a few months to many years.
- About 15% major depressives will commit suicide.
- Patients with depressive illness also have an increased mortality from physical disease, especially carcinoma.
- Alcoholism and drug abuse may be complications of depression.

TREATMENT

1. Depressed patients should always be assessed for diagnosis, contributing factors, severity and risk of suicide.
2. Supportive psychotherapy should always be a part of management. There is some evidence that cognitive therapy is an effective treatment for major depression[3].
3. The major approach to the management of depressive episodes is the use of anti-depressant medication[4] particularly tricyclic anti-depressants such as imipramine and amitriptyline (average effective dosage 150 mg/day, range 100–300 mg/day). Six weeks at an effective dosage should be tried before deciding the drug is not working. The most common side-effects of these drugs are dry mouth, orthostatic hypotension and tremor. The medication is dangerous in overdose, particularly due to cardiac toxicity.
4. Newer anti-depressants such as mianserin which has less cardiotoxicity and risk in overdose, may be effective.
5. Monoamine oxidase inhibitors are used less frequently for depressive illness, and more often for 'atypical depressions' with anxiety.
6. Electro-convulsive therapy (ECT) is generally reserved for those patients who do not respond to tricyclic anti-depressants or who are so ill, either due to a high risk of suicide or stupor, that they require immediate remission. There is good evidence that ECT produces a more rapid remission than drug therapy[4] and is particularly useful in psychotic[5] and endogenous depression.
7. Lithium carbonate is useful for recurrent unipolar and bipolar depression. The serum lithium level should be between 0.5 and 0.8 mEq/l for maintenance treatment. Side-effects may include tremor, nausea and vomiting. Ataxia and confusion develop with toxic doses.
8. When effective, tricyclic anti-depressants should be continued for six months, at reduced dosage, after remission of symptoms.

FOLLOW-UP

Depressed patients should be seen frequently (i.e. every 1–2 weeks) particularly if there is a risk of suicide. Anti-depressants should be continued for six months after remission. Lithium should be monitored with serum levels every 3-6 months for maintenance, depending on the stability of blood levels and mood, and with yearly T_4 assay.

[1] Feighner JP et al. (1972) Arch. Gen. Psychiat., 26, 57.
[2] Lundquist G (1945) Acta Psychiat. Neurol., Suppl. 35.
[3] Rush AJ et al. (1977) Cog. Ther. Res., 1, 17.
[4] Medical Research Council (1965) Br. Med. J., i, 881.
[5] Clinical Research Centre, Division of Psychiatry (1984) Br. J. Psychiat., 144, 227.

Mania

Mania is a disorder characterised by a euphoric or irritable mood in association with: hyperactivity including motor, social and sexual activity; pressured speech; flight of ideas or racing thoughts; grandiosity; decreased need for sleep; and distractability. The illness should last at least 1–2 weeks for the diagnosis to be made. About 10% patients with mania have unipolar mania, i.e. no episode of depression during their lives, but 90% manics have a period of depression at some other time in their lives; thus mania is considered a 'bipolar' affective disorder. Mania is a psychotic disorder, so that delusions and hallucinations are usually present. These are usually mood congruent delusions compatible with the elevated or euphoric mood, but bizarre or typically 'schizophrenic' delusions or hallucinations do not exclude mania. The mean age of onset is about 30 years and 90% cases begin before age 50[1]. The lifetime prevalence is 1%[2]. The sex ratio is 1:1.

PROGNOSIS

- Untreated manic episodes generally last over many months[3], with an average duration of 13 months[4]. It has been found[1] that treated attacks lasted under three months and in those with repeated attacks the length of each episode did not alter in the later attacks. Nearly all manic patients recover eventually, even untreated.
- Manic illnesses often recur and subsequent depression is frequently found (90% cases).
- Estimates of those patients with only a single episode of mania vary from 1–50%.
- The length of remission between episodes becomes shorter up to the third attack, but does not change thereafter[1].

TREATMENT

1. Manic patients should be assessed for diagnosis, contributing factors and severity.
2. Those patients who are psychotic and whose behaviour is likely to lead to harm to others or themselves should generally be hospitalised.
3. Anti-psychotic medication such as phenothiazines (chlorpromazine 300–1200 mg/day) or butyrophenones such as haloperidol (15–60 mg/day) are required for their rapid effect.
4. Lithium carbonate therapy (in dosages to achieve 0.8–1.5 mEq/l blood levels) is used for acute episodes, but may take 10 days to be effective.
5. Some manic patients unresponsive to the above regimen may require electro-convulsive therapy.

FOLLOW-UP

When the manic episode has remitted, the antipsychotic medication can generally be discontinued. Maintenance therapy with lithium carbonate to achieve serum levels of 0.5–0.8 mEq/l has been shown to prevent relapses into both mania and depression[5].

[1] Angst J et al. (1973) Psychiat. Neurol. Neurochi., 76, 489.
[2] Robins LN et al. (1984) Arch. Gen. Psychiat., 41, 949.
[3] Kraepelin E (1921) Manic Depressive Insanity and Paranoia. Edinburgh: E. & S. Livingstone.
[4] Lundquist G (1945) Acta Psychiat. Neurol., Suppl. 35.
[5] Coppen A et al. (1971) Lancet, i, 275.

Anxiety Neurosis

Anxiety neurosis begins before age 40 and is characterised by chronic nervousness with recurrent anxiety attacks manifested by apprehension, fearfulness and a sense of impending doom. Autonomic symptoms characteristic of the attacks include dyspnoea, palpitations, chest pain or discomfort, choking or smothering sensations, dizziness, and parathesiae. The anxiety attacks occur at times other than marked physical exertion or life-threatening situations and in the absence of medical illness that could account for the symptoms. This is a common syndrome with about 5% the adult population being affected[1]. The sex ratio men to women is 1:2.

PROGNOSIS

- The age of risk is from the mid-teens to the early thirties.
- Anxiety neurosis can occasionally be severe, but in the majority of cases the course is mild, and most patients live productively without social impairment. It rarely leads to hospitalisation.
- A group of patients were followed over 20 years[2] and it was found that 12% were well, 35% had symptoms but no disability, 38% had mild disability and 15% had moderate or severe disability.
- If complications occur they are generally in the form of an affective disorder or alcoholism.
- Suicide rarely occurs.
- Dependence on barbiturates and sedatives may occur.
- While anxiety neurotics may worry about developing other illnesses they are no more likely than others to develop stress-related disorders, schizophrenia or other psychiatric illnesses.

TREATMENT

1. Supportive psychotherapy is generally sufficient with brief interviews and reassurance.
2. Treatment of an acute episode of over-breathing is generally by demonstrating that when a patient breathes into a bag the symptoms of parathesiae and carpopedal spasm subside.
3. If drugs are required a benzodiazepine such as diazepam may be given but not beyond a few weeks and should be used as an adjunct to other forms of treatment.
4. Barbiturates should not be used.
5. Beta-adrenoceptor antagonists have limited use unless palpitations are troublesome.
6. Anti-depressant drugs such as tricyclics and monoamine oxidase inhibitors may occasionally be helpful but should be used with caution in view of their side-effects.
7. Relaxation training can be as effective as drugs but requires the patient's cooperation in learning the technique.

FOLLOW-UP

The disorder is chronic and recurrent. Psychotherapy and relaxation therapy will need to be reinforced. Long-term benzodiazepines are to be avoided.

---

[1] Cohen ME et al. (1950) Ass. Res. Nerv. Dis. Proc., 29, 832.
[2] Wheeler EO et al. (1950) J. Am. Med. Assoc., 142, 878.

Phobic Neurosis

A phobia is defined as a persistent and recurring fear which the patient tries to resist or avoid and at the same time considers unreasonable. Onset is before age 40. A patient with phobic neurosis has a significant fear producing symptoms of anxiety, anxious thoughts in anticipation of the anxiety, and avoidance of situations that provoke the fear. Phobias may be divided into: a) simple phobias which include fears of heights (acrophobia), thunderstorms, spiders (arachnophobia), dogs and other animals, and enclosed spaces (claustrophobia); b) social phobias when patients become anxious and avoid situations such as restaurants, canteens, public transport, etc. in which they may be observed by other people; c) agoraphobia occurs when patients become anxious when they travel from home, mix with crowds or are in situations which they cannot leave. Patients are often housebound, and become increasingly dependent on others. The female to male ratio is 2–3:1. The lifetime prevalence of simple phobias in the general American population is estimated to be about 20%[1]. The lifetime prevalence of agoraphobia is 3–7%[1].

PROGNOSIS

- Animal phobias commonly begin in childhood before the age of eight while agoraphobia is rare in childhood and usually begins in young adult life.
- There have been few systematic follow-up studies but clinical experience suggests that simple phobias last many years. A study[2] showed that agoraphobia which has lasted for a year changes little over the following five years.
- At five-year follow-up about 50% phobics had improved, 25% were unchanged and 25% were worse. Isolated phobias had the best prognosis and agoraphobia the worst[3].
- Social, occupational and marital disability and depression are the main complications.

TREATMENT

1. Behaviour therapy is generally the treatment of choice, either by exposure *in vivo* or desensitisation in imagination. These are especially useful for simple phobias.

2. For agoraphobia the treatment of choice is programmed practice in which patients are trained to overcome avoidance behaviour systematically for at least an hour every day.
3. Anxiolytic drugs may be used for immediate relief of symptoms, but care should be taken not to use them long term.
4. Anti-depressant drugs such as tricyclics or monoamine oxidase inhibitors may improve phobias even when depression is not present[4].

FOLLOW-UP

Patients who have only partial response to treatment will require continued supportive psychotherapy.

[1] Robins LN *et al.* (1984) *Arch. Gen. Psychiat.*, **41**, 949.
[2] Marks IM (1971) *Br. J. Psychiat.*, **118**, 683.
[3] Agras S *et al.* (1972) *Arch. Gen. Psychiat.*, **26**, 315.
[4] Zitrin CM *et al.* (1978) *Arch. Gen. Psychiat.*, **35**, 307.

Obsessive Compulsive Neurosis

In obsessive compulsive neurosis, obsessions or compulsions are the dominant symptoms and onset is prior to age 40. Obsessions are defined as recurrent or persistent ideas, thoughts, images or feelings which the person tries to resist, which he finds intrusive and foreign to his personality or nature, and which he recognises as absurd. A compulsion is a recurrent or persistent movement or action which is also intrusive, resisted and ego-alien. Estimates of lifetime prevalence vary from 2–3%[1]. The sex ratio is 1:1.

PROGNOSIS

- Obsessional illness generally begins before the age of 25, and 85% begin before the age of 35.
- Onset may be acute or insidious; the course is generally chronic with varying degrees of remission.
- Obsessionals with mild symptoms have a good prognosis: as many as 60–80% are improved 1–5 years after diagnosis[2].
- Severe cases requiring hospitalisation do less well. Three-quarters remain unchanged 13–20 years later[3].
- 5–10% obsessionals have a course marked by progressive social incapacity[4].
- Favourable prognosis is associated with:

    a) Mild or atypical symptoms.
    b) Short duration of symptoms before treatment is begun.
    c) Good premorbid personality.

- The content of obsessions has no prognostic significance.
- Obsessionals are prone to develop intercurrent depressions and have a higher rate of celibacy than the general population.
- Suicide is uncommon, occurring in fewer than 1% cases.
- While obsessionals often fear they will lose control or become mad these fears are generally unwarranted.

TREATMENT

1. Supportive psychotherapy can be used to reassure the patient that spontaneous improvement can occur and that his impulses will almost certainly not be carried out.
2. If depression is present concurrent treatment of depression will generally improve the obsessions.
3. Anxiolytic drugs give short-term symptomatic relief, but should not be prescribed for more than a few weeks.
4. Anti-depressant drugs such as clomipramine may be effective against obsessional symptoms[5]. However, not all studies found tricyclics to be effective[6].
5. About two-thirds of patients with moderately severe rituals may improve with response prevention and exposure to the environmental cues which provoke rituals.
6. Behavioural treatment is less effective for obsessional thoughts. While thought stopping has been used it has questionable efficacy[7].
7. Exploratory and interpretative psychotherapy seldom helps, and obsessionals are notoriously difficult to treat by psychoanalysts.

FOLLOW-UP

As the disorder is chronic, continued support is often required for years, in the form of counselling for interpersonal problems, anti-depressants for intercurrent depression, and further behaviour therapy if obsessions or rituals become exacerbated. The GP or psychiatrist may provide follow-up, but special experience in behaviour therapy is required for that treatment.

[1] Robins LN et al. (1984) Arch. Gen. Psychiat., 41, 949.
[2] Pollitt J (1957) Br. Med. J., i, 194.
[3] Kringlen E (1965) Br. J. Psychiat., 111, 709.
[4] Rudin G (1953) Archiv. Psychiat. Nervenkrank., 191, 14.
[5] Capstick N (1975) Psychosomat., 16, 21.
[6] Marks IM et al. (1980) Br. J. Psychiat., 136, 1.
[7] Stern RS et al. (1973) Behav. Res. Ther., 11, 659.

Schizophrenia

Schizophrenia is a disorder characterised by delusions and hallucinations, often with disturbances of affect and with illogical thinking (loose associations), in the absence of significant perplexity or confusion and in the absence of organic brain disease, or drug or alcohol abuse sufficient to account for the symptoms. The presence of a manic or depressive syndrome makes the diagnosis questionable and such cases are called 'schizoaffective' or 'schizophreniform'. Onset is before age 45. The delusions are characteristically bizarre, such as delusions of being controlled or having thoughts inserted into the mind, or may be persecutory. The hallucinations are usually auditory, particularly of voices either carrying on a running commentary about the patient, or discussing the patient in the third person. There may also be blunted or inappropriate affect and grossly disorganised behaviour with personality deterioration. The prevalence of the disorder is 2–4 per 1000 of the population, the incidence is about 0.2 per 1000 and the lifetime prevalence is about 1–2%[1]. The importance of the illness is greater than the numbers affected might suggest because of the early age of onset (mean, early 20s), and the lifelong disability and inability to care for themselves of those with the chronic syndrome (defect state).

PROGNOSIS

- Schizophrenia may be divided into forms with a good and poor prognosis.
- Good prognostic features include acute onset, presence of precipitating events, short duration of episode, good premorbid personality, perplexity and confusion present, affective symptoms (such as depression) prominent, being married, family history of affective disorder but not schizophrenia, and older age of onset.
- Poor prognostic factors include insidious onset, absence of precipitating events, an isolated, aloof, poor premorbid personality, absence of perplexity, minimal affective symptoms or the presence of blunted affect, single marital status, family history of schizophrenia but not affective disorder, and younger age of onset.
- The disorder tends to chronicity or periods of remission with frequent relapse. Indeed, many diagnostic systems require chronicity for the diagnosis to be made.
- A 20-year follow-up[2] found that 20% had complete remission of symptoms and 24% were severely disturbed. A good social outcome and adjustment was found in 30%, while 10% required long-term sheltered care. Other studies[3] made similar findings.
- The course is influenced by cultural background, life events, social stimulation, and family involvement.

TREATMENT

1. Treatment of the acute episode characterised by delusions and hallucinations is principally with antipsychotic drugs which have been shown to be clearly effective[4]. Chlorpromazine, fluphenazine, thioridazine, trifluoperazine, haloperidol and others are effective for schizophrenic 'positive' (delusions, hallucinations, loose associations) symptoms. Chlorpromazine and thioridazine have fewer extrapyramidal side-effects, but produce more drowsiness, dry mouth and hypotension, while haloperidol and fluphenazine cause less drowsiness and hypotension, but more frequent extrapyramidal side-effects, such as dystonia and Parkinsonian symptoms.
2. Treatment either orally or depot, with fluphenazine decanoate or flupenthixol decanoate, has been shown to be effective in preventing relapse[5]. It is most important to be certain that the patient has a tendency to relapse before continuing with maintenance therapy. The lowest effective dose should be used to minimise the risk of tardive dyskinesia.
3. Anticholinergic medicines such as procyclidine may be used for the extrapyramidal side-effects.
4. Social treatment, particularly to reduce high expressed emotions in families, has been shown to reduce the risk of relapse[6]. Rehabilitation and occupational therapy to in

troduce the patient back into the community is often required.

5. If symptoms of depression occur during the course of schizophrenia anti-depressant medication or lithium may be used with care, but the value is uncertain. Electro-convulsive therapy is occasionally indicated for schizophrenia with severe depressive symptoms or catatonic stupor.

6. Individual psychotherapy is of doubtful value.

FOLLOW-UP

Chronic schizophrenia requires lifelong follow-up with maintenance medication (usually depot), family support and therapy, and social and vocational rehabilitation. Remitting schizophrenia requires less contact and treatment only on relapse.

[1] Robins LN *et al.* (1984) *Arch. Gen. Psychiat.*, **41**, 949.

[2] Bleuler M (1974) *Psychol. Med.*, **4**, 244.

[3] Ciompi L (1980) *Br. J. Psychiat.*, **136**, 413.

[4] Davis JM (1976) *Am. J. Psychiat.*, **133**, 208.

[5] Hogarty GE *et al.* (1977) *Arch. Gen. Psychiat.*, **34**, 297.

[6] Vaughan CE *et al.* (1976) *Br. J. Psychiat.*, **129**, 125.

Hysteria

Hysteria is a disorder, often classified with the neuroses, in which there are symptoms and signs of disease occurring in the absence of physical pathology and which are produced without the person's conscious awareness. Hysteria has been traditionally subdivided into: a) dissociative hysteria, characterised by amnesia, fugue, somnambulism and multiple personality; and b) conversion hysteria in which there are dramatic symptoms such as paralysis, fits, aphonia, disorders of gait, anaesthesia, blindness and others. A variant of the disorder is called Briquet's syndrome which is defined as a disorder beginning before the age of 30, lasting for many years and in which patients have multiple physical complaints, without evidence of physical disease, of sufficient severity to require the attention of a doctor or to prevent them from carrying out their usual activities. The symptoms emanate from different organ systems and include headaches, shortness of breath, nausea, vomiting, abdominal pain, pseudoneurologic symptoms, multiple pains including back and arm pain, sexual symptoms and affective symptoms[1].

PROGNOSIS

- Most cases with an acute onset seen in general practice or hospital recover quickly. Those symptoms which last longer than a year are likely to persist for many years more.
- A group of patients referred to a nervous diseases hospital diagnosed as having hysteria were followed-up[2] and it was found that one-third of patients developed a definite organic illness within 7–11 years, and a further third developed depression or schizophrenia.
- It has also been found[3] that isolated conversion symptoms tended to result on follow-up in genuine physical illness. Thus the diagnosis of hysteria should be made with care and a tendency to consider it a 'waste basket' diagnosis for unexplained physical symptoms should be avoided.

TREATMENT

1. Supportive psychotherapy with reassurance and suggestion, combined with attempts to help resolve the stressful circumstances leading to the crisis are often successful in alleviating acute cases.
2. For cases lasting longer a behavioural approach to encourage normal behaviour and eliminate factors that are reinforcing the symptoms is helpful.
3. Abreaction either by hypnosis or intravenous sodium amytal allowing the patient to express his or her emotions may be helpful.
4. Exploratory and dynamic psychotherapy may also be used although its value as a therapy is questionable.
5. Medication is not beneficial unless other psychiatric disorders responsive to medication, such as depressive illness, supervene. Electro-convulsive therapy and neuroleptics, such as chlorpromazine, have little value. Long-term neuroleptics especially should be avoided, because of the risk of tardive dyskinesia.

FOLLOW-UP

Patients with isolated conversion symptoms should be followed-up in case of development of physical disease. Continued support over many years may be required for chronic depression, anxiety, marital problems and other complications.

---

[1] Perley MJ et al. (1962) New Eng. J. Med., 266, 421.
[2] Slater E et al. (1965) J. Psychosomat. Res., 9, 9.
[3] Gatfield PD et al. (1962) Dis. Nerv. Syst., 23, 623.

Syndromes Related to Hysteria: Ganser's Syndrome, Munchausen's Syndrome, Compensation Neurosis and Hypochondriasis

Ganser's syndrome is characterised by the giving of approximate answers, somatic or pseudoneurologic symptoms of hysteria, hallucinations, and apparent clouding of consciousness[1]. The condition was first described among prisoners and because hallucinations are often visual and elaborate (uncharacteristic of genuine psychosis) and the approximate answers are plainly incorrect responses to very simple questions, there is a suggestion that Ganser's syndrome is a form of malingering. *Munchausen's syndrome* was first described[2] as patients repeatedly presenting themselves to hospitals with symptoms suggesting serious physical illness. The symptoms and signs are produced deliberately and the patient is consciously trying to deceive his doctors. He often succeeds in having elaborate investigations or physical remedies applied to him. *Compensation neurosis* is used to describe cases in which physical or mental symptoms develop after an alleged injury which has been the subject of an unsettled claim for compensation. Such cases often have a neurotic personality predisposing but the symptoms tend to persist only so long as the claim is under dispute. *Hypochondriasis* is a disorder in which there is excessive concern with one's general health. Hypochondriasis commonly occurs as a symptom associated with anxiety or depressive illness. In particular, elderly depressives may be very concerned with physical functioning, such as abnormal pain or bowel habits, and depressive illness may be missed if not carefully sought. Hypochondriasis, particularly if symptoms are bizarre, may be a symptom of schizophrenia.

PROGNOSIS

- Munchausen's and Ganser's syndromes tend to be chronic. Compensation neurosis tends to last as long as the case is under dispute.
- The prognosis of hypochondriasis is that of the primary disorder; hypochondriacal personality tends to be chronic.

TREATMENT

1. Psychotherapy for *Munchausen's or Ganser's syndrome* is generally ineffective and the patients do not generally cooperate with treatment. Cases should be recognised so that unnecessary procedures are not carried out.
2. Treatment for *compensation neurosis* is with supportive psychotherapy with a discussion and ventilation of the proposed mechanism.
3. Treatment of *hypochondriasis* is that of the primary disorder. Hypochondriacal complaints should be fully explored to rule out depression, anxiety states, schizophrenia and dementia and to ensure that underlying physical illness is not actually present.

FOLLOW-UP

Patients seldom continue with therapy beyond the presenting complaints. Hypochondriasis may require chronic reassurance and treatment of any underlying depressive illness.

[1] Ganser SJ (1965) *Br. J. Criminol.*, **5**, 120.
[2] Asher R (1951) *Lancet*, **i**, 339.

Anorexia Nervosa

Anorexia nervosa is characterised by anorexia with weight loss of at least 25% of the original body weight. There is a distorted attitude towards food, eating and weight: a) denial of illness with a failure to recognise nutritional needs; b) apparent enjoyment in losing weight; c) a desired body image of extreme thinness with overt evidence that it is rewarding to the patient to achieve this state; and d) unusual hoarding or handling of food. There is often associated amenorrhoea, lanugo (a soft down-like hair), bradycardia (resting pulse of 60 or less), periods of overactivity, episodes of bulimia (gorging of food), and vomiting. There is no other medical or psychiatric illness that accounts for the anorexia or weight loss[1]. Most patients are young women, and the age of onset is under 25, most commonly 16–17. The prevalence is approximately 1–2% among adolescent females[2]. The male to female ratio is approximately 1:20.

PROGNOSIS

- Poor prognostic factors are long illness, great weight loss, bulimia, vomiting or purging, difficulties in relationships, and late age of onset.
- Follow-up studies[3,4] find that at 4–10 years approximately 2% had died of starvation, 16% were still under 75% ideal body weight, and 19% were moderately underweight. There was normal food intake in 37%, purgative abuse in 36%, amenorrhoea in 29% and sporadic menstruation in 17%.
- Very long-term follow-ups indicate that premature death occurs in 10–15% cases hospitalised for psychiatric reasons. Death by starvation and the consequences of malnutrition are the most common.
- The illness may involve one lengthy episode lasting many months or it may be marked by many remissions and exacerbations over the course[5].

TREATMENT

1. Thorough clinical and physical assessment should be made.
2. Re-establishment of an adequate body weight is the first priority. A treatment plan should be arranged and agreed with the patient. Admission to hospital is often required so that food intake and activity can be managed, generally by behavioural therapeutic techniques. A programme of eating supervised by nurses to regain body weight should be established. If the patient does not follow the procedure, privileges should be made contingent on weight gain. Allowing the patient to exercise is often a powerful reinforcer of behaviour.
3. Drugs such as chlorpromazine, and occasionally electro-convulsive therapy have been used.
4. Occasionally force feeding is required.

FOLLOW-UP

Supportive and family therapy, particularly involving the spouse, is indicated in the long term.

[1] Feighner JP et al. (1972) Arch. Gen. Psychiat., 26, 57.
[2] Crisp AH et al. (1976) Br. J. Psychiat., 128, 549.
[3] Morgan HG et al. (1975) Psychol. Med., 5, 355.
[4] Hsu LKG (1980) Arch. Gen. Psychiat., 37, 1041.
[5] Kay DW et al. (1954) J. Ment. Sci., 100, 411.

Alcoholism

The World Health Organisation has defined the alcohol dependence syndrome[1] as having seven essential elements: a) the feeling of a subjective compulsion to drink; b) a stereotyped pattern of drinking; c) primacy of drinking over other activities; d) increased tolerance to alcohol; e) repeated withdrawal symptoms (tremulousness, convulsions, sweats, hallucinations, delirium); f) relief (early morning) drinking; g) reinstatement of the syndrome quickly after abstinence. However, there are many people who do not have the full alcohol dependence syndrome, yet have problems with drinking. Such problem drinkers may believe that they drink too much, find that their family object to their drinking, lose friends because of drinking, have arrests for drinking, and have drink-related traffic difficulties, trouble at work and fights. In addition, the presence of physical damage from alcohol, including alcohol withdrawal and medical complications, such as cirrhosis, gastritis, pancreatitis, and alcoholic blackouts (amnestic episodes), are highly suggestive of alcoholism. The disorder is more common in the young. The male to female ratio is 5:1. In the UK psychiatric admissions for alcohol problems account for 10% of all psychiatric admissions. The prevalence of problem drinkers was found to be about 25 per 1000 and of alcohol dependent patients to be about 5 per 1000 in a population survey of Camberwell in London[2].

PROGNOSIS

- About one-quarter of patients may remain abstinent for six months and fewer than 10% for 18 months[3].
- Cirrhosis of the liver is 10 times more common than in the general population[4]. 10% patients with alcohol dependence syndrome develop cirrhosis. The annual incidence of cirrhosis increased threefold in Birmingham from 1959 to 1975[5].
- Central nervous system complications including peripheral neuropathy, epilepsy, cerebellar degeneration, demyelination syndromes, Korsakoff's syndrome and head injury are common in patients with alcohol dependency.
- Anaemia, myopathy, hypoglycaemia, and cardiomyopathy are also recognised complications.
- The mortality rate in alcoholics is twice the expected level overall. Untreated delirium tremens carries a mortality of 50%.
- Alcoholic dementia and personality deterioration are also complications.
- 6–20% alcoholics die by suicide[6].
- The social damage due to alcohol from divorce, job loss, criminality and traffic accidents is also substantial.

TREATMENT

1. A thorough physical and psychiatric assessment should be made and the spouse involved in treatment.
2. Definite, achievable goals should be formulated with the patient.
3. In general total abstinence is preferable to controlled drinking.
4. Withdrawal from alcohol should be carried out carefully, and admission to hospital is required if the patient is severely dependent. Sedative drugs such as chlormethiazole or chlordiazepoxide (50–100 mg every 2–4 hours) are used in reducing dosages over a few days.
5. Thiamine and other vitamins should be prescribed.
6. Long-term treatment involves group therapy and individual supportive therapy, from the doctor who must be willing to tolerate alcoholics' unreliability and tendency to relapse.
7. Medication is sometimes used[7], such as disulfiram (Antabuse) which blocks the oxidation of alcohol leading to an accumulation of acetaldehyde. Flushing, rapid pulse, nausea and vomiting ensue if alcohol is ingested. The treatment may lead to cardiac arrythmias or hypotension and carries some risk. Drugs are generally used only as an adjunct.

Contd.

FOLLOW-UP

Alcoholics Anonymous[8] is a self-help organisation which has a favourable effect in maintaining long-term abstinence. Continued support is required, with treatment of complications such as depression, marital problems and vitamin deficiencies.

[1] Edwards G *et al.* (1977) *Alcohol Related Disabilities.* Geneva: WHO.
[2] Edwards G *et al.* (1972) *Q. J. Stud. Alcohol.*, Suppl. 6, 69.
[3] Armour DJ *et al.* (1976) *Alcoholism and Treatment.* Santa Monica: Rand Corporation.
[4] Williams R *et al.* (1977) *Proc. Roy. Soc. Med.*, **70,** 33.
[5] Saunders JB *et al.* (1981) *Br. Med. J.*, **282,** 1140.
[6] Ritson B (1977) Alcoholism and suicide. In: *Alcoholism: New Knowledge and New Responses* (Edwards G, Grant M eds.). London: Croom Helm.
[7] Goodwin DW (1982) Drug therapy of alcoholism. In *Psychopharmacology* Vol. 1 (Graham-Smith DG *et al.* eds.). Amsterdam: Excerpta Medica.
[8] Robinson D (1979) *Talking Out of Alcoholism: the Self-help Process of Alcoholics Anonymous.* London: Croom Helm.

Drug Dependence

Drug dependence means the repeated, non-medicinal use of a drug causing harm to the user or others. Drug addiction is used in two senses: a) physical addiction refers to a drug-produced condition involving tolerance and physical dependence. Tolerance means that larger doses of drug are required to produce the same effect, and physical dependence means that the drug must be repeatedly administered to prevent the appearance of a stereotyped withdrawal syndrome characteristic of each particular drug; and b) psychological addiction refers to a pattern of compulsive drug use with a high tendency to relapse after withdrawal[1]. Specific types of drug include morphine and its derivatives, heroin and codeine; barbiturates, and similar sedatives and hypnotics. Other drugs include cannabis, amphetamines, cocaine, hallucinogens such as lysergic acid diethylamide (LSD), dimethyltryptamine (DMT), phencyclidine (PCP or angel dust) and solvents. Adolescents and youths are at particular risk of heroin and morphine addiction, solvent abuse, and hallucinogen abuse, while the middle aged and elderly mainly develop dependence on sleeping medication and amphetamines.

PROGNOSIS

- Prognosis depends to a large extent on the type of drug, age, and social and personality characteristics of the patient.
- Follow-up studies of opiate addicts show that after seven years about 25–33% are abstinent, while 10–20% have died due to drug related causes[2]. However, 95% soldiers who became addicted during the Vietnam War were abstinent on follow-up, indicating the importance of personality and social factors on outcome[3].
- Barbiturate dependency is similar to alcoholism in that the course is characterised by relapse and chronicity. Death by accidental overdose or suicide is at higher risk. These medications should not be prescribed to depressed patients.
- Cannabis has no definite withdrawal syndrome or evidence of tolerance and its deleterious effects are principally due to intoxication, but there is some suggestion that it may lead to a psychosis.
- Amphetamines are sometimes prescribed as diet tablets and if taken over a period of time lead to a dependence syndrome that can lead to a paranoid psychosis indistinguishable from paranoid schizophrenia.
- Cocaine, hallucinogens and phencyclidine tend to be recreational drugs whose principal risk is from life-threatening behaviour during the acute intoxication, particularly psychotic episodes leading to suicide.

- Solvent abuse may lead to death through toxic effects and trauma, asphyxia, or inhalation of stomach contents. 140 deaths were reported in the 10-year period 1971–81[4].

TREATMENT

1. Thorough psychiatric and medical assessment should be carried out, with particular attention to depression, psychosis, risk of suicide, and physical complications such as infection, hepatitis and endocarditis.
2. For opiates and barbiturates, the patient should be gradually withdrawn from the addicted drug under medical supervision.
3. Withdrawal from barbiturates carries risk as seizures may develop. It should be carried out whilst an in-patient. The level of addiction is established by giving enough phenobarbitone in divided dose to maintain the patient between intoxication and withdrawal, and then reduce the dosage by 30 mg every other day while avoiding withdrawal symptoms.
4. Withdrawal of opiates is achieved by administering methadone following an initial dose of 20–70 mg depending on the patient's consumption and then reducing by 20–30% every two or three days while avoiding withdrawal symptoms.

Contd.

293

FOLLOW-UP

For those addicts who cannot accept total withdrawal, maintenance therapy with methadone may be provided. Psychological treatment, particularly supportive group therapy, is useful for all forms of addiction and drug abuse. Rehabilitation to help the addict leave the drug subculture, develop new social contacts, find new accommodation and meaningful employment is an important aspect of treatment.

[1] Goodman LS, Gilman A (1965) *Pharmacological Basis of Therapeutics*. New York: Macmillan.
[2] Stimson GV *et al.* (1978) *Br. Med. J.*, i, 1190.
[3] Robins LN *et al.* (1974) *Am. J. Epidemiol.*, 99, 235.
[4] Anderson HR *et al.* (1982) *Human Toxicol.*, 1, 207.

Antisocial Personality

Antisocial personality disorder is a chronic or recurrent disorder beginning before the age of 15 and characterised by lifelong interpersonal difficulties and antisocial behaviour. The person has school problems as manifested by repeated truancy, suspension, expulsion or fighting that leads to trouble with teachers; running away from home overnight; police difficulty as manifested by frequent arrests and convictions; poor work history; marital difficulties with desertion, divorce, frequent separations, recurrent infidelity, physical attacks upon the spouse; repeated outbursts of fighting; sexual problems as manifested by prostitution, pimping or flagrant promiscuity; vagrancy or wanderlust; and persistent and repeated lying[1]. The person tends to have difficulty in making loving relationships, to take impulsive actions, to lack guilt and remorse, and to fail to learn from adverse experiences. The disorder is more common in men, and has an estimated lifetime prevalence of 2–3%[2].

PROGNOSIS

- Patients with antisocial personality generally consult doctors because of complications of their illness or court referral for assessment. 524 people who had attended a child guidance clinic 30 years before as children were followed-up[3]. About one-third of patients diagnosed as antisocial personality improved with age in having fewer arrests, but still had substantial lifelong problems in interpersonal relationships. There was also an increased rate of suicide, alcoholism and injury.

- After the age of 45 patients with antisocial personality behave less aggressively suggesting a spontaneous reduction in such behaviour with age.

TREATMENT

1. Patients with antisocial personality generally do not present themselves for treatment of personality disorder, but rather for its complications such as alcoholism, drug abuse, marital discord, depression, anxiety or trauma.

2. Such patients often cause difficulties for doctors because of their poor compliance and tendency to abuse and exploit the therapeutic relationship.

3. Drugs should be given with care because of the tendency for abuse. It is often more worthwhile to consider specific problems and to provide a supportive yet firm approach in helping the patient to solve those problems.

4. Individual psychotherapy is unlikely to help antisocial personality although group therapy in a therapeutic community may be beneficial in some cases.

FOLLOW-UP

Patients seldom return for treatment beyond immediate relief of symptoms.

[1] Feighner JP et al. (1972) Arch. Gen. Psychiat., 26, 57.
[2] Robins LN et al. (1984) Arch. Gen. Psychiat., 41, 949.
[3] Robins LN (1966) Deviant Children Grown Up. Baltimore: Williams and Wilkins.

Mental Handicap

The diagnosis of mental handicap is generally made by the presence of: a) developmental delay, especially of speech and language; b) delay in acquiring basic living skills such as walking, dressing, reading and writing; and c) an IQ less than 70. Mild mental retardation has an IQ of 50–70; moderate retardation 35–49; severe retardation 20–24; and profound retardation under 20. The prevalence of moderate and severe retardation is about 4 per 1000[1]. The cause of mental handicap was examined in a community survey[2] and it was found that Down's syndrome represented 26%; other inherited conditions or associated congenital malformations 19%; perinatal injury 18%; infections 14%; inherited biochemical errors 4%; others 4%; and undiagnosable 15%. Psychiatric disorder was found to be higher among the mentally handicapped than among the general population. Disturbed behaviour, conduct disorder and psychosis are also more prevalent.

PROGNOSIS

- Certain forms of mental handicap may be treatable, such as a low phenylalanine diet in patients with phenylketonuria.
- Once established however, the prognosis will depend on the degree of impairment and the associated social and family supportive factors.
- Patients with mild mental handicap may be educatable and able to live independently in the community.
- Those with more severe mental handicap will require greater support either by living at home with their parents or with institutional support, particularly for those with severe behavioural problems who cannot be supported at home.

TREATMENT

1. A thorough clinical assessment should be carried out. This will usually be done in childhood when mental handicap is suspected following developmental and intellectual delay.
2. The specific aetiology of the mental handicap should be investigated, such as phenylketonuria, Down's syndrome, other metabolic disorder, tuberous sclerosis, hydrocephalus, or perinatal damage due to infection or intoxications.
3. Any continuing aetiological factors should be reduced or eliminated, if possible, to prevent further damage.

FOLLOW-UP

The doctor may be called upon to provide support for the patient and his family during times of particular difficulty, to serve as liaison between the patient and social services, to give the lead in planning services, and to provide treatment for associated conditions such as behaviour disorders, psychiatric illness, epilepsy, or physical disability.

---

[1] Tizard J (1964) *Community Services for the Mentally Handicapped.* Oxford: Oxford University Press.
[2] Corbett JA *et al.* (1975) Epilepsy. In: *Mental Retardation and Development Disabilities: An Annual Review,* Vol. III (Waters J ed.). New York: Brunner-Mazel.

Suicide and Attempted Suicide

The suicide rate in the UK is estimated to be less than 10 per 100 000 per year. Since 1975 it has been rising, and is highest in the months of April, May and June. Suicide rates increase with age, are higher in men, lowest among the married, and highest in social class 5 (unskilled workers) and in social class 1 (professionals). Mental disorder is the most important cause of suicide. In one series[1] 75% cases had depressive disorder and 15% had alcoholism. Schizophrenia accounts for 3% suicides. The suicide rate is rising among young university students and is higher among doctors than the general population. Attempted suicide is also increasing. Among women it is the most frequent reason for admission to a medical ward and among men it is second only to ischaemic heart disease. Attempted suicide is more common among the young and among women, particularly aged 15–30. Attempted suicide is more prevalent in the lower social classes and among the divorced.

PROGNOSIS

- Between 15–25% patients who attempt suicide will repeat their attempt in the year after the act.
- A repetition of attempted suicide is more common in those with previous attempts, previous psychiatric treatment, antisocial personality, alcohol or drug abuse, low social class and the unemployed[2].
- In repeat attempts the risk of actual completion of suicide is about 1–2%, that is, those who attempt suicide are 100 times more likely to die by suicide than the general population. The risk is greater if other risk factors exist, e.g. being male, depressed or alcoholic, or having suffered a recent disaster, such as divorce[3].

TREATMENT

1. Assessment after attempted suicide is generally carried out by a psychiatrist. Attempts are made to investigate the medical and psychiatric seriousness of the attempt, the presence of psychiatric disorder, and the presence of intentions to die.
2. If there is a continuing risk of suicide, then hospitalisation is generally recommended for treatment of specific disorders, such as depression or alcoholism.
3. For patients with social stress such as unemployment, divorce or marital turmoil, social aid and supportive psychotherapy is indicated.
4. Patients with a depressive illness (p. 280) who attempt suicide should be hospitalised for treatment. Electro-convulsive therapy may be used if patients fail to respond to medication or more rapid response is required.
5. Medications used to treat depression are toxic in overdose (particularly tricyclic antidepressants). If patients who attempted suicide are still depressed and can not be hospitalised, then treatment with tricyclics should be performed with caution, seeing them at least weekly and giving no more than one week's supply of medication. Less toxic drugs, such as mianserin, may be used but they may also be less effective.
6. Patients who attempt suicide because of personality disorders, social stress, attempts at interpersonal manipulation, or alcoholism without depressive illness should not be given anti-depressants as out-patients, because of the risk of further self-poisoning when there is no therapeutic benefit to be gained.

FOLLOW-UP

Patients with depressive illness should be followed-up as p. 280. All patients should receive support and counselling for social and interpersonal problems to reduce the risk of further self-harm.

[1] Robins E et al. (1959) Am. J. Psychiat., 115, 724.
[2] Kreitman N (1980) Medicine, 2nd Series, 1826.
[3] Morgan HG et al. (1975) Br. J. Psychiat., 127, 564.

Acute Organic Syndromes (Confusional States)

Acute organic syndromes have an acute onset, and are generally reversible. They are distinguished from chronic organic brain syndromes (e.g. Alzheimer's disease) which have an insidious onset and are generally irreversible. Acute brain syndromes are characterised by impairment of consciousness with impaired recent memory, disorientation in time, place and person, and confusion. There may also be associated symptoms such as hallucinations (generally visual but also auditory), delusions, depression, obsessions and personality change such that the condition may be misdiagnosed as schizophrenia. Judgement and insight are often impaired. Confusional states may be generally associated with medical, surgical or neurologic disorders or with drug intoxications. Among the many causes are: pneumonia with hypoxia; withdrawal from alcohol, e.g. delirium tremens; drug intoxication with anticholinergics or hallucinogenic compounds; metabolic disorders, such as uraemia, liver failure or disorders of electrolyte balance; intracranial infections, e.g. encephalitis; head injury; nutritional and vitamin deficiency, e.g. thiamin; and epilepsy, e.g. status epilepticus and postictal states[1].

PROGNOSIS

- The prognosis is generally that of the underlying disorder. If the underlying abnormalities are corrected, the brain syndrome will generally subside.

TREATMENT

1. Thorough assessment with mental status examination and physical examination are important. Delusions and hallucinations in the presence of confusion, disorientation and impaired memory are suggestive of brain syndrome and not schizophrenia. Thus recognition of the syndrome is important.

2. Supportive management to prevent suicide or aggressive injury to others may be required. For example it may be necessary to restrain patients with delirium tremens.

3. Medication may be required, for example the treatment of delirium tremens with sedatives and vitamins, or of aggressive or deluded patients with low doses of haloperidol.

FOLLOW-UP

Follow-up will depend on the primary illness.

[1] Lishman WA (1978) *Organic Psychiatry*. Oxford: Blackwell.

Postpartum Depression

Postpartum psychiatric disorders are generally considered not to be a specific illness but the manifestation after a point stress (parturition) of an underlying disorder in a vulnerable individual. Postpartum mental illness may be: a) mild depression such as 'maternity blues'; b) a more severe depressive disorder requiring treatment; or c) a psychotic disorder, which is generally either a depressive or paranoid psychosis. Follow-up studies[1] suggest that subsequent episodes of illness take the form of the postpartum illness, even in the absence of the stress of pregnancy and thus current thinking is that these disorders are not specific to pregnancy. About one- to two-thirds of postpartum women experience brief episodes lasting a few days of lability of mood, episodes of crying generally on the third or fourth postpartum day. About 10% women have a diagnosable depression postpartum which has a severe enough duration and intensity to require treatment by a psychiatrist[2]. The prevalence of postpartum psychosis with delusions or hallucinations is approximately 1 per 500 births. The characteristic clinical picture is of an acute onset affective syndrome with delusions and hallucinations in the presence of significant perplexity and clouding of consciousness.

PROGNOSIS

- Maternity blues resolves spontaneously without treatment.
- The depressive syndrome seen in 10–20% women generally recovers spontaneously after a few months, but about 4% may still be depressed at 12 months after delivery[2]. There are two peaks for postpartum depression, one at 3 months and one at 9–12 months after delivery[3].
- While most patients recover from puerperal psychosis, some (mainly with schizophreniform psychosis), remain chronically ill.
- 50% will suffer a subsequent depressive illness that is not puerperal. Among those who have had a puerperal depressive illness 50% will suffer a subsequent depression not related to birth[1].

TREATMENT

1. No treatment apart from general support is required for 'maternity blues' as the condition resolves spontaneously.

2. Depression of moderate severity may require treatment with psychological and social measures as well as anti-depressant medication.

3. Puerperal psychoses require treatment according to the clinical syndrome, either with antipsychotic or anti-depressant medication. Some cases require electro-convulsive therapy.

FOLLOW-UP

Follow-up depends on the principal illness. None is required for 'maternity blues', regular follow-up is required for moderately severe depression until the condition resolves. See 'follow-up' for *Schizophrenia* (p. 286), *Mania* (p. 282), *Depressive illness* (p. 280) and *Suicide* (p. 297).

[1] Protheroe C (1969) *Br. J. Psychiat.*, **115**, 9.
[2] Pitt B (1968) *Br. J. Psychiat.*, **114**, 1325.
[3] Kendell RE *et al.* (1976) *Psychol. Med.*, **6**, 297.

Abbreviations

ABVD	adriamycin, bleomycin, vinblastine and dimethyl triazeno imidazole carboxamide	**CF**	cystic fibrosis
		CHAD	cold haemagglutinin disease
ACTH	adrenocorticotrophic hormone	**CHD**	coronary heart disease
		ChLVPP	chlorambucil, vinblastine, procarbazine, prednisolone
ACV	acyclovir		
ADH	antidiuretic hormone	**CHOP**	cyclophosphamide, adriamycin, vincristine, prednisolone
ADP	aminodipropylidene diphosphonate		
AF	atrial fibrillation	**CIN**	cervical intraepithelial neoplasia
AHG	antihaemophilic globulin		
AIDS	acquired immune deficiency syndrome	**CMV**	cytomegalovirus
		CNS	central nervous system
AIHA	auto-immune haemolytic anaemia	**CPPD**	calcium pyrophosphate dihydrate
AIN	allergic interstitial nephritis	**CREST**	calcinosis, Raynaud's phenomenon, 'oesophageal' dysfunction, sclerodactyly and telangiectasia
ALS	amyotrophic lateral sclerosis		
ANF	antinuclear factor		
ARF	acute renal failure	**CRF**	chronic renal failure
AS	ankylosing spondylitis	**CSF**	cerebrospinal fluid
ATN	acute tubular necrosis	**CT**	computed tomography
		CTS	carpal tunnel syndrome
		CVA	cerebral vascular accidents
BACOP	bleomycin, adriamycin, cyclophosphamide, vincristine, prednisolone		
		d.c.	direct current
		DDAVP	1-deamino-8-D-arginine vasopressin (desmopressin)
BANS	back, upper arms, neck and shoulder		
BCC	basal cell carcinoma	**DF**	desferrioxamine
BCG	bacille Calmette-Guérin	**DGI**	disseminated gonococcal infection
BCR	British corrected ratio		
bd	two times per day	**DH**	dermatitis herpetiformis
BMT	bone marrow transplant	**DHPG**	dihydroxypropoxy methylguanine
BMZ	basement membrane zone		
BOLD	bleomycin, vincristine, lomustine and dimethyl triazeno imidazole carboxamide	**DHT**	dihydrotestosterone
		DI	diabetes insipidus
		DISH	diffuse idiopathic skeletal hyperostosis
cALL	common acute lymphoblastic leukaemia	**DMSA**	dimercaptosuccinic acid
		DMT	dimethyltryptamine

DNA	deoxyribonucleic acid	**HCG**	human chorionic gonadotrophin
DNCB	dinitrochlorobenzene		
DTIC	dimethyl triazeno imidazole carboxamide	**5HIAA**	5-hydroxyindole acetic acid
DVT	deep vein thrombosis	**HLA**	human leucocyte antigen
DXR	deep x-ray	**HPV**	human papillomavirus
		HS	hereditary spherocytosis
EBV	Epstein–Barr virus	**HSV**	herpes simplex virus
ECG	electrocardiogram	**HTLV**	human T-cell lymphoma/ leukaemia virus
ECT	electro-convulsive therapy		
EDTA	ethylene diamine tetracetic acid	**HUS**	haemolytic uraemic syndrome
EM	erythema multiforme		
ENT	ear, nose and throat	**ICS**	intercellular substance
ESR	erythrocyte sedimentation rate	**IDDM**	insulin dependent diabetes mellitus
ESRF	end stage renal failure	**IHD**	ischaemic heart disease
EVAP	etoposide, vinblastine, adriamycin, prednisolone	**i.m.**	intramuscular
		IM	infectious mononucleosis
		i.u.	international units
FAB	French, American and British	**i.v.**	intravenous
FEV	forced expiratory volume	**JCA**	juvenile chronic arthritis
FFP	fresh frozen plasma		
FSGS	focal segmental glomerulosclerosis	**KCCT**	kaolin cephalin clotting time
FSH	follicle-stimulating hormone	**KS**	Kaposi's sarcoma
		LD	lymphocyte depleted
GBHC	gammabenzene hexachloride	**LFT**	liver function tests
		LH	luteinising hormone
GBM	glomerular basement membrane	**LHRH**	luteinising hormone releasing hormone
GCA	giant cell arteritis	**LMN**	lower motor neurone
GFR	glomerular filtration rate	**LP**	lichen planus (Chapter 7) or lymphocyte predominant (Chapter 8)
GH	growth hormone		
GN	glomerulonephritis		
GP	general practice/ practitioner		
		LSD	lysergic acid diethylamide
GRF	growth hormone releasing factor	**mane**	in the morning
		MBACOP	methotrexate, bleomycin, adriamycin, cyclophosphamide, vincristine, prednisolone
H	isoniazid		
Hb	haemoglobin	**MC**	mixed cellularity
HBSAg	hepatitis B surface antigen	**MCGN**	minimal change glomerulonephritis

MCV	mean corpuscular volume	Pn	coal-workers' pneumoconiosis
MEN	multiple endocrine neoplasia	PPNG	penicillinase producing *Neisseria gonorrhoeae*
MI	myocardial infarction		
MN	membranous nephropathy	prn	*pro re nata* (when required)
MOPP	mustine HCl, vincristine, procarbazine, prednisolone	PTAP	purified toxoid aluminium phosphate
		PTH	parathormone/ parathyroid hormone
MPGN	membranoproliferative glomerulonephritis	PUVA	psoralen plus ultraviolet A radiation
MRC	Medical Research Council		
MS	multiple sclerosis	qds	four times per day
MVPP	mustine HCl, vinblastine, procarbazine, prednisolone	R	rifampicin
		RA	rheumatoid arthritis
MW	molecular weight	RNP	ribonucleoprotein antigen
		RPGN	rapidly progressive glomerulonephritis
NGU	nongonococcal urethritis		
NIDDM	non-insulin dependent diabetes mellitus	RSV	respiratory syncytial virus
nocte	at night	SARA	sexually acquired reactive arthritis
NS	nodular sclerosing		
NSAID	non-steroidal anti-inflammatory drug	SBE	subacute bacterial endocarditis
		SLE	systemic lupus erythematosus
OA	osteoarthritis		
od	once per day	stat	immediately
OI	opportunistic infections	SVC	superior vena cava
PAN	polyarteritis nodosa	tab.	tablet
PCP	phencyclidine	TB	tuberculosis
PCT	porphyria cutanea tarda	tds	three times per day
PDA	persistent ductus arteriosus	TIA	transient ischaemic attacks
PE	pulmonary embolism	TSH	thyroid stimulating hormone
PEFR	peak expiratory flow rate		
PFT	pulmonary function test	TSI	thyroid-stimulating immunoglobulins
PGU	post-gonococcal urethritis		
PID	pelvic inflammatory disease	TTP	thrombotic thrombocytopenic purpura
PMA	progressive muscle atrophy		
PMF	progressive massive fibrosis	UMN	upper motor neurone
		UTI	urinary tract infection
PMR	polymyalgia rheumatica	UVB	ultraviolet B radiation

VAD	vincristine, adriamycin, dexamethasone	**VSD**	ventricular septal defect
		VT	ventricular tachycardia
VF	ventricular fibrillation	**VZ**	varicella/zoster
VIP	vasoactive intestinal polypeptide		
		ZIG	antivaricella-zoster immunoglobulin
VMA	vanillylmandelic acid		

Index

References in *italic* to this volume; in **bold** to *Treatment and Prognosis: Surgery*

References in *italic* to this volume; in **bold** to *Treatment and Prognosis: Surgery*

References in *italic* to this volume; in **bold** to *Treatment and Prognosis: Surgery*

References in *italic* to this volume; in **bold** to *Treatment and Prognosis: Surgery*

References in *italic* to this volume; in **bold** to *Treatment and Prognosis: Surgery*

References in *italic* to this volume; in **bold** to *Treatment and Prognosis: Surgery*

References in *italic* to this volume; in **bold** to *Treatment and Prognosis: Surgery*

Further volumes . . . .

This is one of two volumes published simultaneously in the *Treatment and Prognosis* series. Other titles will appear in the near future. The series includes titles on:

Surgery
Paediatrics
Obstetrics and Gynaecology

Updated editions will also be published from time to time. If you are interested in receiving details of these volumes together with special subscription rates for the entire series, please write to:

Department TP
Freepost EM17
William Heinemann Medical Books
22 Bedford Square
London
WC1B 3BR